More praise for *The Ma~~gnesium Miracle~~*

"Every doctor and patient should read this comprehensive book on the many roles of magnesium. . . . I loved this book. Clearly written and packed with information, it offers a compendium on natural medicine and is an invaluable resource for both practitioner and public alike. It is the most comprehensive and well-referenced guide to the myriad benefits of magnesium published to date."

—CAROLYN DEMARCO, M.D.,
author of *Take Charge of Your Body: Women's Health Advisor*

"Throughout this volume and with utmost clarity, Carolyn Dean presents invaluable recommendations—based on the latest magnesium research. Virtually every American can benefit."

—PAUL PITCHFORD,
author of *Healing with Whole Foods: Asian Traditions*
and *Modern Nutrition*

"Physicians and therapists have paid scant attention to this very important element, which is also involved in maintaining our good health. The massive evidence is here in this important book on magnesium. I am pleased to have been taking magnesium for so many years."

—ABRAM HOFFER, M.D.,
author of *Putting It All Together: The New Orthomolecular Nutrition*

"Excellent research together with valuable inspiration·to empower the doctor within each of us."

—JOSHUA ROSENTHAL,
director of the Institute for Integrative Nutrition,
author of *The Energy Balance Diet*

"An enlightening and practical book. Dr. Dean supplies powerful information for people while trumpeting a reminder to doctors about this essential and often overlooked mineral elixir. *The Magnesium Miracle* should be required reading for living a rich, healthy life."

—EUGENE CHARLES, D.C., DIBAK,
author of *Physician Heal Thy Patient*
and *Becoming Healthy, Wealthy and Wise*

"I have been in complementary medicine for thirty years and I believed I knew all there was to know about magnesium—until I [read] the latest book by Dr. Carolyn Dean. This book is the most comprehensive review on the subject I have ever read. As one can expect from a physician with such vast and diversified knowledge, *The Magnesium Miracle* contains information on allied fields of medicine that makes this book an incredible resource for doctors and patients alike. *The Magnesium Miracle* is a book that is going to be of great service to humanity since, as the author points out, there is so much information on magnesium that has failed to be included in the medical curriculum."

—SERAFINA CORSELLO, M.D.,
Wellness Medical Center for Integrative Medicine,
author of *Ageless Healing*

The Magnesium Miracle

The Magnesium Miracle

SECOND EDITION

(Originally published as *The Miracle of Magnesium*)

CAROLYN DEAN, M.D., N.D.

BALLANTINE BOOKS · NEW YORK

2017 Ballantine Books Trade Paperback Edition

Copyright © 2003, 2007, 2014 by Carolyn Dean, M.D., N.D.
Foreword copyright © 2003 by Dr. Bella Altura and Dr. Burton Altura

Published in the United States by Ballantine Books, an imprint of Random House, a division of Penguin Random House LLC, New York.

BALLANTINE and the HOUSE colophon are registered trademarks of Penguin Random House LLC.

Originally published in hardcover and trade paperback in different form as *The Miracle of Magnesium* by Ballantine Books, an imprint of Random House, a division of Penguin Random House LLC, in 2003 and 2007 respectively.

ISBN 978-0-399-59444-1
Ebook ISBN 978-0-425-28671-5

Printed in the United States of America

randomhousebooks.com

2 4 6 8 9 7 5 3

Book design by Susan Turner

*I dedicate this book to health professionals and practitioners
all over the world who have already embraced the miracle
that magnesium offers and incorporate this essential nutrient
into their recommendations and protocols;
to the "magnesium mavericks," individuals who have already
soaked up this information like they soak up their magnesium
and then pass it along to everyone they meet; and to
all my new readers who are coming to this information
looking for a solution to their particular health challenge.
May this knowledge, combined with effective
magnesium supplementation, transform your health
as it has for countless millions.*

Foreword

"Clearly there is more to life than magnesium" is one of the remarks from Dr. Dean's remarkable, almost encyclopedic, but very readable book. Her book is long overdue, for it gives the lay reader a chance to discover for him- or herself the many needs for this mineral in a healthy diet, and the reasons why this has not been emphasized in the everyday literature.

The requirement for magnesium in our diet is indeed a much-neglected topic, and this book by Dr. Dean brings the message home by her carefully written repetitive emphasis on the subject. That does not mean that there are not many other nutrients necessary in our daily food intake, as stated above, but the point she so clearly makes is that the public in general has not been notified to look for the proper amount of this mineral in the daily diet and the many reasons magnesium is needed in our bodies.

After a cursory overview of the material, the book should be read as one would read an encyclopedia, that is, pick out the parts one is particularly interested in, and then go back and try to read it all. This way the reader will get the gist of how important magnesium really is and how little he or she has been informed, be it from newspapers, magazines, or the rest of the news media. As the old adage says, "An ounce of prevention is worth a pound of cure," and so it is with balanced nutrition, which includes this all-important mineral in adequate amounts. (As to the other interesting parts of the book, our qualifications allow us to comment only on the material pertaining to the scientific basis for the need of magnesium.)

DR. BELLA T. ALTURA
Research Professor of Physiology and Pharmacology
SUNY Downstate Medical Center
Brooklyn, New York

DR. BURTON M. ALTURA
Professor of Physiology, Pharmacology, and Medicine
SUNY Downstate Medical Center
Brooklyn, New York

Acknowledgments

I'd like to thank Daniel Wagner, the translator of the German edition of *The Magnesium Miracle*. Daniel was working on his translation while I was creating this 2017 edition of the book. His many detailed questions assisted me greatly and saved me much time in fine-tuning my own edits.

Contents

Contents

Introduction

I'm pleased to say that since the 2014 revised edition of *The Magnesium Miracle,* magnesium research has skyrocketed. In the past five years, close to 12,000 publications about magnesium appeared in the PubMed database. By the time this book is in your hands there will likely be another 3,000.

It's been wonderful to see a definite public groundswell of interest in magnesium. In commercial terms, magnesium is the fastest-rising product on the supplement market. Sales of magnesium supplements are catching up with and even surpassing calcium supplement sales. Statisticians also analyze what topics are being searched on the Internet, and magnesium is getting its fair share of hits.

There is more than enough proof that people should supplement with magnesium for a myriad of conditions. In fact, I think everyone could benefit from magnesium supplementation, whether you suffer from magnesium deficiency or simply wish to prevent it. I've updated this edition with the latest magnesium research, most of which is online, so you can read it yourself. Through the miracle of the Internet you can find abstracts to most if not all of my references and, in many cases, free access to entire papers. It's so important to educate yourself about the benefits of magnesium since, in spite of all the evidence, researchers continue to call for more studies on the topic, rather than recommending magnesium to the public. That's right—even though research repeatedly proves magnesium deficiency causes dozens of diseases and symptoms, rarely do medical organizations openly endorse magnesium supplementation.

ARRHYTHMIA AWARD

One such rare organization is the Heart Rhythm Society in the United Kingdom. In the fall of 2012 I was given the Arrhythmia Alliance Outstanding Medical Contribution to Cardiac Rhythm Management Services Award. Arrhythmias can be life-threatening, and the only treatment options are to learn to cope with the mild ones or treat the moderate to serious ones with drugs and surgical ablation.

One of my magnesium deficiency symptoms is heart palpitations, so I know how scary and disruptive they can be. It is very distressing to actually feel your heart working improperly. I often tell people, "You don't have a heart problem; you have a magnesium problem." As I've noted many times, the highest amount of magnesium in the body is found in the heart.

I was quite amazed to receive this award because the Heart Rhythm Society is very science- and research-oriented. By honoring me, they acknowledged the important role of magnesium in the treatment of arrhythmia. This award is proof that magnesium research has hit the mainstream, and there is no going back!

It was this award and all the mail I receive about arrhythmias being reversed with magnesium that convinced me to write a book called *Atrial Fibrillation: Remineralize Your Heart*. The fact that serious heart arrhythmias can be affected by such a simple mineral as magnesium makes people more willing to accept its importance in improving health. I'll give you a long excerpt from that book in Chapter 7.

Below I'd like to share a few emails that I've received from people with arrhythmias whose lives have been dramatically improved by using magnesium.

> Dr. Dean, a few months ago I wrote to you regarding my amazing results after using magnesium to suppress PVCs [premature ventricular contractions] and PACs [premature atrial contractions]. It has been almost six months and I still wake up every morning thanking God for this mineral!

Another person, who had almost given up at the age of only thirty-one, wrote a long account that will resonate with many readers:

> I want to thank you so much for your book *The Magnesium Miracle*. It is no overstatement to say that it has changed my life overnight. I'm only thirty-one years old, but for over ten years I have been plagued by premature atrial contractions, premature ventricular contractions, and tachycardia. I was told by multiple doctors that I was fine and to just go home and ignore the arrhythmias. I kept crawling back to the doctors hoping that they could offer me some solution, but all they would do is run more tests and try to put me on Zoloft.
>
> There was one year that I had more echocardiograms than haircuts! Several months ago my palpitations increased from the once-in-a-while range to several times every day. While desperately reading through some posts in an online forum I saw several people singing the praises of your book and the wonders of magnesium, which had worked for them. I purchased some

magnesium and after prayerfully taking my first dose four days ago I have not had a single PVC since! It's truly a miracle.

Even though the first day after starting magnesium I was double slammed with a terrible head cold and the first day of my period, I still had zero palpitations. Ordinarily a day like that would have me kicking out PVCs like a popcorn machine.

I just want to run through the streets kicking up my heels! I have already convinced half a dozen people to read your book and give magnesium a try for various ailments. This supplement has been such a blessing to me and has given me my life back. I am so glad there are people like you out there willing to point patients in a natural direction for good health. I would be honored, flattered, and proud to have you share my story. Please continue in your efforts to bring more light to this miracle.

Why aren't more doctors telling their patients with arrhythmias to take magnesium? Mostly because they never learned about it in medical school—and every doctor is told that if you didn't learn about something in medical school, it isn't important. Also, since some arrhythmias can become fatal, doctors tend to treat all arrhythmias as fatal, justifying the handful of medications they prescribe. I'll say more about magnesium and arrhythmias, especially atrial fibrillation, in Chapter 7.

THERAPEUTIC MAGNESIUM

Unlike most doctors, I'm here to endorse magnesium! In fact, this book is one long, passionate recommendation for supplemental magnesium. With this edition of *The Magne-*

sium Miracle, I find myself on both sides of the discussion, and I want to make this disclosure at the outset. I am a writer and clinical researcher presenting to the public the latest scientific and clinical information about the healing properties of magnesium. I am also an entrepreneur, having invented a superior form of magnesium that is helping thousands of people where other forms of magnesium could not. I'm actually in the position of a scientist who, in the middle of the experiment, realizes that it would be unethical to withhold the data already collected.

Like many experts and researchers who have become intimately familiar with their topic, I have identified a major problem with most if not all of the forms of magnesium recommended by health practitioners—the laxative effect, which often occurs before a person can experience the full therapeutic effect. Because of my own magnesium deficiency symptoms and my inability to take magnesium supplements without the laxative effect, I would like to announce that I have developed a highly absorbed, non-laxative magnesium product called ReMag. Therapeutic levels of magnesium can be achieved with ReMag without the negative impact of diarrhea. I'll talk more about ReMag and my other magnesium recommendations in Chapter 18 and in the Resources section.

In Chapters 3 through 15, I cover the many magnesium deficiency conditions that people suffer. I also provide a treatment protocol for many of these conditions that goes beyond magnesium by including a list of other recommended supplements, making this book a valuable health encyclopedia.

THE IMPORTANCE OF MAGNESIUM

I constantly receive emails from people with questions, stories, and comments about their experience with magnesium.

Every day I learn something new, either from individuals or from the scientific literature. I want very much to give you all this important information. I know I have a whole book to do it in, but I want to impress upon you immediately how crucial magnesium is, the fact that it's no longer readily available in our food, and that you may need a particular kind of magnesium to achieve therapeutic levels.

I know that it's going to take a lot more effort to change erroneous perceptions that the public, other authors, and health care practitioners have about magnesium. Because it has become a very popular topic, there are a handful of new books and hundreds of online articles about magnesium. There are also a plethora of vitamin books that mention magnesium. Unfortunately, they all repeat the same inaccurate information that "you will know you are taking enough magnesium when you reach the laxative effect." However, magnesium oxide is their treatment of choice—even though it is only 4 percent absorbed and therefore highly laxative

These books also repeat the warning that if you have kidney disease, you should be wary of magnesium, and if you have kidney failure, it could be harmful. With the current emphasis on medical testing, people who have even slightly elevated creatinine, BUN, or eGFR levels on their kidney function tests are made to fear magnesium, when in fact they are probably magnesium-deficient.

I have found that kidney patients, even those on dialysis, can safely take a picometer, stabilized ionic form of magnesium (ReMag) for their debilitating leg cramps and heart palpitations. One woman reports that her magnesium levels drop after every dialysis treatment because there is so little magnesium in the IVs they use during the procedure. That means with every treatment she comes closer to a life-threatening magnesium-deficiency heart attack. See the section "Kidneys Need Magnesium" in Chapter 11 for her story.

TOP 10 MAGNESIUM FACTS

As I mentioned earlier, I want to give you a taste of the importance of magnesium at the beginning, and I'll do that with my Top 10 Magnesium Facts, which will be discussed in more detail throughout the book.

1. Magnesium is necessary for the proper functioning of 700–800 enzyme systems in the body—that's why it can be implicated in scores of symptoms and dozens of health conditions. I mention some of these enzyme systems in Chapter 2 in "Magnesium's Many Roles."

2. Most people (70–80 percent) are magnesium deficient, so this book is for you.

3. Calcium depletes magnesium in the body, and many people get too much calcium, either as supplements, in fortified foods, or in dairy products. I cover this in "The Dance of Calcium and Magnesium" in Chapter 1.

4. Magnesium is very deficient in the soil and in the food supply, so it must be supplemented. This information is detailed in Chapter 2.

5. Therapeutic doses of magnesium are impossible to obtain in those who suffer the laxative effect before their symptoms can be relieved. Fortunately, people can get relief from ReMag, a non-laxative form of magnesium that can be taken in therapeutic dosages. See Chapter 18 for more details.

6. Mitochondrial dysfunction is no longer a mystery. Adenosine triphosphate (ATP) energy molecules are made in the mitochondria via the Krebs cycle. Six of the eight

steps in that cycle depend on magnesium. See Chapter 16 for more information.

7. To help you identify your magnesium needs, I've created the list "100 Factors Related to Magnesium Deficiency" in Chapter 1.

8. The definitive test that would tell you your magnesium levels, the ionized magnesium blood test, is not available to the public. A helpful but less accurate test, magnesium RBC, must be used in conjunction with your clinical symptoms. The serum magnesium test is highly inaccurate, yet it is still the standard test used in hospitals, clinics, and most clinical trials—however, it doesn't even appear on an electrolyte panel. See Chapter 16 for more on magnesium testing.

9. Magnesium deficiency is a major factor in chronic disease—diabetes, heart disease, high blood pressure, high cholesterol, migraines, irritable bowel syndrome (IBS), and heartburn. The drugs used to treat all these conditions deplete magnesium, often making symptoms worse. I list many of these unsafe drugs in Chapter 2.

10. Telomeres, which are components of chromosomes, hold the key to aging, as does magnesium, which prevents telomeres from deteriorating. I cover the latest research in Chapter 15.

LONG-STANDING MAGNESIUM DEPLETION

Magnesium deficiency is nothing new, but that information has not been passed on to the general public so that they can take action in their own self-interest. Proof of this can be found more than seventy years ago, in the following statement on soil mineral depletion, which was read into the record of the 74th Congress, 2nd session (Senate document no. 264), 1936:

Do you know that most of us today are suffering from certain dangerous diet deficiencies which cannot be remedied until depleted soils from which our food comes are brought into proper mineral balance? The alarming fact is that foods (fruits, vegetables, and grains) now being raised on millions of acres of land that no longer contain enough of certain minerals are starving us—no matter how much of them we eat. The truth is that our foods vary enormously in value, and some of them aren't worth eating as food.

Our physical well-being is more directly dependent upon the minerals we take into our systems than upon calories or vitamins or upon the precise proportions of starch, protein, or carbohydrates we consume.

Laboratory tests prove that the fruits, the vegetables, the grains, the eggs, and even the milk and the meats of today are not what they were a few generations ago. No man today can eat enough fruits and vegetables to supply his stomach with the mineral salts he requires for perfect health, because his stomach isn't big enough to hold them! And we are turning into a nation of big stomachs.

It's clear to me that since that time, the mineral depletion of our agricultural soil has never been corrected and it's only gotten worse.

WHY HAVEN'T WE HEARD ABOUT MAGNESIUM?

People are more magnesium-aware than they were sixteen years ago when I began my magnesium crusade, so I'm grateful for that. However, the vast majority of schoolchildren are never exposed to nutritional education in school. What about doctors—the people who should know the biochemical workings of the body? Unfortunately, doctors generally do not learn about nutrition or nutrient supplementation in medical school because they are studying disease, not wellness.

I like to talk about my 200 hours of biochemistry in medical school, where I learned about all the nutrient cofactors necessary for every biochemical reaction. But I was likely the only one who recognized their importance because of my extensive study of nutrition before I went into medicine.

When you visit a medical doctor, in your mind you may think you are going there to improve your health or prevent illness, but doctors have little time to educate their patients about how to keep themselves well. What's on their mind is searching for a diagnosis for your symptoms and matching a drug to their diagnosis.

Patients often will not change their lifestyle or improve their nutrition on their own, believing that if diet and supplements were so important, the doctor would have told them. Nutrition is not even a medical specialty. It wasn't a specialty when I went to medical school in the 1970s and it still isn't today! That's why you won't hear most of the information I report in this book from your doctor—because it's outside his or her field of knowledge and expertise.

Basically, doctors only know what they know, and if you ask them anything about health and disease that they don't know, they will simply say it's not important. It's not important because they never learned about it in medical school, which was supposed to teach them everything. Do you see how dangerous this cyclical logic can be?

WHEN ALL YOU HAVE IS A HAMMER

In the first two years of medical school I learned all about diseases; the second two years I studied drug treatments for those diseases. We spent no time on nutrient deficiencies. Have you heard the expression "When all you have is a hammer, everything begins to look like a nail"? That is very much the case with doctors and drug treatments. Even worse, with thousands of drugs in the pharmaceutical compendium, it is quite impossible for doctors to keep up on the latest drugs, and impossible to prevent side effects or serious drug interactions. This is especially true with the polypharmacy practiced today, where medical providers prescribe combinations of drugs that have never been studied together until they reach your body.

Studies show that most doctors are unable to recognize drug side effects, instead confusing them with a need to increase the dose rather than stop the drug. Although allopathic medicine is said to be scientific, most patients are on more than one drug at a time, and there are no studies proving the safety of drug combinations. Let me repeat—there is no science to prove the safety or efficacy of taking more than one drug at a time. Most studies are done using one drug at a time. When a person is on a dozen drugs, all bets are off. There have been a few studies using what's referred to as a "polypill," made up of several drugs for preventing heart disease, diabetes, and hypertension, but in all the studies I have seen, the side effects always outweigh any benefits.

According to magnesium expert Mildred Seelig, M.D., while a tremendous amount of magnesium research has been done in India, Britain, France, and a number of other countries, doctors in the United States use the excuse that not enough research has been done here for them to feel informed enough to prescribe it. Dr. Seelig calls this the "not-invented-here syndrome."

Pioneers such as Drs. Bella and Burton Altura, however, continue to do original magnesium research in the United States. Every year for the past forty years they have produced on average a dozen peer-reviewed journal articles on magnesium and ionized magnesium testing. Their research convinces even die-hard skeptics—when they take the time to become informed—of the clear need for magnesium supplementation and the absolute requirement for accurate testing.

DRUG COMPANIES FUND
MOST MEDICAL RESEARCH

Medical science studies one symptom at a time, in isolation, and generally tries to find one cause for that symptom and one drug that treats it. The bias of medical research is to search for a patentable drug that will eventually pay for the costly studies necessary to bring it to market. There is general agreement that magnesium is indispensable for health, disease prevention, and all life processes, but it has been ignored because there is no profit to be made in selling a common nutrient that cannot be patented.

There is no advertising budget for magnesium compared to the hundreds of millions of dollars spent on advertising prescription drugs, and nutrients do not get media attention. To make matters worse, over the past two decades the bulk of university funding has come from the pharmaceutical industry, which primarily funds drug research.[1, 2]

There is also no incentive for anyone to test magnesium in large clinical trials since they could never recoup the money spent on the trial. Yet doctors seem to be waiting for such a trial, where 20,000 people taking magnesium are followed for life. In a perfect world, that study should have been initiated decades ago. Do we have the luxury of waiting for the results of such a study started now? No, we do not. Do we presently know enough about magnesium to recommend widespread supplementation? Yes, we do.

Doctors may have heard years ago that magnesium offered some promise in heart disease, but they haven't read any new studies, so they assume that the treatment must not have panned out. Drs. Burton and Bella Altura, who wrote the foreword to this book, have published more than 1,000 studies on magnesium. With each passing year, their research recedes further into the past, with the risk of being ignored.

An analysis of seven major clinical studies shows that intravenous magnesium reduced the risk of death by 55 percent after acute heart attack. These results were published in the prestigious *British Medical Journal* and the widely read journal *Drugs*.[3, 4] With such positive scientific results and doctors claiming that they practice "scientific medicine," why isn't IV magnesium being routinely given to everyone who presents in the ER with an acute heart attack?

As noted, Drs. Bella and Burton Altura have been researching magnesium and its clinical application for more than forty years.[5] The ionized magnesium electrode, produced by Nova Biomedical of Waltham, Massachusetts, at the Alturas' urging, and tested at the State University of New York's Downstate Medical Center by the Alturas, has given doctors a reliable magnesium test and taken the guesswork out of diagnosing magnesium deficiency.[6] With such testing in hundreds of clinical trials, the Alturas and groups of other researchers have been able to show that dozens of health conditions are unequivocally related to magnesium deficiency. These are among the conditions listed in the section "Sixty-Five Conditions Associated with Magnesium Deficiency" in Chapter 1.

Dr. Alexander Mauskop, working with the Alturas, has proven the connection between migraines and magnesium many times over and puts magnesium treatment into practice at the New York Headache Center.[7, 8, 9] Dr. Mildred Seelig has contributed comprehensive reviews on magnesium at New York Medical College, the American College of Nutrition, and the Department of Nutrition, University of North Carolina.[10, 11] Dr. Jean Durlach, president of the International Society for the Development of Research on Magnesium (SDRM), editor in chief of *Magnesium Research,* and professor at St. Vincent de Paul Hospital in Paris, has done extensive reviews of ongoing magnesium research.[12, 13]

All these magnesium experts agree that we can no longer sit on the sidelines or reserve judgment on the benefits of magnesium; we need to implement what we know, now.

> I've been saying for many years that you have to take charge of your own health—and one way of doing that is to study all the information I provide about magnesium, find out if you are suffering from magnesium deficiency, and learn what you can do to correct the problem.

MAGNESIUM IS NOT A DRUG

In the past few years I've noticed a mushrooming of medical websites that have decided to treat vitamins and minerals like drugs. Since nutrients aren't drugs and don't act like drugs, and since drugs, by definition, have side effects, such misinformed websites give people the impression that supplements can have side effects and can be dangerous. This is very confusing to the consumer and contrary to the evidence.

In 2003 I wrote a paper called "Death by Medicine,"[14] and later a book called *Death by Modern Medicine: Seeking Safe Solutions,*[15] wherein I enumerated statistics about iatrogenic illness (illness caused by medical treatment) for prescription drugs and for supplements. While there are no deaths from supplements, the *Journal of the American Medical Association* stated that between 90,000 and 160,000 deaths per year occur from using FDA-approved drugs, making drugs the fourth-most-common cause of death. That figure doesn't include medical and surgical mistakes or preventable deaths from smoking, high blood pressure, and being overweight.[16] Tragically, the researcher who reported these findings, Dr. Barbara Starfield, may herself have died an iatrogenic death in 2011.

When anti-supplement critics insist there have been deaths caused by dietary supplements, they are referring to a single batch of tryptophan, tainted with a genetically engineered additive, that was sold in the late 1980s.

The very few reports of magnesium "toxicity" are in hospitalized patients overdosed with IV magnesium. Unfortunately, these reports are constantly repeated inappropriately and irresponsibly. The reality is that there are only certain people with serious health conditions, who are usually already under a doctor's care, who are warned not to take magnesium. There are only four contraindications to magnesium therapy: kidney failure, myasthenia gravis, excessively slow heart rate, and bowel obstruction. You can read more details in Chapter 18.

Medical websites will talk about magnesium's side effect of diarrhea, not understanding that this is the body's mechanism for avoiding a buildup of magnesium. But diarrhea can also happen when anyone takes a large amount of magnesium at one time, causing a relative overload, or if you take magnesium products that are so poorly absorbed they act like laxatives. Read "The Fail-Safe of Magnesium" later in this Introduction. The laxative effect can also happen in people like me who have a sensitive or irritable bowel, but there is a safe non-laxative form of magnesium that you can take; it's called ReMag, and you can read about it in Chapter 18.

The University of Maryland posted an article online about interactions between magnesium and drugs. The ar-

ticle warns people not to use magnesium if they are also taking antacids, laxatives, fluoroquinolone antibiotics, calcium
channel blockers, or medications for diabetes. I won't refute
every statement they make because I'd have to interpret their
illogical approach. Suffice it to say that the warnings do not
take into consideration that magnesium can be a safe substitute for many of these drugs or that these medications can
deplete magnesium. I warn people about taking any of the
drugs in the above list, and if they must take them, to double
or triple their intake of ReMag to counteract the inevitable
magnesium drain.

The tendency for medical practitioners and government
agencies to medicalize nutrients and categorize them as
drugs, playing up rare and sometimes imaginary side effects,
I believe, comes from an organization called the Codex Alimentarius Commission. The commission is run by two
groups that are part of the United Nations, the World Health
Organization (WHO) and the Food and Agriculture Organization (FAO), with disputes being adjudicated by the
World Trade Organization. Codex sets the standards for
food and dietary supplements being shipped across borders.
I've attended Codex meetings in Europe, and I realized that
pharmaceutical companies have taken a great interest in
Codex; their intent is to make sure that nutrient levels of dietary supplements are not high enough to be therapeutic, so
that they will not "interfere" with prescribed medications.
Ultimately they want nutrients to be treated like drugs and
only prescribed by doctors. Many people who take magnesium have been successful in reducing or even eliminating
their medications, which can't please the pharmaceutical
companies. A reputable organization, Alliance for Natural
Health, recognizes the dangers that Codex brings and can
educate you about the problems we face as its worldwide rul-
ings come into effect.[17]

When I attended a nutrition seminar hosted by the National Center for Complementary and Alternative Medicine at the National Institutes of Health (NIH), one of the speakers stated that NIH's mandate was to issue guidelines on the Recommended Daily Allowance (RDA) for nutrients only to prevent deficiency diseases—for example, how much vitamin C we should take to prevent scurvy. She said that the NIH had no interest in or mandate to research supplements for the prevention and treatment of disease. This attitude probably arises from the lack of education about nutrients in medical school. Because doctors know only what they have been taught, they fear what they don't know; this makes it easier for them to box magnesium into the drug category and close the lid.

MAGNESIUM MISINFORMATION

There are hundreds of ways that our bodies utilize magnesium, which makes it impossible for science to identify its "most important function." This approach of looking for the single pivotal function of a supplement is based on the medical model of "one symptom, one diagnosis, one drug." Science depends on this model to isolate one variable at a time for scientific testing. They don't seem to realize that it would be unreasonable and impossible to limit a food nutrient such as magnesium in that way, since it is involved in as many as 800 enzyme systems, affects 80 percent of the body's biochemistry, and interacts with dozens of other nutrients.

There are stacks of papers from researchers all over the world proving the value of magnesium. However, those thousands of papers, including the 1,000 research papers authored by the doctors who wrote the foreword to this book, Drs. Burton and Bella Altura, unfortunately seem to have done nothing to make the public aware of the importance of magnesium. Researchers will just keep getting funding to repeat the same studies and doctors will continue to ignore them because they never learned anything about the clinical application of magnesium in medical school.

I've said it before and I'll say it again: we can't wait for a multbillion-dollar clinical trial to "prove" that magnesium is a necessary nutrient. We have enough research showing its therapeutic value, safety, and efficacy. What's more, people can do their own personal clinical trial by following their magnesium RBC test results and taking magnesium as they watch their symptoms subside. See Chapter 16 for more on magnesium testing and Chapter 18 for my magnesium supplement recommendations.

Magnesium is safe, and people are deficient in it. For every hundred emails I get describing positive responses to magnesium, I get only one that asks if the sender might be having a negative reaction. Since there are essentially no negative reactions to magnesium, please read "When Magnesium Makes Me Worse," later in this Introduction, to learn about the transition symptoms that can occur when you begin to take magnesium or when you take too much too soon.

MAGNESIUM RESEARCH AND REVIEWS

The Magnesium Miracle has been a bestseller since it first appeared in 2003. On Amazon it has occasionally moved into the Top 100 Bestsellers and typically holds the number one position in the "Vitamin and Supplement" book category. It's also received close to 1,000 product reviews from readers. *The Magnesium Miracle* is not just a great book to read; it has helped improve the health of hundreds of thousands of people and saved countless lives. With each new scientific review paper and clinical study, I find it impossible to fathom why doctors don't recommend magnesium as a safe and effective treatment for dozens of conditions.

What impresses me about the current state of magnesium research is the sheer number of review articles and meta-analyses as many groups of investigators summarize what is known about this important mineral. A decade ago science in general didn't give magnesium much thought, but today all of those papers acknowledge the depth and breadth of magnesium's impact on the body. Even so, that information still hasn't made it to the doctor's office or into the patient's treatment plan. As I noted above, most of these reviews are freely available on the Internet, where you can read them and scan their citations to see the extensive web of information about the benefits of magnesium that can no longer be denied. You can even print them out to help educate your doctors and garner their support for your magnesium therapy.

I have to hold myself back from wanting to reference every new publication, which would make this book excessively long and dry. When you come to a heavily referenced section, like the following, you don't have to read every word; you can skim through it and just note the richness of the available magnesium research.

ADD MAGNESIUM TO DESALINATED WATER

I think that the most important study of this decade is a paper titled "Desalinated Seawater Supply and All-Cause Mortality in Hospitalized Acute Myocardial Infarction Patients from the Acute Coronary Syndrome Israeli Survey 2002–2013."[18] One of the coauthors of the study, Dr. Michael Shechter, has been lobbying for magnesium supplementation of the Israeli water supply for many years.

Three-quarters of Israeli water is desalinated and therefore devoid of minerals.

In a July 2016 personal email to me and eleven other magnesium experts, Dr. Shechter described that in this study "we investigated patients with acute myocardial infarction in Israel . . . dividing the patients into 2 areas: those who live in areas with desalinated seawater (almost no magnesium) and those who live in areas with regular tap water (normal magnesium levels)." The results were shocking: "We found an amazing increased 1-year mortality rate in patients who live in a desalinated water area compared to normal water, which was also reflected in their serum magnesium levels."

The results of this study appear to have frightened the Israeli public, spurring a media frenzy. Michael said that "following our preliminary announcement all media in Israel was very busy reporting the results in on-air discussions and for 2 consecutive days I've been interviewed on prime time news on Israel national TV. The result is that our Prime Minister Mr. Netanyahu decided to add magnesium to the desalinated water!"

I heartily congratulated Dr. Shechter, and told him, "I know you put your heart into this study because the government wouldn't accept your request to add magnesium to DSW [desalinated water] years ago. Now you have thoroughly proven them wrong! Already they have changed their minds and are adding magnesium to the DSW!"

This study has huge worldwide implications because in some areas drinking water is filtered extensively, distilled, or subjected to reverse osmosis, which can reduce or remove the good minerals along with the bad. Most bottled water, unless it is mineral water labeled with a list of mineral ingredients, is distilled or treated with reverse osmosis.

It is through our water that we are supposed to receive

magnesium and all our other minerals but we no longer have this luxury. Dr. Shechter has proven beyond a shadow of a doubt that any drinking water that does not contain sufficient levels of magnesium can cause heart attacks!

However, as of February 2017, the pilot project to add magnesium to the desalinated drinking water of Ashkelon, Israel, has become bogged down in bureaucratic bickering over funding. In order to educate the Israeli public about the estimated four thousand Israelis who die annually due to magnesium deficiency, largely because they drink magnesium-deficient desalinated water, Dr. Shechter promoted Magnesium Awareness Week in February 2017. He hopes this will further motivate the government to take action to save lives.

MAGNESIUM REVIEWS

In 2001, at the same time I was writing the first edition of *The Magnesium Miracle,* an excellent review was published by Fox and colleagues, citing sixty-seven references.[19] The investigators stated that three biologic mechanisms could potentially explain how magnesium helps treat hypertension, diabetes, and hyperlipidemia.

- First, magnesium deficiency causes a dysregulation of the sodium-magnesium exchange, resulting in higher intracellular sodium and thus higher blood pressure.
- Second, a relatively low magnesium level creates an intracellular imbalance between calcium and magnesium, which results in increased spasms in the smooth muscle of arteries and therefore increased blood pressure.
- Third, magnesium deficiency causes insulin resistance, which in turn causes hyperinsulinemia, resulting in hypertension, diabetes, and hyperlipidemia.

Fox and his team cite study after study showing the importance of magnesium in many chronic conditions. They report on studies using IV magnesium therapeutically in critical situations such as acute asthma, torsades de pointes (ventricular tachycardia), and preeclampsia. Yet their only conclusion is to call for more funding and more research to see if magnesium supplementation will have a positive effect on hypertension, diabetes, and hyperlipidemia. They conclude: "The clinical implications of replacement therapy, if successful, would have a profound effect on improving the health of the population."

Personally, I think that withholding this vital information from the public has actually reached the point of malpractice.

A 2015 review repeats all the same information in the Fox paper but with additional references; there were 149 citations.[20] Gröber and his team report that 100 years ago the magnesium content of our diet was about 500 mg/day and that today this has plummeted to 175–225 mg/day. I've referenced this fact for years, but I rarely see it mentioned. They also provided the research proof that magnesium deficiency can cause an alarming number of diseases and disease symptoms. It's a laundry list of our chronic diseases, which are occurring in epidemic numbers and cannot be cured by drugs: attention deficit hyperactivity syndrome (ADHS), Alzheimer's, cardiac arrhythmias, asthma, type 2 diabetes, heart disease, heart failure, hypertension, metabolic syndrome, migraine headaches, myocardial infarction, preeclampsia, eclampsia, and stroke. Several conditions for which investigators feel magnesium is promising but which require further research include anxiety, depression, dysmenorrhea, fatigue, fibromyalgia, hearing loss, kidney stones, premenstrual syndrome, osteoporosis, and tinnitus.

After all this great information in their 12,000-word paper about the importance of magnesium, shored up with study after study, what did Gröber and colleagues recommend? I was very disappointed to see that they devoted a mere seventy words to how to treat these serious magnesium deficiency diseases. For dosage, they simply repeat the very lowest recommendation, 4–6 mg/kg/day (220–325 mg daily for a 120-pound person). The first supplement recommendation they make is for the highly laxative magnesium oxide, and the last one on their list is magnesium aspartate, which, according to neurosurgeon Dr. Russell Blaylock, is toxic.[21] (I discuss Dr. Blaylock's concerns about magnesium aspartate in the section "Migraine Mechanisms" in Chapter 4.)

Two other reviews by Volpe, in 2013 and 2015, are titled "Magnesium in Disease Prevention"[22] and "Overall Health and Magnesium and the Athlete."[23] These papers are very similar to the previous reviews, but the citations are for only the ten years prior to publication, as if research from earlier years is now somehow invalid. And these reviews do not list any magnesium supplement recommendations.

The latest study by Drs. Burton and Bella Altura, the brilliant, compassionate, and hardworking doctors who have authored well over 1,000 papers on magnesium, in conjunction with a team of investigators, presents a masterly review of the existing literature on the topic of aging and gives an overview of their entire body of work. I'll give more details about this paper in Chapter 15.[24]

Back in 1999, when I suggested to magnesium expert Dr. Mildred Seelig that I would like the Alturas to write a foreword for *The Magnesium Miracle,* she told me that they were such prominent scientists that they would never be associated with a lay publication. As it turned out, the timing was perfect for our collaboration. The Alturas were completely frustrated because despite all the papers they had written and all the proof they had of the necessity and efficacy of magnesium supplementation in dozens of conditions, their message had never left the ivory tower of the university and reached the public. Each paper that the Alturas have published educates the reader about the incredible potential of magnesium to prevent and treat chronic disease.

Long and Romani wrote a review in order to "advocate for the necessity of identifying easy and reproducible methods to assess serum and cellular magnesium levels and to identify magnesium deficiency in order to alleviate related pathological conditions."[25] Their study acknowledges that serum magnesium is a "poor predictor of tissue magnesium content and availability."

A 2016 review also took up the notion that we aren't using the proper measurement techniques for magnesium, seeking to "present current analytical challenges in obtaining accurate and reproducible test results for magnesium."[26] The investigators presented magnesium as a cation (positively charged ion) of great physiologic importance. They said magnesium exists in two states: a form that is bound with another substance and a free ionized form. The form magnesium is in depends on temperature, pH, ionic strength, and competing ions. It is the free ionized magnesium form that participates in hundreds of biochemical processes and that can be measured by ion-selective electrodes in the ionized magnesium test. The researchers said that "too many magnesium studies use total serum magnesium levels rather than its free bioactive form making it difficult to correlate to disease states." As the authors state, it is the free ionized form of magnesium that participates in the body's biochemical processes. (It is of note that a unique proprietary process transforms the magnesium chloride in ReMag into a stabilized magnesium ion state, allowing the stabilized ions to be completely absorbed at the cellular level and not be automatically bound to another substance.)

The 2015 review "Magnesium in Man: Implications for Health and Disease" provides an extensive and comprehensive summary of magnesium research over the last few decades, focusing on the regulation of magnesium homeostasis in the intestines, kidneys, and bone.[27] I was ecstatic when I read the authors' assertion that magnesium "is involved in over 600 enzymatic reactions including energy metabolism and protein synthesis." (I frequently quote magnesium expert Dr. Andrea Rosanoff, who says the number of such reactions is more likely between 700 and 800. At any rate, we have certainly come a long way from the first reports in 1968 that magnesium is responsible for 325 enzymatic reactions in the body.)[28]

The investigators cover the depletion of magnesium due to drugs and the genetic mutations that can produce magnesium deficiency. This is one of the first papers I've read that thoroughly discusses mutations in genes that code for magnesium-transporting proteins and describes a dozen hypomagnesemia genes, each with additional dozens of genetic mutations.

Isolating these genes, however, may not be such a good thing. With the recent availability of personal genetic testing, I'm concerned that when allopathic medicine finally "discovers" magnesium deficiency, it will come at the topic through the human genome and blame it on the genes. Medicine has no treatment for genetic hypomagnesemia. It barely knows how to treat hypomagnesemia at all, with recommendations swinging between absurdly high doses of IV magnesium and laxative doses of magnesium oxide.

However, while researchers are busy studying the genetic causes of magnesium deficiency, I've found that ReMag does not require magnesium-transporting proteins to bring it to the cells; it doesn't care if a gene alters your magnesium requirements. ReMag's stabilized magnesium ions allow full cellular absorption and assimilation.

"Magnesium in Man" notes that magnesium performs numerous functions that produce, repair, and stabilize DNA and RNA. What if magnesium has the ability to stabilize genes and can prevent mutated gene segments from being turned on? Could therapeutic levels of non-laxative magnesium turn off milder mutations of hypomagnesemia genes?

Will a true genetic defect be treatable with magnesium supplements? A paper in the journal *Gene* began with this statement: "Evidence points to magnesium's antioxidant, anti-necrotic, and anti-apoptotic effects in cardio- and neuroprotection." It concludes that "because of the antagonistic effects of Ca^{++} and Mg^{++} ions in the presence of high Ca^{++} ion concentration at MtHK [mitochondrion-bound hexokinase], MtCK [mitochondrial creatine kinase], and PTP [mitochondrial permeability transition pore], magnesium supplementation may provide cytoprotective effects in the treatment of some degenerative diseases and cytopathies with high intracellular $[Ca^{++}]/[Mg^{++}]$ ratio at these sites, whether of genetic, developmental, drug induced, ischemic, immune based, toxic, or infectious etiology."[29]

A 2012 paper called "Magnesium Basics" references several studies proving that ionized magnesium has the greatest biological activity of all forms of the mineral because it most readily enters into cells.[30] Yet doctors mainly recommend magnesium oxide despite the fact that it is only 4 percent absorbed into the bloodstream and that there are no studies indicating how well it is absorbed by the cells. This paper, featuring an eye-popping 595 references, can be printed out and handed to your doctors to help educate them about the importance of magnesium.

Another 2012 paper, this one by Rosanoff and colleagues, is titled "Suboptimal Magnesium Status in the United States: Are the Health Consequences Underestimated?"[31] The answer is a resounding yes!

Rosanoff's team reports that "low magnesium intakes and blood levels have been associated with type 2 diabetes, metabolic syndrome, elevated C-reactive protein, hypertension, atherosclerotic vascular disease, sudden cardiac death, osteoporosis, migraine headache, asthma, and colon cancer." They speculate that magnesium deficiency in the cells relates to excess calcium that activates inflammatory cascades separate from injury or infection. They call for more research to define how elevated calcium-to-magnesium ratios influence the inflammatory conditions mentioned in their study.

A 2015 paper, "Magnesium and Dialysis: The Neglected Cation," confirms that magnesium requirements need to be reevaluated in the treatment of kidney disease and in dialysis patients.[32] The February 2012 issue of *Clinical Kidney Journal* included an extensive paper called "Magnesium in Disease."[33] I will discuss magnesium and kidney disease and cite these references in more depth in Chapter 11.

A valuable addition to your magnesium education is a free online book from the University of Adelaide called *Magnesium in the Central Nervous System* (2011).[34] I suggest you print out the whole book, or at least several chapters, to present to your doctors to help convince them to give you and your loved ones magnesium when you are under their care. Each chapter is a paper written by a magnesium researcher or expert covering important topics involving the central nervous system. The chapter titles alone show the expanding scope of magnesium research. I've made a list of these chapters in Chapter 5 of this book.

MAGNESIUM REFERENCES

I've updated the scientific citations throughout the book and added several hundred new references, bringing the total to more than 600, proving and confirming the effectiveness of magnesium therapy in a host of diseases: ADHD, anxiety, arthritis, asthma, cancer, cerebral palsy, depression, diabetes, dysmenorrhea, eclampsia, genetic disease, head injury, heart disease, high cholesterol, hypertension, infertility, insomnia, kidney disease, menopause, obesity, osteoporosis, pain, PCOS, preeclampsia, pregnancy, stroke, and syndrome X. So that you can stay current long past the publication date of this book, go to the website of the nonprofit Nutritional Magnesium Association (NMA), www.nutritionalmagnesium.org (I'm on the medical advisory board of the NMA). On that website you will find all the updated references you and your doctor require to prove the safety and efficacy of magnesium therapy.

WHICH MAGNESIUM SHOULD I TAKE?

The past decade has seen an incredible escalation in the number of new magnesium supplements trying to gain market share. The more products there are, the fewer I recommend. In the past five years, a unique form of magnesium that I brought to market has risen to the top of my list. It's called ReMag, a picometer, stabilized ionic magnesium. My second choice is magnesium citrate powder, specifically Natural Calm. I'll describe them both, along with Epsom salts baths, in more detail in Chapter 18.

HOW MUCH MAGNESIUM SHOULD I TAKE?

Some practitioners say to take magnesium until you get diarrhea and then back off by one dose. However, on the basis of this recommendation, I and millions like me would not be able to take any magnesium, so it can't possibly be used as a guideline.

You don't necessarily need a magnesium blood test to determine magnesium deficiency; just look at "Causes of Magnesium Deficiency: The Magnesium Burn Rate" and "100 Factors Related to Magnesium Deficiency," both in Chapter 1, and you will probably find many symptoms that fit your case.

If you do want to do some testing, to prove to your doctor or your family that you are indeed magnesium deficient, I recommend the magnesium RBC blood test. You may repeat it every three to six months, aiming for the optimum value of 6.0–6.5 mg/dL. See Chapter 16 for more on magnesium testing and how to order your own test without a doctor's prescription.

It may take a year or more to build up your magnesium stores in your muscles and bones. However, it usually takes only a few days or a few weeks to notice health improvements, which lets you know you are on the right path. You aren't just looking for symptom relief; it's important to have extra magnesium in reserve for those stressful times that nobody can predict. When your stores are replete and you are no longer magnesium deficient, even the non-laxative ReMag will give you a laxative effect if you take more than your cells need. Read the section "The Fail-Safe of Magnesium" below so that you understand how the body prevents too much magnesium from building up in your body.

Having said that, I must register an official disclaimer

that I can't be responsible in cases where people don't follow these important recommendations:

1. Begin taking magnesium slowly, especially if you have a high toxin load, have a chronic disease, or are on many medications.
2. Don't take copious amounts of magnesium without doing proper testing.
3. Be cautious about taking magnesium if you have any of the four contraindications described in Chapter 18. In those cases, research whether ReMag would be safe for you.
4. Along with magnesium, take a multiple-mineral supplement, like ReMyte, and follow my guidelines for adding sea salt to your drinking water. All of these are necessary to maintain mineral balance.
5. Obtain sufficient calcium (600 mg per day) in the diet or in an absorbable supplement such as ReCalcia.

THE FAIL-SAFE OF MAGNESIUM

Our bodies have a fail-safe mechanism that prevents us from absorbing too much magnesium. If we consume too much magnesium in our diets or from supplements, the body rids itself of the excess by flushing it out through the bowels with diarrhea. This built-in fail-safe makes magnesium, in my opinion, one of the safest nutrients you can take.

This fail-safe was created during our evolution in a culture living near the ocean where most of humanity survived on produce from the sea. Sea water has three times more magnesium than calcium. So the primitive diet was high in magnesium-rich foods (seaweed, fish, and shellfish), and low in calcium. Thus it became important to eliminate too much magnesium via the bowels but grab on to as much calcium as possible via vitamin D.

In current times, we are eating high-calcium foods and calcium-fortified foods, and we're taking far more calcium supplementation than magnesium. We also take high doses of vitamin D, which holds on to calcium, to our detriment. Read more about vitamin D in the section "High-Dose Vitamin D Depletes Magnesium" in Chapter 1.

WHEN MAGNESIUM MAKES ME WORSE

When you take a supplement you have the expectation that it will make you feel better. We know that's not always the case with drugs; in fact, people seem to accept that drugs will give them side effects. But what about supplements?

More people are reading my book and hearing about magnesium, and many are taking magnesium without doing any research. They are surprised to learn that there are over a dozen reasons why you might feel "worse" after taking magnesium. But it's not because magnesium is bad for you—it's the total environment in which you are taking magnesium that can be affecting you. Let me list the reasons why taking magnesium may create a reaction in your body that you may misinterpret as a side effect.

1. **You're not taking enough.** When you feel worse with magnesium, I believe that the hundreds of enzyme systems that require magnesium are being activated—essentially, woken up from a low level of function—and your body simply needs more as they are revving up. Here's how Laura, one of my blog readers, put it: "My obvious magnesium deficiency symptoms, cramping, muscle aches, headaches, etc., are worsening slightly

rather than getting better. Anxiety is the only thing that has gotten better. Is this normal? I'm using magnesium oil and magnesium citrate but not able to tolerate more than 200 mg without getting diarrhea."

Laura woke up her magnesium-dependent enzymes, and they are demanding more magnesium than 200 mg. It's like putting your foot on the accelerator without enough gas in the tank. With each enzyme system pumping away, they quickly use up the little magnesium Laura is giving them, and they simply want more and make her think she is still magnesium deficient. Unfortunately, Laura's body isn't going to get what it needs if she gets the laxative effect on 200 mg. That's one of the main reasons to take ReMag—so you can get the therapeutic effect without the laxative effect.

This doesn't mean that you'll have to keep increasing your magnesium ad infinitum! You will reach a saturation point of magnesium stores and actually be able to decrease your magnesium intake. That might not happen for a year or two. But even ReMag has a fail-safe point, so when you are saturated you will begin to get the laxative effect and you can cut back.

2. **You think you are taking enough but you are burning off magnesium at a rapid rate.** This increased rate of usage can be due to higher stress levels, surges of adrenaline (panic attacks), surgery, medications, yeast overgrowth, or premenstrual syndrome (PMS). Some people are "magnesium wasters"—they can't hold on to magnesium and keep needing to replenish it. Severe forms of this condition are Gitelman syndrome and Bartter syndrome.

3. **You're taking too much too soon.** This usually happens if you have fatigue and weakness from chronic magnesium deficiency. Anyone in this category should

start very slowly on any new supplement or drug. If you take a high dose of magnesium right from the start, it's as though you're giving muscles that are used to walking five minutes a day enough fuel to run a marathon. Your body might be so weak that revving up those hundreds of enzyme systems all at once makes you feel jangled and even anxious. For people with chronic fatigue and adrenal issues, start with one-quarter of the recommended dose of magnesium and work up as your body adapts. Occasionally even ¼ tsp (30 drops) of ReMag is too much, so we advise people to begin with 10 drops in a liter of water sipped through the day. One drop of ReMag contains 2.5 mg of magnesium.

4. **Magnesium is causing a detox reaction.** You are toxic for one or more of the following reasons: a bad diet, prescription medications, heavy metals, stress chemicals, yeast overgrowth, or environmental chemicals. As magnesium enters your cells, it stimulates cellular detoxification and dumps toxins and heavy metals from your cells into the lymphatic system. These are eventually excreted through your skin, kidneys, and colon. Toxins surfacing on the skin can cause skin irritation, inflammation, hives, and rashes.

This type of reaction is not an allergy to magnesium but a simple cleansing reaction, as the body is now better able to do its job because of magnesium. There have only been a few so-called allergy reactions to magnesium. The ones I've studied were due to IV magnesium sulfate, and the reaction may actually be due either to the sulfur trying to get past blocked sulfur pathways or to the aluminum that is found in IV magnesium products. Sulfur is likely the problem, because IV magnesium chloride also contains aluminum and I've not heard of reactions to this form of magnesium. However, I would

advise against chronic administration of these forms of
IV magnesium due to the aluminum content. ReMag is
an excellent substitute for IV magnesium, according to
several case reports. You can read Dana's story in Chapter 18.

5. **You have low blood pressure from long-standing
magnesium deficiency and adrenal fatigue.** You
may have heard that magnesium can lower blood pressure, so you worry because your blood pressure is already
low. This is another instance where you must begin by
supplementing at about one-quarter the recommended
dose of magnesium and slowly build up. You will also
need other minerals. The minerals offered in my formula
ReMyte are important to support the adrenals and the
thyroid. Also, I recommend unrefined sea salt, pink Himalayan salt, or Celtic sea salt (¼ teaspoon per quart of
drinking water) to help improve sodium levels; this will
balance your blood pressure and support your adrenals.
Sea salt contains seventy-two trace minerals, all of which
may be important to the body. I suggest you drink half
your body weight (in pounds) in ounces of water daily.
So if you weigh 150 pounds, you should be drinking
75 ounces of water a day.

6. **You're on heart medications.** As your health improves because of magnesium supplementation, your
meds are becoming toxic. That's because you may not
require them anymore, not because magnesium is bad
for you! For example, magnesium helps lower blood
pressure. If you continue to take the same amount of
blood pressure meds, your blood pressure might become
too low. This is not a side effect of magnesium. It's a side
effect of taking drugs when you don't need them! Check
with your doctor, who can help wean you off your meds.

7. **You've started taking iodine or thyroid medication.** High dose iodine or thyroid meds can increase your thyroid hormones causing mild hyperthyroidism, which can speed up your metabolism and rev you up. If you have a history of heart palpitations, they may increase with this rise in metabolism. There are two keys to recognizing increased thyroid function: your pulse rate is elevated, and the magnesium you normally use to control your heart palpitations is no longer working. Magnesium can independently improve thyroid function and may mean you need to lower your thyroid medication. This can be even more likely if you are taking ReMyte, as nine of the twelve minerals in ReMyte support thyroid function.

8. **You're taking too much vitamin D.** You've been feeling great on your magnesium, and then you begin taking high-dose vitamin D and find yourself experiencing magnesium deficiency symptoms again. Magnesium is required to transform vitamin D from its storage form into its active form and for many other aspects of vitamin D metabolism. That means if you take the extremely high doses of vitamin D that allopathic doctors are now recommending, you can plummet into magnesium deficiency and not know why. For this reason I don't recommend more than 1,000–2,000 IU of vitamin D_3 daily. And never take vitamin D without magnesium. This is such an important aspect of magnesium therapy that it deserves a separate section. Read "High-Dose Vitamin D Depletes Magnesium," which you can find in Chapter 1.

9. **You are taking too much calcium and it's pushing out magnesium.** Read about the competition between calcium and magnesium in "The Failure of Calcium" in

Chapter 2 to understand why calcium is now a pariah. Excessive amounts of this mineral are causing heart disease and many other symptoms of calcification in the women and men who take it.

10. **You're taking fairly high doses of magnesium and not taking trace minerals or drinking enough water.** Trace minerals help your body hold water in the cells. Without minerals your cells can become dehydrated and your tissues can retain fluid—which can show up as, for example, ankle edema. Reread #5 in this list.

11. **You're not taking enough B vitamins.** Vitamin B_6 and B_2 are important vitamins that assist magnesium absorption into cells. A number of papers have reported on the relationship of magnesium and B_6 in the treatment of PMS and kidney stones. Most recently, research has been directed at the benefits of magnesium and vitamin B_6 in autism and ADHD. However, I don't recommend high-dose synthetic B_6 because of the occurrence of peripheral neuropathy in a small percentage of people. This side effect is probably due to magnesium deficiency. Instead I recommend the methylated B vitamins in my product ReAline or the food-based B complex by Grown by Nature. Note that ReMag is so well absorbed that it doesn't require B vitamins, an intact gut, or carrier proteins to bring it directly to the cells.

12. **You are mercury toxic.** In Chapter 13, I state, "Mercury drastically increases the excretion of magnesium and calcium from the kidneys, which may be the cause of the kidney damage seen in mercury poisoning." Removing mercury from the body is important but not the focus of this book; however, taking sufficient amounts of magnesium can help detoxify this dangerous heavy metal.

13. **You're taking a drug that contains fluoride.** Read the section "Fluoride Binds Magnesium" in Chapter 1 to understand why you may be susceptible to magnesium deficiency caused by medically prescribed drugs, fluoride treatments from your dentist, fluoride toothpaste, or fluoridated drinking water.

14. **You have yeast overgrowth.** Your magnesium deficiency symptoms may have been so severe that you didn't realize you have yeast overgrowth. Now that your deficiency symptoms are going away, you may become aware of yeast overgrowth symptoms. Or your magnesium is helping to detoxify yeast toxins or yeast itself, and you are experiencing yeast die-off. The symptoms often manifest as skin rashes, vaginitis, sinusitis, itching ears, and brain fog. The treatment is to do a yeast-free diet, take probiotics, and employ natural antifungal remedies.

PART ONE

The History of Magnesium

The Case for Magnesium

I'll build my argument for magnesium beginning with three case histories of people who successfully overcame their magnesium deficiency.

Mary joked that she felt as though she were constantly being run over by a slow-moving bus. Cramping in her legs startled her awake at night, making her an insomniac, and she had heart palpitations daily. Her doctor also found that she had high blood sugar. It wasn't bad enough for her to need insulin injections. but he prescribed pills to try to stimulate more insulin production. Finally, frightening panic attacks came out of nowhere and made this vibrant, fun-loving woman afraid to go outside.

To try to relieve her leg cramps, Mary began taking calcium at night, having read that it was good for cramps and sleep. At first the calcium seemed to help, but after a week or two the pains got worse. If she yawned and stretched in bed, her calf muscles would seize up and catapult her to the floor, where she would lie frantically massaging her muscles to try to release the spasm. All the next day she would limp about with a very tender, bruised feeling in her calf.

Although Mary's heart palpitations had improved somewhat after she'd given up her three cups of coffee a day, they resumed after a few weeks. Every time the palpitations occurred, which was several times a day, they made her cough slightly and catch her breath. She found it frightening, even though her doctor said her stress tests for heart disease were negative and she didn't need further testing with an angiogram.

Both Mary's parents had suffered adult-onset diabetes, and Mary knew that she should watch her diet, but she was overweight and found sugary and high-carbohydrate foods hard to resist. When the panic attacks hit on top of everything else, Mary knew she had to seek help, and came to my office. She was only fifty-three, far too young to be feeling so ill, and she was worried about her future health.

Sam was just forty-nine and experiencing chest pains. At first he thought they were indigestion, but sometimes the pains would occur in the middle of the night. Concerned, he went to a cardiologist, who found two slightly blocked arteries, not serious enough for bypass surgery. Sam's cholesterol was somewhat elevated, as was his blood pressure, which he attributed to his high-stress occupation and the fact that he had not exercised regularly for the past six months, when he was sidelined with back pain.

The cardiologist warned Sam that his arterial blockage would almost inevitably worsen over time and eventually necessitate surgery. The doctor offered him medication for his high cholesterol and slightly elevated blood pressure, told him not to eat butter or eggs, and gave him nitroglycerine to take whenever he had the pain. He said that if the symptoms got worse, he would prescribe more medications. Sam couldn't imagine taking pills for the rest of his life and waiting to have surgery when he got worse! He knew there must be something he could do to avoid surgery, and came to me for advice.

At thirty-five, Jan had actually begun to look forward to menopause. That's how bad her PMS symptoms were every month. And as soon as those horrible PMS feelings lifted, she was hit by the sledgehammer of menstrual cramps. She also had migraines, which for years had come before her period but now were occurring once or twice every week. She was so miserable that she was considering a complete hysterectomy, with removal of her hormone-producing ovaries, but wondered whether the migraines were not actually hormonal, since they were happening all month.

Different as their symptoms were, Mary, Sam, and Jan were all suffering from magnesium deficiency. While women and men seem equally susceptible to magnesium deficiency, women, pound for pound, have less magnesium. Women have fewer circulating red blood cells, which carry magnesium, and perhaps less magnesium available, but they seem to utilize the magnesium they do have more efficiently than men.

There are a few other gender differences. Because of magnesium's effect on hormonal regulation and vice versa, women appear to have more problems with low magnesium because they can suffer deficiencies during pregnancy, when breast-feeding, with premenstrual syndrome, and with dysmenorrhea (painful periods).

Osteoporosis, which affects more women than men, is evidence of an imbalance of calcium and magnesium. An overactive thyroid, which afflicts more women than men, increases the metabolic rate, which uses up magnesium-requiring ATP (adenosine triphosphate), the energy packets made in each cell in the body. Without magnesium, ATP would not be produced. However, women's efficient use of magnesium may explain why prior to menopause they are more protected from heart attacks than men.

Let's follow Mary, Sam, and Jan and see how they overcame their magnesium deficiencies.

When Mary visited me, I charted her health history in detail, according to procedures commonly used by naturopathic doctors, and found several symptoms of magnesium deficiency. In her case it had been made even worse by too much calcium, however, so simple magnesium supplementation wouldn't be enough for Mary. Her diet and lifestyle needed a complete overhaul. I explained that calcium appears to help leg cramps, at least initially, because excess calcium forces magnesium to be released from storage sites. But if someone is magnesium-deficient, the excess calcium will eventually cause more problems.

I gave Mary a list of magnesium-rich foods that she needed to start eating, which included nuts, beans, greens, and seeds such as sunflower and pumpkin. Mary realized that she'd been avoiding almost all of these foods: she thought nuts were fattening, beans gave her gas, and greens never seemed fresh enough at the supermarket. She had never even thought about eating seeds.

After a week of enthusiastically eating a lot more magnesium-rich foods, Mary felt somewhat better. To make sure she could get fresh organic greens regularly, she tracked down a local CSA (community-supported agriculture) program and bought a share from a neighboring organic farm. Mary also learned how to soak and cook beans to prevent them from causing gas, and began eating nuts and seeds rich in magnesium and healthy oils, such as almonds, walnuts, pecans, sunflower seeds, and pumpkin seeds.

After her second visit I recommended that Mary begin taking magnesium supplements. Starting with a dosage of 75 mg a day, we added another 75 mg every two days to build slowly to 600 mg. I cautioned her that it could take months to eliminate magnesium deficiency symptoms and that not all her symptoms would necessarily respond quickly. Mary, excited by the improvement she felt by just increasing magnesium-rich foods, expressed impatience and wanted to know if she should have intravenous magnesium to saturate her tissues more quickly. I explained that IV magnesium would indeed do just that, but a more effective and much less expensive way would be to stay with her picometer ionic magnesium (ReMag) and use Epsom salts regularly in baths, including foot baths.

Within one month Mary was singing the praises of magnesium. Her palpitations and panic attacks had disappeared. Her cravings for sweets were fewer, she was able to control her blood sugar with diet alone, and tests for blood sugar were normal. Her leg cramps were gone, and with them her insomnia. At three months we added calcium-rich foods along with magnesium supplements to keep a 1:1 ratio between the two. Mary's internist was quite surprised at her improved health and told her to keep up the good work with her diet and supplements.

Sam had an inquiring mind, and I encouraged him to start reading about heart disease and magnesium. He found that up to 30 percent of angina (chest pain) patients do not have badly blocked arteries but may be suffering from an electrical imbalance that is driven by mineral deficiency, most commonly magnesium.[1] An astonishing 40 to 60 percent of sudden deaths from heart attack may occur in the complete absence of any prior artery blockage, clot formation, or heart rhythm abnormalities, most likely from spasms in the arteries (magnesium is a natural antispasmodic).[2, 3, 4, 5] Moreover, he found that magnesium deficiency has been linked to sudden cardiac death.

Sam didn't want to wait around for a heart attack to

happen; he was determined to find out what was causing his problem. The more he read, the more intrigued he became. When he read that magnesium deficiency is also associated with muscle pain, especially back pain, that really got his attention, since he started having back pain four or five months before he developed chest pain.[6]

With a packet of information on magnesium, Sam went back to his cardiologist. After Sam had been waiting impatiently for the doctor a full thirty minutes, a nurse took his blood pressure; it was elevated, even though at home it was usually only a few points above normal. (Doctor-induced hypertension, often called "white coat syndrome," is commonly reported by patients.) After hearing the blood pressure reading from his nurse, the cardiologist swept into Sam's room and immediately began talking about blood pressure medication. Sam countered with magnesium. The cardiologist visibly cooled and said that magnesium was used to control hypertension that occurred in pregnant women because there were no side effects, but that there were plenty of effective drugs for everyone else. When Sam said he would rather not have side effects either, the cardiologist gathered up his file and told him to come back when he was ready to take medications for his heart disease.

When Sam came back to see me, he was still pretty upset by this encounter; he didn't like the specialist refusing to discuss a possible magnesium deficiency as part of the picture. Sam and I agreed that magnesium seemed to be the best treatment for him to initiate at this time since he was not willing to take medications. Sam began adding magnesium to his diet by eating magnesium-rich foods. After a week he felt much calmer, but he still had chest and back pain. So he added magnesium supplements, and in about three months he felt almost normal.

Among the studies Sam read was one that looked at the correspondence between type A personalities and magnesium deficiency. From the description, Sam realized he was a type A, an aggressive guy who lived on adrenaline, time pressure, and stress. This type of behavior drains the body of magnesium and can lead to disorders such as heart disease, muscle spasms, hypersensitivity, and irritability.[7]

Prolonged psychological stress raises adrenaline, the stress hormone, which depletes magnesium.[8] Both Sam's back and chest pain would hit when he was under stress. Sam worked on ways to control his stress and added more magnesium when he knew he couldn't avoid it. On days when he exercised, Sam added an extra 150–300 mg of magnesium to his regime, since sweat loss during heavy exercise (cycling and jogging) and working in the heat deplete magnesium. Drinking plain water won't replace the minerals lost. And electrolyte drinks contain mostly sodium and sugar. By paying attention to the many factors that affected his mind-body health, Sam lowered his cholesterol and stress levels and reduced his chance of a heart attack and of needing surgery to unblock his arteries.

Jan heard that yoga might help her PMS and painful periods, and she really needed to learn to relax, so she took classes at a local health club. The teacher also ran regular detox and cooking classes, which Jan decided to join when she realized she didn't have to "give up everything" and become a vegetarian.

One of the first things Jan learned in the detox class was the importance of having regular bowel movements. Jan felt she was lucky if she had one a week. If the bowel doesn't empty once a day, toxins can be reabsorbed back into the body from the colon. The longer debris sits in the colon, the more fluid is reabsorbed, making stools more solid and difficult to pass. PMS and endometriosis, which causes painful periods, are considered by some natural-health experts to be triggered by constipation and toxicity.[9]

During cooking classes, Jan faced the fact that she was a junk food addict. Magnesium is necessary in hundreds of enzymes in the body but is almost totally lost during the processing of packaged and fast foods. The older women in her class were suffering from a variety of problems that included cancer, heart disease, and osteoporosis. Jan wondered if that was how she would end up in ten or twenty years if she didn't take care of her health now. Learning how many basic nutrients she lacked in her diet made her marvel that she wasn't even more ill.

Her new diet included greens, beans, nuts, and seeds, which cleared up her constipation and almost eliminated her PMS and painful periods. When she came to see me on the advice of her yoga teacher, it was clear she was on the right track. I recommended that she begin taking a magnesium supplement and a multimineral supplement, as well as increasing her dietary calcium. With all her lifestyle changes, Jan soon felt like a new person.

CAUSES OF MAGNESIUM DEFICIENCY: THE MAGNESIUM BURN RATE

It is quite a shock to see all the ways that magnesium can become depleted or burned off. I'll talk about most of these magnesium deficiency factors throughout the book in more detail. I've also listed "100 Factors Related to Magnesium Deficiency" later in this chapter. However, the following list of twenty-six major causes of magnesium deficiency is a good summary and bears repeating so you can truly understand what we are up against in our magnesium-depleted world.

Causes of Magnesium Deficiency

1. Athletic performance causes sweat loss of magnesium.
2. Alcohol causes magnesium depletion due to its diuretic effect.
3. Antacids counteract stomach acid, decreasing magnesium absorption.
4. Acid rain is high in nitric acid, which draws calcium and magnesium out of the soil to try and neutralize the acidity and consequently depletes the soil of these minerals.
5. Caffeine causes magnesium depletion with its diuretic effect. It also stimulates the adrenal glands, causing adrenaline surges and magnesium loss.
6. Most drugs cause magnesium depletion; this is especially true of drugs containing fluorine atoms.
7. Fertilizers do not replace necessary minerals but are high in phosphorus, potassium, and nitrogen. Excess potassium and phosphorus are preferentially absorbed into plants, inhibiting magnesium absorption.
8. Fluoride and fluorine in water, from dental procedures, in toothpaste, and in drugs bind magnesium, making it unavailable to the body. Magnesium fluoride (MgF_2), called sellaite, is an insoluble compound and replaces magnesium in bone and cartilage with a brittle, unstable crystalline substance.
9. Food processing and cooking decrease magnesium levels.
10. Herbicides such as Roundup bind with magnesium, making it unavailable for plants to utilize for decades.
11. Pesticides kill worms and bacteria and thus their function of processing the soil and breaking down minerals is lost, which means fewer minerals are absorbed by plants.
12. Intestinal disease, including irritable bowel syndrome (IBS), leaky gut, gluten and casein sensitivities, funguses, and parasites, interferes with magnesium absorption.

13. Junk foods, especially sugar products, drain magnesium. The liver needs twenty-eight atoms of magnesium to process one molecule of glucose. Fructose requires fifty-six atoms of magnesium.
14. Meat from animals eating magnesium-depleted food is low in magnesium.
15. Oxalic acid (found in rhubarb, spinach, and chard) and phytic acid (found in cereal grains and soy) block absorption of magnesium.
16. Low potassium levels can increase urinary magnesium loss.
17. High-protein diets can decrease magnesium absorption and require more magnesium for digestion and assimilation.
18. Refining grains, especially rice and wheat, reduces magnesium.
19. Sauna therapy for weight loss, to detox, or just to stay healthy can cause enough mineral loss through sweating to create magnesium deficiency symptoms.
20. Soil on farmland is woefully depleted of magnesium.
21. Soil erosion makes it easier for heavy rain or irrigation to wash away soil, leading to a loss of minerals, including magnesium.
22. Stress or trauma of any type—physical, mental, emotional, environmental—can cause magnesium deficiency.
23. Stomach acid deficiency due to stress results in decreased absorption of magnesium.
24. Tannins in tea bind and remove minerals, including magnesium.
25. Trans fatty acids and mineral deficiency alter cell wall integrity, making the cell walls more rigid, which affects receptor site function and prevents the flow of nutrients in or out of cells.
26. Water softening treatment reduces magnesium.

THE CLINICAL IMPACT OF
MAGNESIUM DEFICIENCY

Magnesium was first discovered in huge deposits near a Greek city called Magnesia. Magnesium sulfate, known today as Epsom salts, was used in ancient times as a laxative, and still is to this day. A 1697 medical paper titled "Treatise on the Nature and Use of the Bitter Purging Salt Contained in Epsom and Such Other Water" recommended magnesium for health problems as varied as skin ulcers, depression, vertigo, heartburn, worms, kidney stones, jaundice, and gout. Most of these problems are still treated with magnesium, and current research supports its use for many of those conditions along with a long list of other ailments that you will read about below.

SIXTY-FIVE CONDITIONS ASSOCIATED WITH
MAGNESIUM DEFICIENCY

In the introduction to the first edition of *The Magnesium Miracle*, I listed twenty-one conditions that have a direct clinical correlation with magnesium deficiency and respond to magnesium treatment. From more recent magnesium research and clinical experience, I've expanded this list to sixty-five conditions. What follows is an overview of these conditions, some of which I will develop further in the text.

1. **Acid reflux.** Spasm of the lower esophageal sphincter at the juncture of the stomach can leave the sphincter open, causing acid reflux, gastroesophageal reflux disease (GERD), or heartburn. Magnesium relieves esophageal spasms.
2. **Adrenal fatigue.** Adrenal fatigue follows after a time of chronic stress, anxiety, and panic attacks, and it seems to be occurring in epidemic proportions in recent years.

Adrenaline, noradrenaline, and cortisol (elevated in chronic stress) deplete magnesium. Stress causes excess elimination of magnesium through the urine, further compounding magnesium deficiency. "Stress" is such an overworked word, but we all suffer physical, emotional, and mental stress every day, and every bit of it drains magnesium.

3. **Alzheimer's disease.** Magnesium blocks the neuroinflammation caused by the inappropriate deposition of calcium and other heavy metals in brain cells. Magnesium is at work even before the inflammation appears, guarding cell ion channels and not allowing heavy metals to enter. Picometer, stabilized ionic magnesium (ReMag) easily enters cells and can help eliminate heavy metals and solubilize calcium.

4. **Angina.** The pain of angina is caused by severe spasms in heart muscles, which are caused by magnesium deficiency. The heart ventricles have the highest levels of magnesium in the whole body; this is why magnesium is so important for the pumping function of the heart.

5. **Anxiety and panic attacks.** When the adrenals are no longer protected by sufficient magnesium, the fight-or-flight hormones adrenaline and noradrenaline become more easily triggered. When they surge erratically, they cause rapid pulse, high blood pressure, and heart palpitations. The more magnesium-deficient you are, the more exaggerated is the adrenaline response. Magnesium calms the nervous system, relaxes muscle tension, and lowers the pulse rate, helping to reduce anxiety and panic attacks.

6. **Arthritis.** Magnesium can help dissolve calcium that builds up in joint spaces. It also can treat the pain and inflammation of arthritis as a safe substitute for pain medication.

7. **Asthma.** Histamine production and bronchial spasms (in the smooth muscles of the bronchial tract) both increase as a result of magnesium deficiency.

8. **Atherosclerosis with calcium deposits.** Magnesium is necessary to help dissolve calcium and keep it soluble in the bloodstream. Magnesium, along with vitamin K_2, helps direct calcium to the bones, where it belongs.

9. **Blood clots.** Magnesium does not act like a blood-thinning drug. Instead, it prevents the calcium buildup that triggers clots. Magnesium naturally balances the clotting factors in the blood.

10. **Bowel disease.** Magnesium deficiency slows down bowel peristalsis, causing constipation, which can lead to toxicity as well as symptoms of colitis, microscopic colitis, IBS, diverticulitis, and Crohn's disease.

11. **Brain dysfunction.** You can obtain a free copy of the 355-page book *Magnesium in the Central Nervous System* (2011) online and read an extensive overview of the beneficial effects of magnesium on the brain.[10] (See Chapter 5 for a list of chapters in that book.)

12. **Bruxism (teeth grinding).** Up to 80 percent of cases of bruxism occur during sleep, and your dentist may be the first to notice that your teeth are being gradually worn down. Bruxism is related to clenching of the jaw muscles during the day and is usually associated with stress or anxiety. Any muscle tension can be the result of magnesium deficiency.

13. **Cholesterol elevation.** When I was in medical school in the mid-1970s, normal cholesterol levels were considered to be around 245 mg/dL. In the first edition of *The Magnesium Miracle* I reported allopathic medicine's "normal" value of cholesterol at 180–220 mg/dL. Now doctors are advising that cholesterol should be below 200 mg/dL (5.2 mmol/L) to be considered normal.

What doctors don't seem to know is that magnesium, bound to ATP (Mg^{2+}-ATP), is the controlling factor for the rate-limiting enzyme in the cholesterol biosynthesis sequence that is targeted by the statin pharmaceutical drugs.[11] Thus magnesium is responsible for naturally slowing down HMG-CoA reductase activity when cholesterol is present in sufficient quantities. To repeat, this is the same enzyme that statin drugs target for destruction, while creating magnesium deficiency.

14. **Chronic fatigue syndrome (CFS).** I write about CFS in Chapter 12. It is remarkable how magnesium, especially ReMag, can help people increase their energy and get back on track. We still don't know what causes CFS, but in my discussion about the interaction between calcium and magnesium, I consider whether calcium excess and magnesium deficiency could be the underlying cause of mitochondrial dysfunction that many natural medicine practitioners say can trigger chronic fatigue syndrome and other chronic diseases.

15. **Cystitis.** Magnesium deficiency causes bladder spasms, which can cause urinary frequency often misinterpreted as a bladder infection. Magnesium deficiency can also allow calcium to build up in the lining of the bladder and urethra, causing irritation that mimics cystitis. We've had reports from elderly women who have thrown away their adult diapers because, apparently, ReMag dissolves bladder tissue calcification and eliminates incontinence.

16. **Depression.** Serotonin, a neurotransmitter that elevates mood, depends on magnesium for its production and function, whether it's made in the brain or in the intestines. Dopamine, a neurotransmitter that helps control the brain's reward and pleasure centers, utilizes magnesium in several steps in its biochemical pathway. A

magnesium-deficient brain is also more susceptible to allergens and foreign substances, which in some instances can cause symptoms similar to mental illness.

17. **Detoxification.** Magnesium is crucial for the removal of toxic substances and heavy metals such as mercury, aluminum, and lead from the cells. Magnesium is a cofactor in both the production of glutathione and the function of the P450 detoxification pathways in the liver.

18. **Diabetes.** Magnesium is necessary to make and secrete insulin, facilitates carbohydrate metabolism, and allows insulin to transfer glucose into cells. Otherwise, glucose and insulin build up in the blood, causing various types of tissue damage. Tyrosine kinase, an enzyme that allows glucose entry into the cell (along with insulin), is magnesium dependent. Seven of the ten enzymes needed to metabolize glucose in the process called glycolysis are also magnesium dependent. All these factors mean that magnesium helps to overcome insulin resistance.

19. **Fatigue.** Magnesium-deficient patients commonly experience fatigue because hundreds of enzyme systems are underfunctioning. The most important factor in energy production is ATP, which must be bound to a magnesium ion in order to be biologically active. Mg^{2+}-ATP is produced in the Krebs cycle, which requires magnesium in six of its eight steps. The Krebs cycle begins by using pyruvate from the glycolysis cycle and functions exclusively in the mitochondria.

20. **Headaches.** Muscle tension and spasms in neck and head muscles can be alleviated with magnesium therapy. Magnesium can be either applied locally or taken orally.

21. **Heart disease.** The heart, specifically the left ventricle, has the highest amount of magnesium in the whole body. Magnesium deficiency is common in people with heart

disease, and taking magnesium can reduce that risk. IV magnesium can prevent heart muscle damage and cardiac arrhythmia if given at the onset of a heart attack. Most drugs used in treating heart disease drain magnesium from the body.

22. **Hypertension.** With insufficient magnesium and too much calcium, the smooth muscles lining blood vessels can go into spasm and cause high blood pressure. If cholesterol is elevated, which can also be due to magnesium deficiency, cholesterol can bind with calcium, causing atherosclerosis in the blood vessels and worsening high blood pressure.

23. **Hypoglycemia.** Magnesium regulates the production of insulin so that inappropriately large amounts aren't released, which would cause the blood sugar to drop suddenly, resulting in symptoms of low blood sugar.

24. **Indigestion.** The gastric proton pump that acidifies the contents of the stomach for proper digestion is dependent on magnesium.

25. **Inflammation.** Most drug companies are now embracing inflammation and not cholesterol as the cause of heart disease. They don't know what causes inflammation, but that doesn't stop them from producing drugs to suppress it. Drug companies don't acknowledge that calcium is extremely proinflammatory and magnesium is very anti-inflammatory. The entire inflammatory cascade (which involves substance P, interleukins, tumor necrosis factor, chemokines, and cytokines) escalates when magnesium is deficient.[12] The bottom line is that inflammation is triggered by magnesium deficiency and relative calcium excess.

26. **Insomnia.** Magnesium relieves the muscle tension that can prevent restful sleep. Also, sleep-regulating melatonin pathway production is disturbed without sufficient

magnesium. Magnesium is so effective as a sleep aid that if someone is taking magnesium and their sleep is not improved, I say, "Take more magnesium." You may have to take ReMag to get the therapeutic effect without the laxative effect.

27. **Irritable bowel syndrome.** In my book *IBS for Dummies,* I describe the importance of magnesium in the treatment of pain and spasm in IBS.[13]

28. **Kidney disease.** Magnesium deficiency contributes to atherosclerotic kidney failure because calcium builds up in the renal (kidney) arteries. Magnesium deficiency leads to abnormal lipid levels and worsening blood sugar control in kidney transplant patients. It's important for kidney patients to receive picometer, stabilized ionic magnesium (ReMag) that is absorbed directly into cells and therefore does not build up in the blood to cause electrolyte imbalance and rhythm disturbances.

29. **Kidney stones.** See Chapter 11 for evidence of magnesium's ability to prevent and treat kidney stones, especially when combined with its partner, vitamin B_6.

30. **Migraine.** Deficiency of serotonin can result in migraine headaches and depression. Serotonin depends on magnesium for proper balance. Also, tiny blood clots can block capillaries in the brain, leading to migraines. Magnesium prevents calcium from causing inappropriate blood clotting. It is well known that IV and oral magnesium can treat and prevent migraine headaches.

31. **Musculoskeletal conditions.** Insufficient magnesium and the relative excess of calcium will cause sustained muscle contraction in any muscle group in the body. The following musculoskeletal conditions are amenable to magnesium therapy:
    a. Muscle cramps
    b. Fibrositis

    c. Fibromyalgia

    d. GI spasms (chronic pain from undiagnosed spasms can lead to inappropriate exploratory surgery)

    e. Tension headaches

    f. Muscle spasms in any muscle of the body

    g. Chronic neck and back pain

    h. Jaw tension

32. **Nerve problems: neuralgia, neuritis, neuropathy.** Insufficient magnesium and the relative excess of calcium will cause sustained nerve excitation in any nerve cells in the body. Magnesium alleviates the following nerve disturbances that can occur:

    a. Burning pain

    b. Muscle weakness

    c. Numbness

    d. Paralysis

    e. Pins-and-needles sensations

    f. Seizures and convulsions

    g. Skin sensitivity

    h. Tingling

    i. Twitching

    j. Vertigo

    k. Confusion

33. **Obstetrical and gynecological problems.** Magnesium helps prevent or treat the following:

    a. Premenstrual syndrome

    b. Dysmenorrhea (cramping pain during menses)

    c. Female infertility (by relieving fallopian tube spasm)

    d. Premature contractions (which can be triggered by magnesium-deficiency muscle spasms)

    e. Preeclampsia and eclampsia in pregnancy (fluid retention, high blood pressure, and seizures)

    f. Cerebral palsy

    g. Sudden infant death syndrome (SIDS)

    h. Male infertility (magnesium and zinc are present in significant quantities in healthy semen)

34. **Osteoporosis.** Low magnesium in the presence of elevated calcium, with or without vitamin D, triggers a cascade of events leading to bone loss.

35. **Parkinson's disease.** Dopamine deficiency results in Parkinson's disease, and magnesium is a required cofactor in the production of dopamine. Magnesium blocks the neuroinflammation caused by calcium deposits in the brain.

36. **Raynaud's syndrome.** Magnesium helps relax the spastic blood vessels that cause pain and numbness of the fingers.

37. **Sports injuries.** Pain, inflammation, muscle spasm, muscle tension, and scarring can all be treated with magnesium.

38. **Sports recovery.** Magnesium reduces lactic acid buildup and replaces loss of magnesium in sweat, which otherwise can result in postexercise pain.

39. **Temporomandibular joint syndrome (TMJ).** This hinge joint connects the jawbone to the cheekbone. The joint can become irritated and inflamed due to arthritis, excessive gum chewing, injury to the teeth or jaw, misalignment of the teeth or jaw, poor posture, stress, and teeth grinding. Most of these factors are aggravated by magnesium deficiency.

40. **Tongue biting.** In a magnesium-deficient person, the muscles of the tongue and the muscles lining the inside of the mouth can go into spasm while the person is eating, causing the teeth to suddenly and inadvertently clamp down on the tongue or the lining of the inside of the mouth.

41. **Tooth decay.** Magnesium deficiency causes an unhealthy balance of phosphorus and calcium in saliva, which damages the teeth.

If you tell me you are taking magnesium and are still having magnesium deficiency symptoms, it usually means you aren't taking enough or you aren't taking the right kind of magnesium. I encourage you to find out if you are absorbing magnesium by ordering a magnesium RBC test. See Chapter 16 for more on magnesium testing. If you are not absorbing magnesium, the solution is to take picometer, stabilized ionic ReMag, which is completely absorbed at the cellular level.

If your doctor doesn't realize that the above sixty-five conditions can be due to magnesium deficiency and are treatable with magnesium, you will be prescribed drugs. Unfortunately, drugs such as painkillers, diuretics, antibiotics, and cortisone further deplete magnesium and other minerals, allowing symptoms to get completely out of control.

A study conducted by the Mayo Clinic made the headlines with the following sensational title: "Study Shows 70 Percent of Americans Take Prescription Drugs."[14] Based on the prescription records of 147,377 patients, Mayo Clinic researchers found that almost 70 percent of Americans are on at least one prescription drug, and more than 50 percent take two. Twenty percent of patients are on five or more prescription medications, and one in four women between the ages of fifty and sixty-four is on antidepressants.

According to the Centers for Disease Control and Prevention, the percentage of people using at least one prescription drug in the past month increased nearly 50 percent between 2007 and 2010. Prescription drug spending is likely to only continue to increase in the future. While the Mayo Clinic study reported that payment for prescription drugs reached $250 billion in 2009 and accounted for 12 percent of total personal health care expenditures, in 2015 the IMS Institute for Healthcare Informatics found that drug spending in the United States had reached $310 billion annually—that was a 24 percent increase in just six years.

WHO IS DEFICIENT?

The questions I'm most frequently asked about magnesium are "How do I know if I need more magnesium?" and "Should I take magnesium supplements?" I have come to the conclusion that everyone could benefit from magnesium supplementation. You can find out if you are magnesium deficient by identifying your magnesium deficiency symptoms and/or having your blood tested. I talk about the three magnesium blood tests in Chapter 16. However, a blood test and your clinical symptoms together, or your clinical symptoms alone, can give you your answer.

There is a long list of possible symptoms and behaviors that can confirm your need for magnesium. The following one hundred factors in sixty-eight categories will help you recognize why you may be magnesium deficient. There's no way of knowing how many factors correlate with any one person's magnesium deficiency. But if you find yourself ticking off a dozen or more, you may want to see how many of your symptoms improve after you take magnesium supplements.

100 Factors Related to Magnesium Deficiency

   1. Alcohol intake—more than seven drinks per week
   2. Anger
   3. Angina
   4. Anxiety
   5. Apathy

6. Arrhythmia of the heart
7. Asthma
8. Blood tests
    a. Low calcium
    b. Low potassium
    c. Low magnesium
9. Bowel problems
    a. Undigested fat in stool
    b. Constipation
    c. Diarrhea
    d. Alternating constipation and diarrhea
    e. Irritable bowel syndrome
    f. Crohn's
    g. Colitis, microscopic colitis
10. Brain trauma
11. Bronchitis, chronic
12. Caffeine (coffee, tea, chocolate), more than three servings per day
13. Chronic fatigue syndrome
14. Cold extremities
15. Concentration difficulties
16. Confusion
17. Convulsions
18. Depression
19. Diabetes
    a. Type 1
    b. Type 2
    c. Gestational diabetes
20. Fibromyalgia
21. Food cravings
    a. Carbohydrates
    b. Chocolate
    c. Salt
    d. Junk food

22. Food intake imbalances
    a. Limited in green leafy vegetables, seeds, and fresh fruit
    b. High-protein diet
23. Gagging or choking on food
24. Headaches
25. Heart disease
26. Heart—rapid rate
27. High blood pressure
28. Hyperactivity
29. Hyperhomocysteinemia
30. Hyperventilation
31. Infertility
32. Insomnia
33. Irritability
34. Kidney stones
35. Medications
    a. Digitalis
    b. Diuretics
    c. Antibiotics
    d. Steroids
    e. Oral contraceptives
    f. Indomethacin
    g. Cisplatin
    h. Amphotericin B
    i. Cholestyramine
    j. Synthetic estrogens
36. Memory impairment
37. Menstrual pain and cramps
38. Mercury amalgam dental fillings
39. Migraines
40. Mineral supplements
    a. Taking calcium without magnesium
    b. Taking zinc without magnesium

     c. Poorly absorbed forms of magnesium block iron absorption; well-absorbed forms assist iron absorption

41. Mitral valve prolapse
42. Muscle cramps or spasms
43. Muscle twitching or tics
44. Muscle weakness
45. Numbness of hands or feet
46. Osteoporosis
47. Paranoia
48. Parathyroid hyperactivity
49. Polycystic ovarian disease
50. Pregnancy
     a. Currently pregnant
     b. Pregnant within the past year
     c. History of preeclampsia or eclampsia
     d. Postpartum depression
     e. Have a child with cerebral palsy
51. Premenstrual syndrome
52. Radiation therapy, recent
53. Raynaud's syndrome
54. Restlessness
55. Sexual energy diminished
56. Shortness of breath
57. Smoking
58. Startled easily by noise
59. Stressful life or circumstances
60. Stroke
61. Sugar, high intake daily
62. Syndrome X
63. Thyroid hyperactivity
64. Tingling of hands or feet
65. Transplants
     a. Kidney
     b. Liver

66. Tremor of the hands
67. Water that contains the following
    a. Fluoride
    b. Chlorine
    c. Calcium
68. Wheezing

MAGNESIUM AND JANE'S TOP TEN IMPROVEMENTS

One woman in her early fifties, whom I'll call Jane, filled out my patient symptom survey. The survey has seventy questions, each scored on a scale of 0 to 10. A healthy person would have a very low score, from 0 to 30. Jane, however, scored an incredible 275!

After three months with only the addition of magnesium, Jane sent me a list of the top ten improvements she had already seen.

1. **Less knee pain.** Our knees take the brunt of our weight. The knee is just a simple hinge joint that is held in place by the thigh and leg muscles. If those muscles are tight or in spasm, that alone can cause a slight displacement of the knee, which over time can turn into what medicine calls knee arthritis. However, instead of immediately going on pain medication or undergoing knee surgery to clean out the joint, magnesium supplementation to relax the muscles is the treatment of choice.

2. **Carbohydrate/sugar cravings reduced.** On a scale of 0–10, Jane saw her level of cravings drop from 9 to 0.5. Magnesium is a necessary cofactor in the proper metabolism of carbohydrates. It also helps insulin work properly to put sugar inside cells, where it belongs, and

not leave it in the bloodstream, where it can continue to cause sugar cravings.

3. **Facial wrinkles and crevices diminishing.** This is a new benefit of magnesium that I hadn't heard before, but Jane is a very observant lady. I'm sure others are receiving the benefit of magnesium in this way but aren't taking note. It's likely to do with tissue integrity, cellular hydration, and cell health, all of which are important effects of magnesium balance.

4. **Dramatic reduction in migraines.** Migraines can cause the most severe pain known to humans. They are debilitating and said to be incurable. Lifelong use of pain medication seems to be the only option that doctors can offer. However, Jane and thousands of other readers of *The Magnesium Miracle* have found relief from migraines and headaches by using magnesium. In Chapter 4, I talk about also using a combination of methylated B vitamins (B_2, B_6, B_{12}, and folate), in a product called ReAline, if magnesium alone doesn't give full relief.

5. **Periods went from dark to bright red, and from severe clots to minimal.** Magnesium works in several ways to lessen the intensity of menstrual flow. It facilitates the oxygenation of the blood and detoxifies it, changing a dark toxic flow to a bright red one. It also thins the blood naturally, breaking up clots.

6. **Able to exercise intensively for the first time in years.** Prior to this, Jane would be exhausted for at least three days after any exercise. In Jane's case, it was probably a combination of things. She likely didn't have enough magnesium to neutralize the lactic acid she was building up, so instead she got aches and pains. Also, one of the first symptoms of magnesium deficiency is fatigue. Adenosine triphosphate (ATP) is the energy molecule

that is created with the help of magnesium. When you don't have sufficient ATP, you just don't have the oomph that you need to exercise.

7. **Sleep has improved.** When your body is magnesium deficient, it's as if your cells and nerves are all on edge. They are tight and contracted and ready to snap. If you lie down in that state, your body can't relax, your mind can't relax, and you toss and turn. Simply having the proper amount of magnesium turns off that tension, relaxes your muscles, and allows you to slip into sleep.

8. **Able to keep going past 6:30 p.m.** Without enough magnesium, the energy the body gets from ATP is diminished and people have no staying power.

9. **Less sound sensitivity/hypersensitivity.** Studies done on pilots showed an increased sound sensitivity in the face of magnesium deficiency. A woman phoned into a talk show I was appearing on and asked about her son, who was in a rock band. She said that her son had developed a tic below one eye and wondered if it could be magnesium deficiency. I said it absolutely could.

10. **Better able to concentrate when someone is speaking to her.** Jane had been finding that her concentration was hampered, especially if there was a lot of background noise. Poor concentration is not something you will find in a list of symptoms of magnesium deficiency. However, it makes sense that if your body is tense and irritable and you are sound sensitive, then you can have trouble concentrating.

MAGNESIUM AND BLEPHAROSPASM

A dentist from Mexico wrote to tell me about the twenty symptoms that improved when she took magnesium. The most dramatic was her "incurable" eye blinking. I'll let her tell her own story.

Hello, Dr. Dean. I'm a Mexican dentist, forty-two years old. In June 2002, I started feeling something like sand in my eyes and went to an ophthalmologist, whose diagnosis was allergic dermatoconjunctivitis, and I was prescribed some ointments and drops for my eyes. They didn't work, so I went to see another four ophthalmologists, and they changed the diagnosis to keratitis.

In the meantime, I started to develop eye blinking that got worse and worse until it became such a severe spasm that I couldn't open my eyes. I also started having tetany [muscle spasms]. From the first doctor until this point, two months had passed.

Needless to say, I was desperate and very depressed. I couldn't work, drive, or even walk! Then I went to see a neuro-ophthalmologist who gave me the terrible diagnosis of essential blepharospasm [eyelid twitching], which means that they don't know what causes it and of course there is no cure. He also told me that this was known as "Meige syndrome," and he offered me three options:

1. To take neurological prescriptions (sedatives) for life. The prescriptions would have to be changed every three months because they lose their effect.
2. Botox injections, with the risk that the eyelid could droop.
3. A facial nerve blockage (the motor part) in my face. The treatment is horrible: they give you shots all around the forehead and eyelids with an alcohol-derived substance; the injections go to the depth of the bone.

He recommended that I try number three first, so I accepted the treatment. This was in August 2002. Let me tell you that it was a horrible experience. My face was swollen to at least five times normal size, and he definitely did something wrong, because he left me with facial paralysis on the left side. So my right eye couldn't close and my left eye was still closed because it didn't respond to the shots. He prescribed me cortisone and told me that we had to wait and see what happened. I was feeling miserable.

And then the miracle happened: I needed something to be fixed in my kitchen, and the person who came to do the job brought your book about magnesium. It caught my attention because I had started to take a calcium-magnesium supplement because someone told me that it was very good for stress. By this time I couldn't read because the eye drops I was using caused mydriasis [excessively dilated pupils]. He saw my interest and obvious need for magnesium and brought me a copy of the book the next day.

Since I could do absolutely nothing else, I made a huge effort and started to read the book, line by line. As I got further and further, I realized that almost everything that I was reading was about the health problems I've had my whole life, so I started to take magnesium.

I got magnesium chloride in drops and started to take it in November 2002. I began to improve week by week. Four weeks later the injection paralysis was gone and the blepharospasm was improving beautifully. Besides the blepharospasm and paralysis, these are all my other symptoms that are diminishing day by day:

1. Chronic fatigue syndrome
2. PMS
3. Excessive emotional stress
4. Joint pain

5. Back and neck pain
6. Constipation
7. Anxiety
8. Nervousness
9. Arrhythmia
10. Cystitis
11. Colitis
12. Bad circulation
13. Cold hands and feet
14. Feeling disoriented in space and time
15. Depression without apparent cause and inability to cope with everyday things
16. Flatulence
17. Mood swings
18. Hormonal imbalance

My symptoms are not 100 percent gone, but almost! The "incurable" blepharospasm has almost disappeared, and I feel that it will very soon be gone completely. I'm taking 800 mg of magnesium per day (400 mg in the morning and 400 mg before going to bed). I'm also taking flaxseed oil and a multivitamin for women. I'm telling you my story because if someone has the same diagnosis, I want them to know that there is hope, that this is curable with the miracle of magnesium. Thank you very much!

DRUGS AND MAGNESIUM DEFICIENCY

Drugs often play a big role in creating magnesium deficiency. Unfortunately, this drug side effect usually goes undiagnosed and is frequently mistreated with more medication. When you realize your magnesium deficiency may be escalating because of the medication you are taking, it adds to your overall anxiety. Perhaps the reason you are trying to find relief with magnesium is that you are not feeling well on your medications.

Therefore, if you begin taking magnesium because you don't feel well, I caution you to stay on your medication while increasing your magnesium. Then, as you start feeling better and your health improves, slowly wean off your drugs under a doctor's supervision.

Ironically, one of the foremost magnesium experts, Mildred Seelig, M.D., began her research career in the 1960s working for a drug company. That's when she first noticed that many drug side effects were actually magnesium deficiency symptoms. It seemed to her that many drugs cause increased demand for and utilization of magnesium—for example, by creating acidity in the body, which then draws on available magnesium from the cells to try to neutralize the acid and minimize its toxic effects. She said that some drugs seemed to deplete magnesium from the body or, conversely, manifest their positive effects because they pulled magnesium from storage sites and increased the level of magnesium in the blood.[15]

Dr. Seelig later informed me that when she mentioned this anomaly to her employers, they were not interested in pursuing her findings. At a certain point Dr. Seelig realized that this temporary increase in blood levels of magnesium, triggered by the ingestion of drugs, could be what makes drugs appear to be working in the initial few weeks of intake. When this information was rebuffed as well, Dr. Seelig quit her job and eventually became a prominent magnesium expert, writing dozens of research papers on magnesium throughout her career.

Magnesium is quite safe to take with any medication—as long as it's not being used as a laxative. However, as I've mentioned before, drugs tend to deplete magnesium, so you could say that it's not safe to take medications because they deplete magnesium. The 2015 review paper "Magnesium in Man" describes the science behind drugs that deplete magnesium. The paper names diuretics, epidermal growth factor receptor inhibitors, calcineurin inhibitors, and proton pump inhibitors as the greatest offenders. The *Physicians' Desk Reference* has identified the following commonly used drugs as magnesium robbers for many years.[16] But there is much more to the story, which I will detail below.

Magnesium Robbers

- Birth control pills
- Bronchodilators, such as theophylline (for asthma)
- Cocaine
- Corticosteroids (for asthma)
- Digitalis (for some heart conditions)
- Diuretics (for high blood pressure)
- Fluoride-based drugs (see below)
- Insulin
- Nicotine
- Proton pump inhibitors (for acid reflux)
- Statins (for cholesterol)
- Tetracycline and certain other antibiotics

In spite of warnings about the danger of using antibiotics when not needed, they are the most-prescribed drugs. In spite of the fact that antidepressants work only 40 percent of the time, they are the second-most-prescribed drugs. In spite of the fact that painkilling opioids are highly addictive, they are the third-most-prescribed drugs. And in spite of the fact that statin drugs don't let you live any longer, they are the fourth-most-prescribed drugs.

HEARTBURN DRUGS INHIBIT MAGNESIUM

Proton pump inhibitors (PPIs) have a long history of causing magnesium deficiency, which can lead to heart disease. From the literature, it appears that the same may be said for statin drugs, painkillers, and asthma medications. But since medicine doesn't pay attention to the effect of magnesium on the body, doctors miss these important facts, and the morbidity and mortality statistics from drug side effects escalate.

Whole classes of drugs are now being given warning labels identifying them as magnesium wasters. Hypomagnesemia was first recognized as a complication of proton pump inhibitors in 2006, and one of those drugs that is frequently used, Nexium, received a warning label in March 2011. In the 2013 paper "Effects of Proton Pump Inhibitors and Electrolyte Disturbances on Arrhythmias," investigators concluded, "There is a statistically significant association between PPI use, magnesium levels, and the occurrence of cardiovascular events."[17]

The investigators concluded that patients receiving PPIs should be followed closely for magnesium deficiency, especially if they experience acute cardiovascular events, because this may contribute to worsening arrhythmias and further complications. By 2015 enough patients had been followed for the researchers to title their paper "Hypomagnesemia Induced by Long-Term Treatment with Proton-Pump Inhibitors."[18]

A 2015 study from researchers at Houston Methodist and Stanford University reported that adults who take proton pump inhibitors for heartburn and other gastrointestinal ailments are between 16 percent and 21 percent more likely to experience a heart attack than those who do not.[19] Researchers claim they don't have a clue why there is this correlation between PPIs and heart attack; they are just reporting the statistics. However, when you look at these studies through the lens of magnesium deficiency, it's obvious that the increasing magnesium deficiency caused by chronic use of PPIs is causing heart attacks. Since doctors do not acknowledge magnesium in any way, they are unable to accept magnesium deficiency as a cause of heart disease.

DIURETICS DEPLETE MAGNESIUM

A paper written more than thirty years ago shows that the medical community has long known that common diuretics eliminate magnesium from the body as well as potassium, leaving a person susceptible to arrhythmias.[20] However, it is only potassium depletion that is acknowledged, and patients on diuretics are routinely told to drink their orange juice. Most OJ these days is fortified with calcium, so a person may unwittingly deplete the body's magnesium even further by simply trying to supplement potassium. The premise of this paper was to investigate why patients on antihypertensive treatment were at a higher risk for sudden death.

The investigators commented that increased urinary excretion of potassium was a well-established complication of diuretics. They noted that hypokalemia (low levels of potassium) and hypomagnesemia (low levels of magnesium) can be induced by the same mechanisms and are often clinically correlated with each other. They also established that the reported incidence of hypomagnesemia is greater than that of hypokalemia, that there is a significant interrelationship between plasma concentrations of magnesium and potassium, and that there is evidence that magnesium deficiency plays a critical role in the creation of cardiac arrhythmias.

The paper calls for routine measurement of magnesium during diuretic therapy, but to this day that is not done. If you are taking diuretics and your doctor isn't testing you for magnesium, I strongly recommend that you order your own magnesium RBC test periodically to guide your magnesium intake. See Chapter 16 for more on magnesium testing. However, clinical symptoms of magnesium deficiency, as noted above, are of even greater importance than blood testing alone, especially if the test is for serum magnesium.

Other drugs interact with magnesium in specific ways.[21] For example, magnesium is a muscle relaxant, so it enhances the actions of prescription muscle relaxants such as tubocurarine (used in surgery), barbiturates, hypnotics, and narcotics. These medications can be decreased under a doctor's supervision if you are on magnesium. In other words, you may not need as much muscle relaxant because magnesium is a natural relaxant. Tell your anesthesiologist before surgery if you are taking magnesium supplements.

Magnesium protects the kidneys, so supplementation may be beneficial during treatment with aminoglycoside antibiotics such as gentamicin and immunosuppressant drugs such as cyclosporin and cisplatin, which result in magnesium loss. Discuss this with your doctor. I am saying discuss this with your doctor to make sure you realize that I cannot give you medical advice. However, I am very much aware that most doctors know nothing about magnesium therapy and will just tell you to stop taking magnesium and to continue taking your drugs.

According to drug interaction research, magnesium inhibits the absorption of the following drugs: tetracycline, ciprofloxacin, vancomycin, isoniazid, chlorpromazine, trimethoprim, nitrofurantoin, and sodium fluoride. The mechanism of interaction with ciprofloxacin has been identified as competition for magnesium receptor sites. The solution is to take these medications two to three hours before or after magnesium supplements. Of course, my advocacy of magnesium encourages me to ask why your doctor doesn't prescribe magnesium for your osteoporosis, not sodium fluoride. Tak-

ing magnesium may be a wiser choice—especially since fluoride (discussed later in this chapter) binds with magnesium
and makes it unavailable to the body. (See Chapter 11 for
more on osteoporosis.)

In general, I do not recommend that people stop taking
their medications in order to take magnesium. I say you can
take magnesium along with your drugs because taking magnesium is like taking food—only our food no longer has
enough magnesium to sustain us. As your magnesium deficiency symptoms improve and your body no longer needs
medication, you should work with your doctor to wean off
your drugs. This process works very well when you are using
ReMag because you can take therapeutic amounts without
causing a laxative effect.

FLUORIDE BINDS MAGNESIUM

The element fluorine is number 9 on the periodic table.
Fluoride is the negative ion of fluorine. When fluorine combines with another element, a fluoride compound is created.

When the fluoride compounds in fluoridated water, dental products, and drugs release toxic fluorine ions, the tissue
and cell damage begins. Besides directly damaging cells and
tissues, fluorine ions bind with magnesium, making magnesium unavailable to the body. In a population that is already
80 percent magnesium deficient, this is a medical emergency.

According to many concerned scientists and laypeople,
fluoridation of tap water is a disaster afflicting the population with an epidemic of chronic disease, including arthritis
and cancer. Online, go to the Fluoride Action Network's
website for research updates on fifteen diseases associated
with fluoride ingestion.

Most of Europe and half of the United States have completely abandoned the use of fluoride in the water supply.

However, it still remains in the other half of the United States and many parts of the world.

Fluoride toothpaste and fluoride gel painted on teeth by dentists are supposed to protect teeth from decay. That erroneous supposition was based on a small study showing that natural fluorides in drinking water prevented dental decay in a narrow age range in children.

The Wikipedia entry on fluorine informs us that about 30 percent of agrichemical herbicides and fungicides are fluoride compounds containing fluorine ions. Many insecticides contain sodium fluoride. Perhaps the worst abuse of fluoride compounds can be attributed to the pharmaceutical industry, because fluorine is hidden in many drugs as part of the chemical formula and it's never discussed as a possible cause for concern. Drug companies found that fluorine has unique properties that are ideal for prolonging the active presence (or half-life) of a drug in the body. So they have put that principle to use in most of the well-known drugs on the market.

Fluorine is the most electronegative element in the periodic table and it can substitute for hydrogen in drugs, making the compound stronger, more stable, more acidic, and more fat-loving. These qualities increase the bioavailability of the drug and its ability to cross cell membranes (which are made of fat) and attach to binding sites on cell receptors and enzymes in the body. Drug companies may think fluorine is only intensifying the effects of the drug, but it's also magnifying the number and intensity of the drug's side effects.

As I mentioned above, fluorine ions seek out magnesium and bind with it, making magnesium unavailable to the body and unable to do its work. The magnesium fluoride compound produced is called sellaite (MgF_2). It is almost insoluble and ends up taking the place of magnesium in hard tissues such as bone and cartilage, but its brittleness makes the bone susceptible to fracture. The magnesium-fluorine bond is so tight that magnesium is irrevocably lost to the body, interfering with its hundreds of biochemical interactions and decreasing enzymatic action.[22] Remember, magnesium is responsible for the optimal functioning of as many as 800 enzyme systems in the body. Any or all of them could be impaired.

On the website of the Fluoride Toxicity Research Collaborative, you can click on fourteen common classes of drugs that contain fluorine to see the lists of specific drugs. There is no listing for anti-arrhythmia drugs. Yet my least favorite anti-arrhythmia drug is flecainide, with six fluorine atoms. How ironic—a drug that is supposed to suppress arrhythmia may actually be destroying your magnesium, which can only make your arrhythmia worse.

The side effects of flecainide read like a poster on magnesium deficiency symptoms:

Heart: Fast, irregular, pounding, or racing heartbeat or
    pulse
Lungs: Shortness of breath, tightness in the chest,
    wheezing
Nerves: Burning, crawling, itching, numbness, prickling,
    pins and needles, tingling feelings, chest pain

The Fluoride Toxicity Research Collaborative, on its website, is careful to say that "it is unclear to what extent, if any, the fluorinated drugs listed here may increase the body burden of inorganic fluoride." Researchers may argue that in the test tube these fluoride drugs do not appear to release their fluorine component. However, anyone familiar with the Human Microbiome Project knows that the trillions of microorganisms in the gut can make short work of drugs that reach the intestines by completely dismantling them into their individual components. I learned this in personal communication with toxicologists and gastroenterologists. This activity of gut flora would help explain the increasing toxicity we are seeing from fluoride drugs such as ciprofloxacin, which I discuss below.

In addition to its interactions with magnesium, fluoride has other harmful effects in the body. When I interviewed Dr. Paul Connett from the Fluoride Action Network on a radio show in September 2005, he reported that Harvard grad student Elise Bassin, in her Ph.D. thesis, found a strong correlation between water fluoridation and osteosarcoma, a type of bone cancer. Bassin found a 700 percent increase in osteosarcoma in young men who had been exposed to fluoridated water from ages six to eight. According to the U.S. Department of Health and Human Services, "subsets of the population may be unusually susceptible to the toxic effects of fluoride and its compounds. These populations include the elderly, people with magnesium deficiency, and people with cardiovascular and kidney problems."[23] It bears repeating that with about 80 percent of the population being magnesium deficient, most of us are unusually susceptible to the toxic effects of fluoride.

Neurosurgeon Dr. Russell Blaylock, medical director for Second Look, a nonprofit that examines public policy on water fluoridation and fluorinated drugs, confirmed to me that people taking fluorinated drugs are at higher risk for developing magnesium deficiency and suffering severe side effects. I asked Dr. Blaylock what percentage of drugs are fluorinated, as I've heard figures ranging from 20 to 55 percent.

Dr. Blaylock said that what's more important than the percentage is the fact that most of the commonly used drugs harbor this toxin. These include Prozac, Paxil, Cipro, Diflu-

can, Celebrex, Prevacid, Propulsid, Lipitor, Advair, and steroids. Every day you take one of these drugs you are robbing
your body of magnesium, and the true cause of magnesium
deficiency symptoms such as anxiety and depression goes
unrecognized. Not only are you lacking magnesium because
it's not in your food, but any magnesium in your body is destroyed by fluorine in your drugs. How crazy is that—taking
a drug for a problem that is made worse by taking that drug!

FLUOROQUINOLONES ROB MAGNESIUM

Fluoroquinolones, including the widely used antibiotic Cipro
(ciprofloxicin), can cause disabling tendon rupture, which
the FDA warned about in 2008. In May 2016 the FDA
strengthened its black box warning for these drugs, saying
that their serious side effects outweigh the benefits for the
treatment of sinusitis, bronchitis, and uncomplicated urinary
tract infections. It seems to me that they should just remove
these drugs from the market altogether.

I think it's obvious that the brittleness that MgF_2 imparts
to cartilage may be one of the reasons Cipro can cause tendon rupture after an escalation of side effects that begin with
muscle pain, sore joints, and muscle spasm. Cipro can also
be an unrecognized cause of fibromyalgia. The danger from
Cipro is that it is cumulative, so although the first prescription may not affect you, the next one might cause symptoms.

Therapeutic levels of magnesium (especially ReMag)
can be an effective treatment for the side effects of Cipro,
especially when taken soon after ingesting the drug. However, many people have been suffering from Cipro toxicity
for years, and recovery can take a long time and can be
hampered by other imbalances, symptoms, and toxic conditions. For such severe conditions, I recommend my Total
Body ReSet program mentioned as #10 of my Personal Recommendations under Resources.

HIGH-DOSE VITAMIN D DEPLETES MAGNESIUM

Vitamin D is the newest sexy supplement, but it's being prescribed in druglike doses. What you are not being told is that vitamin D requires magnesium in order to transform it into its active form. The relationship between vitamin D and magnesium is crucial and has been ignored by doctors and the media alike. The important lesson is to make sure you are taking enough magnesium before supplementing with vitamin D. You can do that by following your magnesium RBC levels and targeting an optimal level of 6.0–6.5 mg/dL. See Chapter 16 for more on magnesium testing.

Optimal vitamin D levels are actually more toward the low normal end of the range (around 40 ng/mL), not the high end. The normal range for 25-hydroxy vitamin D (25(OH)D) is from 30.0 to 74.0 ng/mL. The paper "Magnesium, Vitamin D Status and Mortality" in the journal *BMC Medicine* displays a detailed flow chart of vitamin D metabolism, which shows that magnesium is required in eight crucial steps.[24] This is vital information that every doctor prescribing vitamin D and every person taking vitamin D needs to know and act upon.

The investigators said, "Our preliminary findings indicate it is possible that magnesium intake alone or its interaction with vitamin D intake may contribute to vitamin D status." They reveal that the increased mortality associated with low serum 25(OH)D is modified by the level of magnesium ingestion. They call for more studies, but this information is enough for me to recommend that you must take magnesium if you are taking supplemental vitamin D. I recommend only 1,000–2,000 IU of vitamin D per day and some daily sun exposure if you can, along with supplemental magnesium.

From the existing literature, we know that low vitamin D

increases the risk of mortality and morbidity and that magnesium plays an essential role in vitamin D metabolism. Putting these two facts together, researchers in a 2015 study investigated whether magnesium intake modifies the serum $25(OH)D_3$ concentration and its association with mortality in middle-aged and older men.[25] The study included 1,892 men ages forty-two to sixty without cardiovascular disease or cancer. They concluded that low serum $25(OH)D_3$ concentration was associated with increased risk of death mainly in those with lower magnesium intake.

Here's a common scenario that I have observed. You feel great on your magnesium supplements. Then you add high-dose vitamin D (anything from 5,000 IU to 50,000 IU), and you begin to feel worse and think you have magnesium deficiency all over again, or you assume your magnesium is no longer working, or you just feel terrible and don't know why.

I've had emails from people who can't seem to take even 1,000 IU of vitamin D without negative reactions. Yet vitamin D is supposed to make you feel better. Even worse, you aren't taking supplemental magnesium and begin taking high doses of vitamin D and start having all sorts of unidentifiable symptoms.

Let me repeat—magnesium is required for many steps along the pathway of vitamin D metabolism, including transformation of vitamin D from its storage form (which is also the supplement form) to its active form. That means if you take extremely high doses of vitamin D, you can plummet into magnesium deficiency and not know what's happening.

To make matters worse, calcium is a mineral that vitamin D grabs from the diet and holds on to for dear life. When you start taking high doses of vitamin D, you can accumulate so much calcium that it overrides your magnesium and forces it out of your body. In short, too much vitamin D can overutilize magnesium, block magnesium, purge magnesium, build up calcium (causing calcification), and propel people into serious magnesium deficiency. I discussed this calcium-magnesium dynamic in the section "The Fail-Safe of Magnesium" in the Introduction.

Magnesium expert Andrea Rosanoff, Ph.D., is one of the very few people who understand this dynamic between vitamin D, magnesium, and calcium. She makes this the topic of her 2016 paper called "Essential Nutrient Interactions: Does Low or Suboptimal Magnesium Status Interact with Vitamin D and/or Calcium Status?"[26] Andrea lists the problems encountered when trying to define this interaction. At the very least, she is opening a conversation that may be alien to allopathic medicine and its tendency to identify one drug or one therapy for one condition. Andrea's paper shows the intricate interaction of magnesium, calcium, and vitamin D and the many ways they affect one another.

An even more controversial aspect of vitamin D is that it is actually a hormone. Hormone levels are regulated through a biochemical feedback system. For example, one of the main jobs of vitamin D is to grab calcium from the diet and put it in the bloodstream. When you have enough calcium, then vitamin D levels should go down because no more calcium is required at that time and so vitamin D is no longer necessary. But if you regard vitamin D as a vitamin, you might think it's not good for a vitamin to be low and you should take more of it.

In our current state of too much calcium and not enough magnesium in our diet and supplements, perhaps we are supplementing a hormone that the body doesn't need in such high doses.

I began investigating this aspect of vitamin D when people told me they were experiencing adverse reactions on high doses. These reactions included seizures, kidney stones, month-long migraines, palpitations, angina, and anxiety. People who had been happy on their magnesium supplements until they started taking vitamin D would say all their magnesium deficiency symptoms came back and didn't go away until they stopped taking vitamin D and added more magnesium.

Here are excerpts from letters sent to me about experiences people have had with taking high doses of vitamin D.

I experienced high blood pressure and rapid heartbeat when taking even just 500 IU of vitamin D, I can't imagine what would happen if I took 50,000 IU!

I started taking omega-3s and 5,000 IU of vitamin D in October 2010 and I did great! I could walk without a limp again, my knees stopped hurting and my feet stopped hurting. But I had a scary episode of angina in March 2012 and that's when I started taking more magnesium. I believe now I was taking too much vitamin D and it may have caused the angina.

I've been using vitamin D supplements for around six months, and experienced heart palpitations during this period. I never connected the two until I heard Dr. Dean on the *Coast to Coast* radio show and did some research. I'm taking magnesium supplements now and the palpitation problem is much improved. Apparently the vitamin D was interfering with my magnesium levels.

When I take a 1,000 IU vitamin D supplement daily, my elbows start to hurt, my knees start to hurt, my lower back starts to hurt and feels stiff, and I have angry thoughts. When I take magnesium, I feel relaxed and peaceful.

I have been taking magnesium for a long time and every time I take vitamin D, I get a very bad reaction. I am now taking 600 mg of magnesium and only 1,000 IU of vitamin D. I also spray on magnesium oil.

I know I developed angina because of high vitamin D. When I read an article by Dr. Dean, I cut back and took more magnesium. I am so frustrated with the way I was treated by the doctors while I was in the hospital. They were no help in solving my angina symptoms. All they could say is, "This is stress related." And they prescribed an angina medication for me while leaving me scared for my life for the two weeks between my hospital stay and finding your website. I am such a believer in magnesium now, you just don't know. I'm so thankful for you and your work. I just cannot thank you enough (with tears, really, with tears).

As I mentioned above, I only recommend 1,000–2,000 IU of vitamin D daily along with supplemental magnesium. I do receive reports from people who say they take high amounts of vitamin D and achieve great benefit. I wonder if these people are already well supplied with magnesium, if the benefits are short-term, or if they don't realize they are developing magnesium deficiency symptoms. After the initial honeymoon and rave reviews about the benefits of high-dose vitamin D, the more recent studies are more sobering. Unfortunately, most researchers have not yet recognized the need for magnesium to be taken in conjunction with vitamin D supplementation.

As for the dosage of magnesium to take along with vitamin D, that is very individual; some people need more than others. I recommend getting a magnesium RBC test and using ReMag, a source of magnesium that will enable you to take enough magnesium to help assimilate vitamin D without the laxative effect, which can actually deplete your magnesium. See Chapter 16 for more on magnesium testing and Chapter 18 for more on ReMag.

For the proper functioning of vitamin D, calcium, and magnesium, I recommend vitamin K_2. Dr. Weston Price, the inspiration for the Weston A. Price Foundation, discovered the X factor, which turned out to be vitamin K_2. Vitamin K_2 helps guide calcium into the bones, where it is needed, instead of leaving it circulating to calcify blood vessels and other soft tissues.

We are supposed to create our own vitamin K_2 in the gastrointestinal tract from vitamin K_1, found in leafy green vegetables, but most people are deficient. Vitamin K_2 is fat soluble, like vitamin A and vitamin D, and benefits from associating with good fats such as olive oil and coconut oil. Other sources of vitamin K_2 are animal products, including egg yolks and butter from animals raised on green pastures. The only vegetarian source of vitamin K_2 is natto, a Japanese fermented soy product that some find difficult to tolerate because of its unique taste. In my practice, I recommend Blue Ice Royal (fermented cod liver oil plus butter oil) from Green Pasture as the perfect combination of all three fat-soluble vitamins.

Let me be clear. I do not know all the answers and you do not have to listen to me, but neither do you have to listen to anyone else. You have to listen to yourself and what makes sense to you and your body. Allopathic medicine is about taking big guns and shooting them off indiscriminately. For them, vitamin D is the new calcium; they will promote it very widely and wait a few decades before acknowledging any negative fallout. I'm writing about the downside of vitamin D so you can start asking questions now. I don't want you to wake up in ten or twenty years and find out you made a big mistake by overdosing with vitamin D.

NUTRIENTS THAT NEED MAGNESIUM

It's likely there are interactions among all vitamins and minerals and we just haven't done enough research to uncover all the associations. But here is what we know so far about magnesium and its associations with other nutrients.

- Both calcium and magnesium are required in order for either mineral to work properly in a variety of functions.
- Magnesium is necessary to convert the storage form of vitamin D into the active form.
- Magnesium enters cells with the support of vitamin B_1 (thiamine) and vitamin B_6 (pyridoxine).
- Selenium helps magnesium stay inside cells, where it belongs.
- Zinc helps the absorption of magnesium.
- Vitamins D, A, and K, along with zinc and boron, work with magnesium for balanced bone health.
- Boron is essential for magnesium and calcium metabolism.
- Magnesium deficiency exacerbates a potassium deficiency.
- Magnesium along with iodine, selenium, zinc, molybdenum, boron, copper, chromium, and manganese support thyroid function by providing the mineral building blocks for thyroid hormone. My formula ReMyte contains twelve minerals, nine of which are these thyroid-supporting minerals.

Magnesium: The Missing Mineral

In a poetic reference to magnesium's crucial role in evolution, Dr. Jerry Aikawa of the University of Colorado calls magnesium the ur-mineral, the most important mineral to human beings and all other living organisms.[1] I call magnesium "the spark of life."

Magnesium is critical to the metabolic processes of lowly one-celled living organisms, and it is the second-most-abundant element inside human cells. Magnesium existed at the beginning of life and was involved with all aspects of cell production and growth. When plants evolved to use the sun as their energy source, magnesium played a pivotal role in the development of chlorophyll. So in both plants and animals, magnesium became an essential mineral involved in hundreds of enzyme processes affecting every aspect of life.

Presently, nineteen minerals are considered essential for human life, and it is quite possible that more will be found to be indispensable as we take more time to study life's mineral connection. Minerals make up 4 percent of the body by weight. Nine macrominerals account for 99 percent of the body's mineral content: sodium, potassium, calcium, phosphorus, magnesium, manganese, sulfur, cobalt, and chlorine. Ten trace minerals constitute the remaining 1 percent.[2]

As with most minerals, the element magnesium occurs in nature combined with other elements. It joins naturally with sulfur to make Epsom salts (magnesium sulfate), with carbon to make magnesium carbonate, and with calcium to make dolomite. Magnesium is also found in partnership with silica in talc and asbestos. Like calcium, it is an alkaline mineral that neutralizes acid; therefore, some magnesium compounds are antacids, used to treat heartburn.

My first encounter with magnesium was in high school chemistry. Each student was given a thin strip of magnesium and told to light one end carefully. The previous week we had learned that magnesium is the eighth-most-abundant element, constituting approximately 2 percent of the earth's crust and 0.13 percent (1,272 parts per million, or ppm) of seawater. By comparison, calcium makes up 3 percent of the earth's crust but only 0.04 percent (440 ppm) of seawater. The website of the NIH's Office of Dietary Supplements informs us that "an adult body contains approximately 25 g magnesium, with 50 to 60 percent present in the bones and most of the rest in soft tissues." But none of the facts we were told about magnesium prepared us for the dynamic effect of lighting the magnesium strip. It flared up like a sparkler and disappeared in a flash. This incendiary property serves as an important reminder of magnesium's versatility as the spark of life, constantly igniting metabolic reactions throughout the body.

THE BODY IS ELECTRIC

The impulses for any and all movement in the body arise from electrical transmission. These microcurrents of electricity that pass along the nerves were first measured in 1966. Scientists soon discovered that the conductor for these bodily electrical currents is calcium and that magnesium is necessary to maintain the proper level of calcium in the blood and the cells.[3]

More recent research indicates that calcium enters the cells by way of calcium channels that are jealously guarded by magnesium. Magnesium, at a concentration 10,000 times greater than that of calcium inside the cells, allows only a certain amount of calcium to enter to create the necessary electrical transmission or muscle firing, and then immediately helps to eject the calcium once the work is done. Why? If calcium accumulates in the cell, it causes hyperexcitability and eventually calcification that disrupts cell function. Too much calcium entering cells can cause symptoms of heart disease (such as angina, high blood pressure, and arrhythmia), asthma, or headaches. But if there is enough magnesium, it acts as the body's natural calcium channel blocker.[4, 5, 6]

About 60–65 percent of all our magnesium is housed in our bones and teeth. The remaining 35–40 percent is found in the rest of the body, including muscle and tissue cells and body fluids. Our blood contains only 1 percent of the body's total magnesium, which is why blood serum is a very poor measure of total body magnesium. The highest concentrations are in the heart and brain cells, so it is no wonder that the major symptoms of magnesium deficiency affect the heart and brain. These are also the two organs that have considerable electrical activity, measured by EKG (electrocardiogram) and EEG (electroencephalogram).

Magnesium mostly works inside our tissue cells; one major function is to bond with adenosine triphosphate (ATP) as Mg^{2+}-ATP to produce energy packets for our body's vital force. That happens after magnesium activates six of the eight steps of the Krebs cycle in the mitochondria. Not enough can be said about the importance of this energy-producing function of magnesium. The combination of ATP and magnesium triggers production of the body's protein structures by revving up messenger RNA. This combination is also a requirement for the production of DNA, our genetic code.

Understand that both basic building blocks of life, RNA and DNA, are dependent on ATP and magnesium to maintain stable genes.[7] Magnesium is required as a cofactor for production of DNA polymerase.[8] The DNA polymerases are enzymes that create DNA molecules by assembling nucleotides, the building blocks of DNA. These enzymes are essential to DNA replication. In addition to its stabilizing effect on DNA and the structure of chromosomes, ATP and magnesium are essential cofactors in almost all enzyme systems involved in the processing of DNA. Research shows that without sufficient magnesium, DNA synthesis becomes sluggish. Because of these roles, I'm convinced that therapeutic magnesium can keep gene mutations and single-nucleotide polymorphisms from creating health problems. I'll write more about magnesium's effect on our genes in Chapter 15 in the "Treating Telomeres" section and in the section "The Magnesome" in the introduction to Part Three.

THE DANCE OF CALCIUM AND MAGNESIUM

You can see from the above discussion that calcium and magnesium share equal importance in our bodies. To fully understand magnesium, you have to know where calcium fits into the picture. Appropriating Newton's law of physics that says "for every action there is an equal and opposite reaction," neither calcium nor magnesium can act without eliciting a reaction from the other. Magnesium and calcium antagonize each other in absorption, reabsorption, cell cycle regulation, inflammation, and many other physiologic activities.[9]

At the biochemical level, magnesium and calcium are known to act antagonistically toward each other. Many enzymes whose activities critically depend on a sufficient amount of intracellular magnesium will be detrimentally affected by small increases in levels of cellular calcium. Growth of cells, cell division, and intermediary metabolism are also absolutely dependent on the availability of magnesium, which can be compromised if excess calcium is present.[10]

To understand how you can create a calcium/magnesium imbalance in your own body, try this experiment in your kitchen. Open a capsule of calcium powder and see how much dissolves in 1 ounce of water; a goodly amount settles in the bottom of the glass. Then open a capsule of magnesium powder and slowly stir it into the calcium water. When you introduce the magnesium, the remaining calcium dissolves; it becomes more water-soluble. The same thing happens in your bloodstream, heart, brain, kidneys, and all the other tissues in your body—except your bones.

If you don't have enough magnesium to help keep calcium dissolved, you can develop muscle spasms, fibromyalgia, calcified arteries, dental cavities, and calcium deposits (including breast tissue calcifications). Another scenario plays out in the kidneys and bladder. If there is too much calcium in the kidneys and lining the renal (kidney) arteries, and not enough magnesium to dissolve it, you can get kidney stones. Calcium deposited throughout the bladder can make it rigid, lower its capacity, and lead to frequent urination. A 2015 study confirms that magnesium has a major role in dissolving calcium crystals in calcified arteries.[11] We know that coronary artery calcification leads to heart attacks, and carotid artery calcification leads to stroke; don't forget about renal artery calcification, which can initiate the process of kidney failure.

All muscle cells, including those of the heart and of the smooth muscles lining the blood vessels, contain more magnesium than calcium. If magnesium is deficient, calcium floods into the smooth muscle cells of blood vessels and causes spasms, leading to constricted blood vessels and therefore higher blood pressure, arterial spasm, angina, and heart attack.[12] A proper balance of magnesium in relation to calcium can prevent these symptoms.

Calcium excess stimulating the cells in the muscular layer of the temporal arteries (located over the temples) can cause migraine headaches. Excess calcium can constrict the smooth muscle surrounding the small airways of the lungs, causing restricted breathing and asthma. Finally, too much calcium, without the protective effect of magnesium, can irritate delicate nerve cells of the brain. Cells that are irritated by calcium fire electrical impulses repeatedly, depleting their energy stores and causing cell death.

THE CALCIUM DISTRACTION

The irony of the calcium-magnesium story is that without magnesium, calcium will not work properly in the cells, but it will inappropriately precipitate out into soft tissues. However, our high-calcium diet and tendency to take calcium supplements make getting enough magnesium almost impossible. Research shows that the ratio of calcium to magnesium in the Paleolithic or caveman diet—the ancient diet consumed by our earliest ancestors as the human body evolved to its current form—was 1:1, compared with a ratio of anywhere between 5:1 and 15:1 in present-day diets.[13]

With an average of ten times more calcium than magnesium in our diet in modern times, there is no doubt about widespread magnesium deficiency. The emphasis on calcium supplementation has diverted our attention from any other mineral, even though all minerals are crucial to the proper functioning of the body. In our society we tend to look for "the best," "the most important," "the star," and forget that it takes a team and teamwork to get anything accomplished, including body processes. Calcium, because it is the most abundant mineral in the body, therefore became "the star." Even though research has accumulated on magnesium over the past four decades, it has never been adequately publicized and discussed.

THE FAILURE OF CALCIUM

I talk about the "dance" of calcium and magnesium, but it's more like a "dance competition" between these two important minerals. It's finally been proven that calcium supplements can increase the risk of heart disease. However, researchers simply blame calcium without realizing that it's the imbalance of calcium and magnesium that's actually causing the problem. It's not sufficient to just stop supplementing with calcium. We must begin supplementing with magnesium and focus on getting our calcium from foods or from a completely absorbed calcium supplement such as ReCalcia.

Researcher Dr. Diane Feskanich found in 2003 that too much calcium can cause some forms of arthritis, kidney stones, and osteoporosis, in addition to calcification of the arteries (leading to heart attack and cardiovascular disease).[14] Her study, published in the *American Journal of Clinical Nutrition*, reported that neither milk consumption nor a high-calcium diet appears to reduce the risk of hip fractures. Dr. Feskanich missed the magnesium connection.

Following Dr. Feskanich, five studies published in several prestigious journals between 2008 and 2015 by lead author Dr. Mark Bolland provide even more evidence that an excess of calcium produces an increased risk of heart disease in women.[15, 16, 17, 18, 19] To impress upon you the importance of Bolland's research and the conclusions that many doctors have not yet embraced, you must read the online abstract from Dr. Bolland's fourth paper, "Calcium Supplements and Cardiovascular Risk: Five Years On." The paper acknowledges that calcium supplements have been in widespread use, recommended to help prevent bone fractures. However, in the past decade that recommendation has changed because of the increased risk of heart disease associated with calcium supplementation and the conclusion that "calcium supplements with or without vitamin D marginally reduce total fractures but do not prevent hip fractures" for the majority of people.

Bolland's 2015 paper "Calcium Intake and Risk of Fracture: Systematic Review" concluded that increasing calcium intake from diet or supplements did not result in a clinically significant reduction in risk of fracture. Not only did calcium not help, but in fact it hurt—Bolland found that calcium supplements can cause kidney stones and acute gastrointestinal events (constipation, abdominal distress, and abdominal pain requiring hospitalization) and can increase the risk of myocardial infarction and stroke. Bolland concluded that any benefit of calcium supplements in preventing fracture is outweighed by an increased risk for cardiovascular events. They said that while there is little evidence to suggest that dietary calcium intake is associated with cardiovascular risk, there is also little evidence that it is associated with fracture risk. Therefore, for the majority of people, dietary calcium intake does not require close scrutiny. Bolland and his team concluded that because of the unfavorable risk/benefit profile, widespread prescribing of calcium supplements to prevent fractures should be abandoned.

I want to emphasize the fact that many more diseases than just heart disease have at their core an excess of calcium. Dr. Bolland mentions kidney stones and acute gastrointestinal events as well as an increased risk of stroke. We can widen the scope to include calcium as a direct cause of inflammation. Any disease with a name ending in -*itis* means an inflammatory condition, which also means magnesium deficiency.

However, I must stop here and emphasize that it's not just a matter of stopping calcium supplements. To truly heal the effects of calcium supplementation, you require therapeutic levels of magnesium. The finding that calcium in the diet does not prevent hip fractures may be disconcerting to some who still feel that calcium should be the answer to fragile bones; however, the fact is that magnesium and calcium work together to protect the bones.

The most recent study showing that calcium supplements make people more prone to plaque buildup in arteries, which contributes to the risk of heart attack, was published in October 2016.[20] The researchers recommend that people try to get their calcium from foods such as dairy products, leafy green vegetables, fortified cereal, and juices. The scientists said they wanted to build on previous research findings that the calcium in supplements never actually makes it to a patient's bones and instead accumulates in soft tissue and muscles, including the heart.

Three hormones—parathyroid hormone, calcitonin, and vitamin D—are involved with the level and location of calcium in the body. Furthermore, all three of these hormones depend on magnesium for their activation and regulation. I will discuss hyperparathyroidism below because it can cause elevated calcium in the body and exacerbate mag-

nesium deficiency symptoms but the condition is often misdiagnosed.

The body doesn't take the threat of excess calcium lying
down. Dr. Guy Abraham detailed how the body protects itself.[21] He said that in order to protect the fluid inside the cell
from becoming saturated with calcium, there is a magnesium-
dependent mechanism that shunts calcium into the mitochondria. However, this is a short-term solution that can
backfire because if too much calcium is taken up for too
long, the excess calcium in the mitochondria inhibits ATP
synthesis. Mitochondrial calcification without the intervention of sufficient magnesium eventually results in cell death.
Could calcium excess and magnesium deficiency be the underlying cause of mitochondrial dysfunction that many natural medicine practitioners say can trigger chronic fatigue
syndrome and other chronic diseases?

Another of these chronic diseases is age-related macular
degeneration (AMD). A 2015 study reported on the association of calcium supplement intake with AMD.[22] This is an
important paper because AMD is a leading cause of blindness around the world. Using the public National Health
and Nutrition Examination Survey (NHANES) database
from 2007–2008, investigators followed 3,191 participants.
They matched photographs of the back of the eye with calcium intake. AMD was found in 248 or (7.8 percent) of the
study participants. Of these 248 patients with AMD, 146
(59 percent) took calcium supplements. Investigators concluded, "Self-reported supplementary calcium consumption
is associated with increased prevalence of AMD. The stronger association in older individuals may be due to relatively
longer duration of calcium supplementation."

Posts on various medical forums about this study and
other similar ones try to downplay the findings, commenting
instead about the importance of calcium and how people

shouldn't just stop taking it. However, I and many other doctors have grave concerns about poorly absorbed calcium supplements increasing the incidence of heart disease and creating soft tissue calcification. It's possible that patients with AMD are developing soft tissue calcification in the macula of their eyes. If that's the case, AMD patients should increase their intake of magnesium and focus on getting their daily 600 mg of calcium from dietary sources, or from ReCalcia, and not from poorly absorbed calcium supplements. Actually, that's the same advice I have for most people suffering magnesium-deficiency symptoms.

CALCIUM PRECIPITATION

Let me summarize the extent of the problems that result when calcium precipitates in the soft tissues of the body.

- In the large intestine, calcium interferes with peristalsis (the waves of muscle contractions that push food through the bowels) by causing magnesium deficiency and also because it is physically "binding," which results in constipation.
- When calcium settles out in the kidneys and combines with phosphorous or oxalic acid, kidney stones form.
- Calcium can deposit in the lining of the bladder and prevent it from fully relaxing, and therefore from filling completely with urine. This leads to urinary frequency and infections, especially in older people.
- Calcium can precipitate out of the blood and deposit in the lining of arteries, causing hardening of the arteries (arteriosclerosis); the new term for this is *vascular calcification*. Vascular calcification in the coronary arteries can lead to heart attack; in the carotid arteries, it can lead to stroke; and in the renal arteries, it can lead to kidney failure.

- Calcium can even deposit in the brain. Many researchers are investigating it as a possible cause of dementia, Alzheimer's, and Parkinson's disease.
- Calcium can deposit in the smooth muscle lining the bronchial tubes and cause symptoms of asthma.
- Calcium precipitation in the cell membranes can impair their permeability. This makes it increasingly more difficult for glucose (a very large molecule) to pass through the cell membrane to be converted into ATP in the cells' mitochondria. High glucose levels created by excess calcium may be misdiagnosed as diabetes.
- According to Dr. Guy Abraham, in order to protect the cell, in acute situations, from taking on too much calcium, resulting in excessive cell spasms (either muscle or nerve), a magnesium-dependent mechanism shunts calcium into the mitochondria. Chronic uptake of calcium in the mitochondria will inhibit ATP synthesis and eventually result in cell death.

CALCIUM-TO-MAGNESIUM RATIO

I've always been wary of calcium supplements, and I went out on a limb when I wrote in the first edition of *The Magnesium Miracle* that we should be getting equal parts of calcium and magnesium (a ratio of 1:1) in our diets and if we take supplements. Back in the late 1990s when I was reading everything I could about magnesium, there was an unexplained consensus that you had to take 2 milligrams of calcium for every milligram of magnesium. This 2:1 ratio is still evident in the composition of most calcium-magnesium supplements and in every health book and article I read.

I traced this 2:1 calcium to magnesium ratio back to a 1989 report in the journal *Magnesium Research* by the famous French magnesium scientist Dr. Jean Durlach.[23] His actual words, mistranslated from French, were that we should never exceed the 2:1 ratio of calcium to magnesium intake from all sources (food, water, and supplements). This was obviously misunderstood as a recommendation, not as an absolute cut-off point.

Calcium excess coupled with magnesium deficiency only exacerbates the symptoms of calcification. As I mentioned earlier, the average diet today has a shocking 10:1 ratio of calcium to magnesium. I've described this ratio as a time bomb leading to impaired bone health and heart disease. To reiterate, an ideal dietary ratio is 1:1.

CALCIUM-TO-MAGNESIUM RATIOS	
Seawater	1:3
Squash	1:1
Milk	7:1
Yogurt	11:1
Calcium-fortified orange juice	27:1
Antacids	100:1

Note that I'm saying there should be a 1:1 ratio of calcium to magnesium not just in supplements but in a combination of diet, water, and supplements. Also, I feel that people who eat dairy can get their 600 mg of calcium in their diet. However, many people avoid dairy and don't get enough calcium. Since most sources say we only obtain about 200 mg of magnesium from food, we then need to take at least 400 mg of elemental magnesium in supplement form.[24]

I often recommend taking more magnesium than calcium for people who are burning through their magnesium. In some cases people have to reverse the ratio and take twice the amount of magnesium to undo damage from calcium buildup, drug intake, stress, heavy athletic activity, surgery, and inflammation. I would like to get my calcium from food, but I must admit that I don't often get around to making bone broth and I can't eat yogurt every day without mucus building up. For myself and many other people who require a safe calcium supplement, I've created a picometer, stabilized ionic calcium formula called ReCalcia.

While I was in the midst of writing this edition of *The Magnesium Miracle*, a woman told me about her husband's uphill battle with his doctor about what minerals she would allow him to take. Angela said:

> My husband just had his yearly physical at the VA hospital. His physician asked what supplements he was on. We told her magnesium, calcium, and potassium (500 mg per day of both calcium and magnesium and 99 mg potassium) and an additional 250 mg of magnesium per day in another tablet.
>
> The doctor asked why he was taking these supplements, and I told her that research shows they will help with his high blood pressure (now under control), restless leg syndrome (gone), back pain (still working on this), and other health problems. She said he should not be taking any of them and they could be dangerous if he got too much!
>
> His magnesium and potassium were tested and the doctor said they were both high and he should stop taking them. In your book, however, you mention that the normal magnesium blood tests usually show inaccurate amounts of magnesium, especially if the patient has other stress factors and ailments, which my husband does. Do you have any other suggestions of how to find out his true level of magnesium? Do you think he truly is getting too much of these, or could it be just inaccurate testing?

I wrote back and told Angela that her husband should obtain a magnesium RBC test, either at the VA hospital or at RequestATest.com. I pointed out that the reference range is considered to be 4.2–6.8 mg/dL, but that this is based on a population where at least 80 percent of individuals are magnesium deficient. The optimal level, I stressed, is 6.0–6.5 mg/dL. (See Chapter 16 for details.)

The VA probably performed the serum magnesium test, however. Getting a high level on that test is a good thing. The magnesium in serum has to be in a very tight range to keep the heart beating properly. If the serum magnesium level goes down, the body immediately responds by pulling magnesium out of storage in the bones or muscles and putting it into the blood. If the serum magnesium test is in the low normal range, it actually indicates a serious magnesium deficiency.

High calcium in the blood is not good. See my discussion about hyperparathyroidism directly below. For one thing, most labs perform the ionized calcium test, which is quite accurate. As I'll discuss below, if your ionized calcium levels are high, you must be tested for hyperparathyroidism. I also told Angela that I don't recommend calcium supplements. When people take too much calcium, it can precipitate in soft tissues (including arteries); it also increases the likelihood of magnesium being neutralized by calcium.

I received a very appreciative email back in which Angela admitted that she was frustrated that the VA doctor refused to recognize that a lot of her husband's symptoms were from magnesium deficiency and that they were actually improving with magnesium supplementation. When she reread *The Magnesium Miracle* and many of my online articles, she was convinced that the doctor just didn't know enough about magnesium to be giving advice and that if her husband went off magnesium his ailments would only get worse.

In a March 2012 press release from the nonprofit Nutritional Magnesium Association (where I sit on the Medical Advisory Board), titled "High Calcium–Low Magnesium Consumption Poses Health Risk," I quoted the National Institutes of Health's "2011 Dietary Supplement Fact Sheet on Calcium," which stated that 43 percent of the U.S. population (and 70 percent of older women) take calcium supplements. However, the NIH admits that less than half of that calcium is absorbed in the gut; the rest is either excreted through the large intestine, causing constipation, or through the kidneys, potentially forming kidney stones. Or it is transported to other soft tissues, where it can form gallstones, heel spurs, atherosclerotic plaques, fibromyalgic calcifications, and breast tissue calcifications.

What the NIH fact sheet does not say is that magnesium in adequate amounts is essential for the proper absorption, metabolism, and distribution of calcium and the proper metabolism of vitamin D. Magnesium converts vitamin D supplements or vitamin D in storage form (calcidiol) into its active form (calcitriol), which can be properly absorbed in the gut. Magnesium also activates the hormone calcitonin, which helps to preserve bone structure and draws calcium out of the blood and away from soft tissues and into the bones. This necessary action lowers the risk of osteoporosis, some forms of arthritis, heart attack, and kidney stones. Read the section "High-Dose Vitamin D Depletes Magnesium" in Chapter 1.

ELEVATED CALCIUM AND HYPERPARATHYROIDISM

My resource for information on hyperparathyroidism is the Norman Parathyroid Center and its extensive website Parathyroid.com. A reader of my blog, who successfully had a benign parathyroid adenoma removed at the center, referred me to the site.

Hyperparathyroidism appears to be relatively common, affecting 1 in 100 people, including 1 in 50 women over the age of fifty. Hyperparathyroidism is diagnosed by finding high levels of calcium in the blood. Ninety-nine percent of all cases of elevated blood calcium are due to a small benign tumor of the parathyroid glands, called an adenoma or simply hyperplasia, causing elevated levels of parathyroid hormone (PTH). Parathyroid adenomas are not cancerous tumors.

Something is stimulating the parathyroids to produce more parathyroid tissue, which lumps up inside the parathyroid gland, causing an adenoma. So my question is, what is stimulating the parathyroid to enlarge? Is it similar to how a thyroid that lacks iodine enlarges into a goiter so that it can make more thyroid hormone? Is it like the prostate that is missing zinc and enlarges into prostate hypertrophy? Doctors say they don't know why parathyroid tissue overgrows. But when it does, it produces excess PTH, which grabs on to calcium, elevating it in the blood, causing calcification throughout the body, depleting magnesium, and causing all kinds of calcium excess/magnesium deficiency symptoms.

There is certainly a general deficiency of magnesium and an elevation of calcium in the population, which must have something to do with stimulating the parathyroids. But because medicine does not study minerals in a scientific way, there is no research looking into the calcium/magnesium balance and its effect on the parathyroid glands.

A 2013 study out of Denmark says that hyperparathyroidism in Denmark is epidemic.[25] The most dramatic increase in incidence is seen among women over the age of fifty. They also admit that they do not know the cause.

Most patients with hyperparathyroidism are symptomatic, but they are very often misdiagnosed. "Moans, groans, stones, and bones" summarizes the symptoms: kidney stones, frequent headaches, fatigue, high blood pressure, heart palpitations, GERD, osteoporosis, depression, and poor concentration. All these are the same as symptoms of magnesium deficiency. Hyperparathyroidism and magnesium deficiency are related because if your parathyroid hormone is elevated, then your calcium is elevated, which pushes down your magnesium—ergo, magnesium deficiency symptoms on top of hyperparathyroid symptoms.

If hyperparathyroidism is not diagnosed and treated with surgical removal of the overactive parathyroid gland or glands, patients eventually die of heart failure, stroke, heart attack, kidney failure, breast cancer, or prostate cancer. Hyperparathyroidism promises a slow death as symptoms of excess calcium and magnesium deficiency build in a dramatic example of what happens in cases of extreme calcium and magnesium imbalance.

The parathyroids are four small endocrine glands located behind the thyroid in the neck. They range in size from that of a grain of rice up to the size of a pea. Tiny though they may be, these glands are extremely important because they control the calcium in your bones and blood. When they aren't working properly, calcium becomes elevated—but doctors don't look at the other nutrients that are also affected—magnesium, vitamin D, and vitamin K_2.

Medical textbooks say that the only purpose of the parathyroid glands is to sample the calcium in the blood and regulate it in the body within a very narrow range, keeping the nervous system and muscular system functioning properly. If the calcium levels drop, PTH is secreted and attacks the bones to release calcium into the blood. When the glands perceive that the calcium in the blood is high enough, they shut down and stop making PTH.

Doctors don't know why parathyroid adenomas form— maybe they are a reaction to the imbalance of calcium, magnesium, vitamin D, and vitamin K in our current diet. For example, if there isn't enough vitamin D to help absorb calcium from the diet, your calcium becomes low and the parathyroids are stimulated to produce more PTH, which breaks down bone to release more calcium into the blood. Also, if you are magnesium deficient, PTH production is diminished. You can have low vitamin D, which should force PTH to rise, but with magnesium deficiency PTH will be in the normal range. Could the constant seesaw stimulation of the parathyroids trigger an overreaction that results in adenoma?

The following list identifies the important role that magnesium may play in the creation of hyperparathyroidism.

- Adequate levels of magnesium are essential for the absorption and metabolism of calcium, so in the face of magnesium deficiency, calcium absorption may also be low and trigger PTH production.
- Magnesium stimulates the body's production of calcitonin, a hormone that helps to preserve bone structure and draws calcium out of the blood and soft tissues and sends it back into the bones, preventing some forms of arthritis and kidney stones. But in magnesium deficiency, this action is curtailed.
- Magnesium has a complex relationship with PTH. It suppresses PTH when it is elevated, preventing it from breaking down bone, but it is also necessary for PTH production.
- Magnesium converts vitamin D into its active form so that it can help calcium absorption.

Please pay attention to elevated blood calcium levels if you are having symptoms that seem to be related to magnesium deficiency but don't entirely clear with magnesium therapy. If your levels of ionized calcium are elevated, have your PTH levels checked. If your doctor is not willing to perform these tests, in the United States you can obtain them from the website RequestATest.com—ionized calcium testing is $49 and PTH testing is $59. (Note: This type of testing is not available in all states.) You can also order a magnesium RBC test because low magnesium can make your PTH low and confuse the diagnosis, since doctors expect to see high calcium and high PTH in hyperparathyroidism.

If calcium and PTH are both high, or even if your calcium is high and you have symptoms of hyperparathyroidism, you need to have tests that visualize your parathyroids. According to the Norman Parathyroid Center, adults over age thirty-five should not have calcium levels higher than 9.9, even though the laboratory range for normal is 8.8–10.7 mg/dL.

You can ask for a parathyroid MRI or the more definitive sestamibi scan. Sestamibi is a small protein labeled with technetium 99. They call it a very mild and safe radioactive agent, which is injected into a vein and absorbed by an overactive parathyroid gland. There are no medications to treat hyperparathyroidism created by benign adenomas. Surgical removal by an experienced surgeon is curative. The Norman Parathyroid Center has a 99 percent success rate with their twenty-minute outpatient parathyroid surgery.

I apologize if this discussion about hyperparathyroidism seems complex, but you do have to know this information because most doctors do not. You can go directly to the Parathyroid.com website and contact the Norman Parathyroid Center if you have more questions. And I would like to put the incidence of hyperparathyroidism and my recommendations into perspective. As I noted earlier, hyperparathyroidism occurs in 1 percent of the general population and in 2 percent of women over fifty. By contrast, magnesium deficiency affects 80 percent of the population. So it's far more likely that your symptoms are the result of magnesium deficiency rather than hyperparathyroidism.

CALCIUM AND INFLAMMATION

Calcium overload is one of the main causes of body-wide inflammation. Inflammation is an important topic in the earlier edition of *The Magnesium Miracle* because magnesium is one of the most important anti-inflammatory nutrients. But I didn't emphasize enough that calcium is the major cause of inflammation and that you can neutralize calcium with magnesium, dramatically reducing your levels of inflammation.

The FDA and drug companies are aware of the importance of treating inflammation, but regrettably they are using drugs, with all their side effects, as the primary treatment instead of recommending magnesium. Even worse, anti-inflammatory steroids and many nonsteroidal anti-inflammatory drugs are often fluoride compounds, which means they bind up magnesium. Treating inflammation with ineffective and unsafe drugs inevitably creates more inflammation.

Where is all this calcium coming from? Recommendations for calcium intake vary greatly. In the United States, women over fifty are told by doctors and health publications to take up to 1,500 mg daily. However, in the United Kingdom, the RDA is set at 700 mg daily, while the World Health Organization recommends only about 500 mg.

When osteoporosis clinics advise 1,500–2,500 mg of calcium, they don't consider the amount that people are already getting in their food and water. Many people, especially those consuming dairy products, have very high-calcium diets. This can lead to escalating amounts of unabsorbed calcium.

As mentioned earlier, food and water have higher amounts of calcium than magnesium, with the standard American intake approaching a 10:1 calcium-to-magnesium ratio. Levels of all minerals have been diminishing because farmers don't use mineral fertilizers and because many of the chemicals used as herbicides and pesticides bind up minerals, especially magnesium. However, the amount of calcium in the soil is still higher than that of magnesium.

You can find a list of the amount of calcium in common foods in Appendix B. You'll see that a mere 7 sardines (with bones), half a can of salmon (with bones), or 20 oysters give you between 284 and 393 mg of calcium. A cup of bok choy nets you 252 mg. When someone tells me they don't eat dairy, I send them a recipe for bone broth, something your grandmother probably made all the time. I've included a basic Bone Broth Recipe in Appendix C. You can find more recipes for chicken, beef, and fish bone broth by searching the Weston A. Price website. It's difficult to determine the actual number of milligrams of calcium in a serving of bone broth, as every batch will be different, but taking it along with several servings of high-calcium vegetables, nuts, seeds or dairy should cover your daily requirements for calcium. But if that's not enough, or if making bone broth is too much work to fit into your busy schedule, you can use my ReCalcia mineral formula.

I've proven to myself the power of calcium in the diet. When I go on a yogurt or goat cheese binge, I'll begin experiencing some of my old heart palpitations and leg cramps and know that I need more magnesium to balance the extra calcium in my diet!

MAGNESIUM'S MANY ROLES

Now that we've gotten calcium sorted out, let's get right into the magic of magnesium. My original list of the roles of magnesium covered only five general functions: (1) catalyzing most chemical reactions in the body, (2) producing and transporting energy, (3) synthesizing protein, (4) transmitting nerve signals, and (5) relaxing muscles. That list has expanded to fourteen major magnesium functions, and it's very likely there are many more. Over the years I've realized that magnesium is much more complex than I ever thought possible.

Fourteen functions of magnesium are brilliantly described in the magnesium chapter of a textbook called *The Atlas of Diseases of the Kidney*.[26] Some of the language is very technical, so feel free to skim through it, but I want to give you a sense of the sophistication of this simple mineral. As you read what magnesium is capable of doing, just imagine how many necessary functions are interrupted when a person is magnesium-deficient.

Fourteen Functions of Magnesium

1. **Energy.** Magnesium's most important function is the creation of energy in the trillions of cells making up our body. Magnesium is a cofactor in the production of ATP via ATP synthase. ATP is manufactured in the mitochondria, and it must be bound to a magnesium ion (Mg^{2+}-ATP) in order to be biologically active. There are 1,000–2,000 mitochondria in each human cell, and ATP is made in each one through a series of eight steps called the Krebs cycle. What's remarkable about magnesium is that it is indispensable in six of those eight steps.[27, 28]

   We think of the Krebs cycle as a pathway for the breakdown of glucose, but it takes pyruvate from the glycolysis cycle and makes ATP energy molecules. The Krebs cycle is necessary for the breakdown of all metabolites: sugars, amino acids, and fatty acids. Each of these groups of molecules has a pathway that leads into the Krebs cycle. In addition, intermediates from the Krebs cycle can go the other direction and be used to synthesize amino acids and fatty acids. With the help of magnesium, the Krebs cycle in the mitochondria is our basic life force. Mitochondrial dysfunction is being investigated by both allopathic and alternative medicine, but any treatment must begin with therapeutic levels of magnesium.

ATP has many other functions besides being an energy source. Transmembrane ATPase imports substances necessary for cell metabolism and exports toxins and wastes across cell membranes. A hydrogen-potassium ATPase creates the gastric proton pump, which acidifies the contents of the stomach. Many other pumps and transporters are all directed by ATPases, with magnesium as a necessary cofactor.

2. **Membrane stabilizer.** Magnesium is an important membrane-stabilizing agent. Stabilization decreases excitation of nerves and excessive contraction of muscle cell membranes.

3. **Protein production.** Magnesium is required for the structural integrity of numerous body proteins. To date, 3,751 magnesium receptor sites have been found on human proteins.

4. **RNA and DNA.** Magnesium is required for the structural integrity of nucleic acids. Consequently, magnesium is a requirement for RNA and DNA production.

5. **GTPase.** Magnesium is a cofactor for the enzyme guanosine triphosphatase. GTPase has many functions: (a) signal transduction, or "switching" on specific receptor proteins located on cell membranes and transmitting that signal to trigger taste, smell, and perception of light;

(b) protein biosynthesis; (c) control and differentiation of cell division; (d) translocation of proteins through cell membranes; and (e) transport of vesicles within the cell and assembly of vesicle coats.

6. **Phospholipase C.** Magnesium is a cofactor for phospholipase C, which is a class of enzymes that split phospholipids at the phosphate group, creating signal transduction pathways. The most important one allows calcium to enter cells.

7. **Adenylate cyclase.** Magnesium is a cofactor for the enzyme adenylate cyclase. This enzyme converts ATP to cyclic adenosine monophosphate (cAMP) and pyrophosphate. cAMP is used for intracellular signal transduction of the effects of hormones such as glucagon and adrenaline into cells because the hormones can't pass through cell membranes. It is involved in the activation of protein kinases and regulates the effects of adrenaline and glucagon. It also binds to and regulates the function of ion channels or gateways into the cell.

8. **Guanylate cyclase.** Magnesium is a cofactor for the enzyme guanylate cyclase. This enzyme synthesizes cyclic guanosine monophosphate (cGMP) from guanosine triphosphate (GTP), keeping cGMP-gated ion channels open, which allows calcium to enter the cell. Cyclic GMP is an important second messenger that transmits the message across cell membranes from peptide hormones and nitric oxide, and it can also function in hormone signaling. It can trigger changes requiring protein synthesis. In smooth muscle, cGMP is the signal for relaxation, which can regulate vascular and airway tone, insulin secretion, and peristalsis.

9. **Up to 800 enzyme processes.** Magnesium is a required cofactor for the activity of hundreds of enzyme

processes. I quoted the standard number of 325 enzymes when I wrote the first edition of *The Magnesium Miracle*. However, that number is far too low. Dr. Rosanoff says, "While it was estimated in 1968 that magnesium was a required cofactor for over 300 enzyme processes, that number is now more reliably estimated at 700 to 800."[29] The authors of "Magnesium in Man: Implications for Health and Disease" put the number of magnesium enzymatic reactions at over 600.[30]

10. **Regulates ion channels.** Magnesium is a direct regulator of ion channels, most notably via the other key electrolytes potassium, calcium, and sodium. Magnesium is intimately involved in potassium transport.[31] Magnesium and potassium depletion cause similar damaging effects on the heart. Furthermore, it is impossible to overcome potassium deficiency without replacing magnesium. That's why hospitals seem to have such a difficult time finding the right electrolyte balance of sodium, potassium, calcium, and chloride, because they ignore magnesium and do not routinely measure it in their electrolyte panels, and when they do test for it, they use the inadequate serum magnesium test.

Magnesium is intimately involved in calcium channels. I write about magnesium guarding the ion channels that allow calcium to enter and leave the cell, orchestrating the exact amount of calcium that's required to cause a muscle or nerve cell to contract and then flushing that extra calcium out to prevent excessive contraction. Thus, magnesium is a natural calcium channel blocker. But instead of using magnesium to modify the effect of calcium on body physiology, allopathic medicine insists on using calcium-channel-blocking drugs that have many side effects, including magnesium deficiency.

11. **Intracellular signaling.** Magnesium is an important intracellular signaling molecule itself. I've mentioned signaling several times; the role of cell signaling cannot be underestimated. Without intercellular communication the cells of the body would not be able to function at all.

12. **Oxidative phosphorylation.** Magnesium is a modulator of oxidative phosphorylation, during which electrons are transferred from electron donors to electron acceptors such as oxygen in redox reactions, using magnesium as a cofactor. These redox reactions, called electron transport chains, form a series of protein complexes within the cell's mitochondria that release energy as ATP.

13. **Nerve conduction.** Magnesium is intimately involved in efficient nerve conduction. Above, you have read about the detrimental effects of excess calcium. Although calcium is vital for proper nervous system function, too much calcium is dangerous. Excess calcium is proinflammatory and can excite nerves to the point of cell death.

14. **Muscle function.** Magnesium is intimately involved in efficient muscle function. The mechanisms are varied and include oxygen uptake, electrolyte balance, and energy production. Magnesium makes muscles work properly, allowing calcium to cause muscle contraction and then pushing calcium out of the muscle cells to allow the relaxation phase. In the same way that nerve cells can be "excited to death," muscle cells stimulated by too much calcium can go into uncontrollable spasm, resulting in tissue damage such as occurs in a heart attack.

MAGNESIUM: THE MISSING MINERAL

Who or what stole magnesium from the dinner table? A 1988 U.S. government study concluded that the standard American diet failed to provide the daily requirement of magnesium.[32] That was almost two decades ago, and you can be sure that most people get even less today. Junk food—that is, nutrient-poor foods such as soft drinks, sweets, salty snacks, and alcoholic beverages—makes up about 25 percent of the average American diet.[33] And food items that are processed in some way—which means they may contain added salt, sugar, or some of the 5,000 recognized food additives—make up about 70 percent of the average diet.[34]

Dr. Mildred Seelig and many other magnesium experts have come to the inescapable conclusion that the typical American diet, which is rich in fat, sugar, salt, synthetic vitamin D, phosphates, protein, and supplemental calcium, not only is deficient in magnesium but actually increases the need for magnesium in the body.

Unfortunately, it is impossible to find studies that tell us the actual incidence of magnesium deficiency. This stems from there being no accepted medical standard for measuring whole-body magnesium status. As will be discussed in Chapter 16, blood testing for magnesium relies on inadequate measurements, since only 1 percent of the body's magnesium is in the blood and only 40 percent is in the tissues.

The National Academy of Sciences found that most Americans are possibly magnesium-deficient. When men on average obtain only 80 percent of the minimum requirement of magnesium to run innumerable body functions, and when women, at 70 percent, get even less of what they absolutely need, then our bodies are just not able to function properly.[35]

Let's look at some of the reasons you may be lacking in magnesium—and it begins with what's missing from the soil.

MAGNESIUM-DEFICIENT SOIL

The mineral depletion of our farmland, described in the 1936 Senate document quoted in the introduction to this book, is probably the most important reason most Americans are magnesium deficient. Unfortunately, the issue of depleted soils has not been addressed in America. As Kirkpatrick Sale expressed in *The Nation*, the war on our farmland began in earnest after World War II, when war technology was retrofitted for use in agriculture. Tractors were modeled on battle tanks; instead of spraying bullets, wartime planes sprayed pesticides and herbicides, which were cousins of chemical weapons. "It was a war on the land, sweeping and sophisticated as modern mechanization can be, capable of depleting topsoil at the rate of 3 billion tons a year and water at the rate of 10 billion gallons a year."[36]

DEAD SOIL

The present state of our soil is not just deficient, it's dead! Kirkpatrick Sale talks about the war waged on the land and all its inhabitants by farmers lured into believing that killing weeds and pests was far superior to living in harmony with nature. The whole experiment backfired when it became clear that the poisons could not be controlled—they killed indiscriminately. Without living worms, which break up the earth, leave their own form of compost behind, and chop up minerals into the proper size particle to be absorbed by plants, the soil becomes hard and less porous, so rainfall simply washes away more topsoil. Without nitrogen-fixing rhizobacteria in the soil, which make it possible for plants to absorb certain nutrients, those plants are weaker and less nutritious.

That the experiment has failed has not deterred big agrochemical companies such as Monsanto. Monsanto continues to promote genetically engineered seeds and a glyphosate herbicide called Roundup that binds magnesium, removing 50 percent of what little is left in the soil. Research further suggests that Roundup can have a very long half-life, as much as twenty-two years, in the soil.[37] (Note: In late 2016,

Bayer AG agreed to buy Monsanto for $66 billion, creating the world's largest seed, pesticide, and herbicide company.)

GRASS TETANY

Observing animals can teach us important lessons about our environment—if we only pay attention. One man who did was André Voisin, a French biochemist and farmer born in 1903. In 1963 Voisin wrote a book called *Grass Tetany*.[38] Grass tetany is a metabolic disease of cattle and goats caused by a deficiency of magnesium in the soil. When animals eat magnesium-deficient grass they develop irritability, staggering, tremors, and spasms. Most dramatically, the animals fall down in convulsions when they hear sudden loud noises or if they are frightened or excited. Voisin reported in the 1930s that magnesium deficiency was the cause of grass tetany, since low levels of magnesium were found in suffering animals and the condition was miraculously reversed by injections of magnesium.

Chapter 1 of Voisin's book says it all: "Modern Farming Methods Favour the Development of Grass Tetany." As a farmer, Voisin observed that intensive grazing and the overuse of mineral-deficient commercial fertilizers were common practices. Voisin identified Holland as the country that used the most commercial fertilizer on its pastures and also suffered the most grass tetany.

High-potassium potash has been the fertilizer of choice since the 1930s. It's cheap, is easily obtained, is readily absorbed by plants, and makes plants look green and healthy. Potassium is so easily absorbed that plants favor its uptake above magnesium and calcium, which are relatively harder to absorb. Crops grown with excessive amounts of potash have a low content of magnesium and calcium and high potassium levels. However, you will never know that since there is no minimum amount of minerals required in our grains, fruits, or vegetables—the nutrients in such foods are not routinely measured and never labeled.

Even if the magnesium content of soil is high, using potassium fertilizer can prevent its absorption into the plant. But because most agricultural land in America has been overworked for decades and fertilizers don't replace this important mineral, magnesium is rarely found in our soils. Doctors talk about the metabolic nightmare of trying to balance blood electrolytes in patients in the hospital. I think the nightmare begins on the farm where magnesium is not used on the soil. Thus we develop magnesium deficiency diseases from deficient plants. And it continues in the hospital wards when patients are admitted with magnesium deficiency diseases but magnesium is not even tested as part of the electrolyte panel, or if it is tested, the inferior serum magnesium test gives an inaccurate reading.

SOIL EROSION

Paul Mason, owner of a magnesium-rich spring in California, shows us what happens to magnesium that is being leached from cultivated soil.[39] Based on measurements of the dissolved magnesium in the Mississippi River, estimates are that the annual loss of magnesium from midwestern soils is an incredible 7.1 million kilograms at least, and likely more, since some of the magnesium is undissolved and embedded in dirt carried away by the river.

BURNING OFF MAGNESIUM WITH ACID RAIN

Acid rain provides yet another attack on the magnesium in soil; it occurs in industrial and urban areas that experience excessive air pollution. Atmospheric scientist William Grant, during his study of air pollution, concluded that an accumulation of acid rain, which contains nitric acid, can change the chemistry of the soil in which trees grow.[40] This abnormal soil acidity creates a reaction with calcium and magnesium in the soil to neutralize the excess nitric acid. He found that eventually these minerals are depleted, leaving the nitric acid to react with the aluminum oxide in the soil. The reactive aluminum builds up in the plant, replacing the calcium and magnesium and making it difficult for the plant to survive.

Calcium is beneficial to trees and plants because it strengthens the walls of the cells that combine to shape the tree, so without it plants weaken. Magnesium is an essential component of the chlorophyll necessary for photosynthesis, during which organic chemicals are produced with exposure to sunlight. While calcium and magnesium deficiencies weaken plants, the excess nitrates from acid rain cause plants to grow faster. The lack of calcium and magnesium, however, means that this early growth cannot be supported, and the plants may be too weak physically to survive.

If we eat plants that are grown on soil contaminated with acid rain, they may be very deficient in calcium and magnesium. On the farm, soil acidity is tested, and if the soil is too acid it is usually treated with lime—a calcium oxide product, which further depletes magnesium by competing with it for absorption.

DEFICIENT FOOD FROM DEFICIENT SOIL

When you walk into a grocery store and pick up your produce, for the most part you just want it to look nice. You reject bruised, wilted, or misshapen vegetables or fruit. This emphasis on superficial appearance, not nutritional content, is what drives the industry. There is no labeling law that requires that the level of magnesium be displayed.

Foods that commonly contain magnesium are leafy green vegetables, nuts, seeds, whole grains, and chocolate. However, unlike vitamins, which can be manufactured by plants if they have sufficient sunlight and water, minerals must be present in the soil to show up in plants. If there is no magnesium in the soil, plants will have none; they cannot manufacture it out of thin air. So don't believe it when someone says that you can get all your nutrients in a good, balanced diet. That may be true only if you eat organic food, and then only if the organic farmers use a full spectrum of minerals in their fertilizer. I'm convinced that to get enough magnesium today, you need to take supplements.

PROCESSED FOOD LACKS MAGNESIUM

During the refining and processing of food, significant amounts of magnesium can be lost. The process of extracting oils from magnesium-rich nuts and seeds strips away this essential mineral. Nearly all the magnesium in grains is lost during the milling process when the bran and germ are removed from whole grain to make white flour. For example, one slice of whole-wheat bread provides 24 mg of the mineral, while a slice of white bread has only 6 mg. And yet magnesium is never considered in the fortification of refined foods. Finally, in the kitchen, when vegetables are boiled, magnesium leaches out into the cooking water. Of note is the fact that less calcium than magnesium is lost due to food processing and cooking, another reason the average diet is higher in calcium than magnesium.

PERCENTAGE OF MAGNESIUM LOST DURING FOOD PROCESSING

Refining of flour from wheat	80 percent
Polishing of rice	83 percent
Production of starch from corn	97 percent
Extraction of white sugar from molasses	99 percent

What can we do to defend our magnesium sources? It is best to buy organic foods, but encourage your farmer to fertilize the soil with minerals. Eat as many raw vegetables as possible, and when you do cook vegetables, quickly steam them for only a few minutes, until they are slightly cooked but still crisp. You must also save the nutrient-filled water to use as soup stock. Chapter 17 presents the Magnesium Eating Plan, which focuses on whole grains, nuts, seeds, and greens.

MAGNESIUM-DEFICIENT DIETS

In the past few years I've seen a major public focus on healthy diets. Young people are "going raw" and drinking green smoothies every day. In the opposite extreme, the Paleo diet is reaching cult-like status. Families are growing vegetable gardens, going to local farmers markets, and shopping for organic produce. People are actively seeking diet solutions for their health problems.

I think all these efforts are commendable—except, unfortunately, it's a little too late to do much good. There has been a gradual decline of dietary magnesium in the United States, from a high of 500 mg/day at the turn of the century to barely 175–225 mg/day today.[41] I've already noted that the National Academy of Sciences has determined that when it comes to magnesium intake, most American men obtain only about 80 percent of the recommended daily allowance (RDA), and women average only 70 percent.[42] Most magnesium experts agree that the current RDA is inadequate to prevent magnesium deficiency, but most men and women don't even get this minimal amount of magnesium.

The current Fact Sheet on Magnesium for Health Professionals on an NIH website confirms that the problem of magnesium-deficient diets continues.[43] This document says,

"Magnesium dietary surveys of people in the United States consistently show that intakes of magnesium are lower than recommended amounts." An analysis of data from the National Health and Nutrition Examination Survey (NHANES) of 2005–2006 found that a majority of Americans of all ages ingest less magnesium from food than their respective Estimated Average Requirements (EAR).

The RDA is defined as the amount of a nutrient necessary to meet the daily requirements of a healthy individual. There are no guidelines for the amounts to use if someone is not healthy or on medications. Furthermore, nutrients are not regarded by allopathic medicine as being able to treat disease. In fact, it's not even legal to say so. If a supplement manufacturer defines a nutrient as being able to treat a disease, that supplement is automatically recategorized as a drug and must undergo enormously expensive drug trials, costing upward of $5 billion, in order to make such claims.

You may ask if any of the current fad diets are closing the gap on magnesium deficiency. I say no, because even if the produce is organic and even if you eat a lot of it, you can still be magnesium-deficient if the food comes from magnesium-deficient soil. Let's take a closer look at the current diet fads.

PALEO DIET PROBLEMS

The Paleo diet has a huge following, but the Paleo gurus don't mention that in order to digest a high-protein diet, more magnesium is required. And you get less magnesium in a Paleo diet because you avoid grains that can potentially offer some magnesium. A cup of chicken has 32 mg of magnesium compared to 160 mg in a cup of amaranth—but only if that amaranth was grown on magnesium-rich soil.

When protein breaks down, it produces homocysteine. On a high-protein diet you will produce lots of homocysteine. Homocysteine oxidizes cholesterol, and oxidized cholesterol is the kind that damages blood vessels. The major enzymes involved in breaking down and getting rid of homocysteine are magnesium dependent. Thus more oxidized cholesterol is created from homocysteine that builds up when there is a lack of magnesium. I discuss hyperhomocystein-emia in Chapter 6.

A Paleo diet could be setting you up for more problems if you don't have enough magnesium. Drs. Michael and Mary Dan Eades, authors of *Protein Power,* state that if they had only one supplement to offer their patients, they would choose magnesium above all others.[44]

PUT SUGAR ON PAUSE

A diet high in sugar and other simple carbohydrates also puts you at risk for magnesium deficiency. Natasha Campbell-McBride, N.D., in her book *Gut and Psychology Syndrome,* says that twenty-eight atoms of magnesium are required to process one molecule of glucose.[45] If you are trying to break down a molecule of fructose, you need fifty-six atoms of magnesium. That's an extremely unbalanced and unsustainable equation that drains magnesium.

Even the raw-foodists and green-juicers are not immune to magnesium deficiency. For one thing, they eat way too much fruit. They think they can eat all they want "because it's natural." I recently received an email from a young man who asked if there was anything wrong with him eating sixteen bananas a day on his vegan diet! I told him to do the math. One medium-sized banana has about 27 grams of carbs, so sixteen bananas give him a total of 432 grams. A good diet should only offer 100–150 grams of carbs a day.

This person is using up his magnesium stores to metabolize fruit sugar. Raw-foodists also give themselves permission to lace their green drinks with lots of pineapples, bananas, apples, and berries to try to overcome the bland or bitter taste of greens. High intake of fruit sugars can trigger type 2 diabetes (partly as a result of magnesium deficiency) and can also cause dental caries. *Sugar: The Bitter Truth,* with about seven million views, is a must-see YouTube video by a pediatric endocrinologist, Dr. Robert Lustig, who explains the dangers of fructose sugars and how much worse they are than sucrose (table sugar).[46]

Magnesium is the central mineral in "plant blood," or chlorophyll, much as iron is the central mineral in hemoglobin. You would think a diet high in green vegetables would have you covered. Not so. I have consulted with people who are drinking more than 40 ounces of organic green juice a day, yet they are still magnesium deficient, with symptoms such as heart palpitations and leg cramps, which were relieved when they took ReMag. Let me repeat this fact: if the food you are eating is not grown on soil replenished with minerals, the food will automatically be mineral deficient—even if it is organic.

MAGNESIUM AND YEAST OVERGROWTH SYNDROME

The consequence of too much sugar in the diet—either table sugar or fruit sugar—is yeast overgrowth. It is not widely known that yeast (*Candida albicans*) in the human body produces 178 different chemical by-products in its normal life cycle. When yeast overgrows due to antibiotics, steroids, birth control pills, or a high-carb diet, these chemical by-products can be absorbed into the bloodstream and set up a never-ending inflammatory cascade.

I'll give you an example of how a yeast toxin drains magnesium. Acetaldehyde is one of the powerful toxic by-products of yeast, and the enzyme that breaks it down (acetaldehyde dehydrogenase) depends on magnesium for its

function. When excess acetaldehyde overworks the dehydrogenase enzyme, using up stored magnesium, the enzyme can
no longer metabolize acetaldehyde. A buildup of this chemical can cause many problems. Free acetaldehyde is toxic to
the brain, liver, and kidneys and can cause depletion of B
vitamins. It can also block hormone receptors for the thyroid, adrenals, and pituitary.

Symptoms of thyroid imbalance are very common today,
partly because thyroid hormones, which may appear normal
in blood tests, cannot get inside cells to do their work as a
result of chronic acetaldehyde poisoning. The same happens
with female hormones, especially estrogen—it's blocked
from getting into cells, even though blood estrogen levels
may be normal.

Apart from *Candida albicans*, exposure to acetaldehyde
occurs due to alcohol consumption, inhaling exhaust from
cars and trucks, cigarette smoke, and the use of high-fructose
corn syrup.

STOMACH ACID AND MAGNESIUM ABSORPTION

That stomach acid is essential for magnesium absorption
was a true statement when I first researched magnesium in
the late 1990s, and it's true for magnesium found in food and
most magnesium supplements. However, in my own search
for a non-laxative, fully absorbed magnesium I found that
stabilized ions of magnesium (specifically those in ReMag)
can bypass the need for stomach acid or even the need for an
intact gut. So in spite of having low stomach acid, a leaky
gut, or even gastric bypass surgery, you can still obtain optimum levels of magnesium with ReMag.

When you are under serious physical or emotional stress,
your body might not produce sufficient stomach acid, which
is required for digestion and for chemically changing miner-

als into an absorbable form. Minerals are usually bound to another substance to make a mineral complex; for example, magnesium bound to citric acid creates magnesium citrate, and bound to the amino acid taurine it becomes magnesium taurate. When a magnesium complex hits the stomach, it needs an acidic environment to help break the two substances apart, leaving magnesium in the ionic form and ready for action in the body. However, magnesium ions are very unstable and bind with another compound immediately. Fortunately, there is a proprietary process that can stabilize magnesium ions and that process is used to create ReMag.

Inefficient stomach digestion and faulty intestinal absorption can lead to incomplete food digestion, poor absorption of minerals, and consequently, magnesium deficiency. What's worse, when magnesium is deficient, gastric acid production is diminished, hindering magnesium absorption even more.

The elderly as well as people with arthritis, asthma, depression, diabetes, gallbladder disease, osteoporosis, or gum disease are often deficient in hydrochloric acid.[47] All these conditions are also associated with magnesium deficiency.

Another disruption to digestion is America's addiction to antacids—the number one over-the-counter drug group. Heartburn and indigestion, the result of bad eating habits, plague the nation. But the "cure" in this case is no better than the disease. The roiling and burning in the gut from sugary junk food and greasy fast food is being inappropriately blamed on too much stomach acid. In many cases, heartburn is due to sugar fermentation in the stomach and a backflow of pancreatic enzymes from the small intestine.[48] By neutralizing normal stomach acids, antacids make it impossible for us to digest our food or absorb minerals properly.

Our magnesium can be even further depleted if we use calcium carbonate antacids because the calcium they contain causes more magnesium to be lost.

It's also important to understand the grave effects low stomach acid and low magnesium have on calcium absorption. I've already talked about calcium's inability to dissolve in water, making it entirely dependent on stomach acid to put it into solution. However, when calcium leaves the stomach's highly acidic environment it enters the alkaline environment of the small intestine and precipitates out of solution unless sufficient magnesium is present. Without magnesium to keep it in solution, calcium quickly deposits in soft tissues throughout the body.

ACID-ALKALINE BALANCE

A common saying in natural medicine circles is that a healthy body is an alkaline body. Some people take this message too far and eat mostly alkaline foods, drink alkaline water, and even take baking soda, which is alkaline. However, excessive alkalinity in the stomach first reduces stomach acidity and then causes a rebound reaction, with the production of more gastric acid to maintain the proper acidic stomach pH. This increased stomach acid production requires more magnesium, which it pulls away from other functions.

Stomach acidity is vital for proper protein digestion, helps the absorption of minerals from our food, and kills unwanted organisms (parasites, bacteria, yeast, fungi, and viruses) that find their way into our food and water. I have concerns about the practice of using baking soda to manipulate internal pH. When you drink baking soda in water, you are neutralizing stomach acids—much like an antacid. Incomplete digestion of food molecules turns them into fodder for yeast and intestinal bacteria, leading to dysbiosis and leaky gut.

In order to assess the body's pH, a number of alternative practitioners recommend doing saliva and urine pH testing several times a day. When I experimented with this practice several decades ago, I found it very unwieldy and highly inaccurate. My saliva and urine pH would bounce around every time I ate or drank, so I found it impossible to draw any conclusions or formulate a treatment plan.

The more important pH is that of our blood. But the blood pH stays within a very tight range and you can't get a measurement of it without an arterial blood sample, which just isn't practical. So saliva and urine pH act as inaccurate proxies for the blood. I know there is much more to this system and that some practitioners still rely on pH testing, but I'm just not one of them.

Instead of becoming obsessive about pH testing and trying to manipulate your diet and supplements in a constant teeter-totter to achieve a certain pH, I tell people to eat lots of vegetables and make sure they are taking enough magnesium, which stockpiles our alkaline reserves and also helps maintain gastric acid. Magnesium acts as a buffer so the body can maintain an alkaline pH while performing metabolic chores that constantly shift the blood pH by small increments. When you are magnesium deficient, your body has a more difficult time achieving this goal.

ABSORPTION OF DIETARY MAGNESIUM

In general, magnesium is ultimately absorbed into the bloodstream from the small intestine. However, I've been able to circumnavigate that rule with ReMag, which is absorbed directly into cells starting with the mouth, then the esophagus, the stomach, and the small intestine. ReMag does not have to be bound to a carrier protein and ferried through the intestinal lining.

Otherwise, at the best of times, only about one-half (or as little as one-third) of the magnesium that is contained in food and water is absorbed; the rest is eliminated in the stool or urine. Add to this the fact that very little magnesium exists in the majority of farmland in the United States and thus in the food supply, plus the recent widespread recognition of the condition called leaky gut and the disruption of the intestinal microbiome, and you have a magnesium deficiency disaster. All this is happening at a time when 80 percent of the U.S. population does not even obtain the meager RDA of magnesium, making magnesium deficiency symptoms epidemic.

Fortunately, ReMag is not hampered by poor absorption because it exists in a stabilized ionic form and represents a breakthrough in magnesium therapeutics. However, most people don't take ReMag and they depend on the little magnesium they get in their diets. Therefore, I'll continue with the discussion about absorption of dietary magnesium that I wrote about in the first edition of *The Magnesium Miracle*.

INTESTINAL MINERAL ABSORPTION

A study reported in *Metabolism* used radioactive magnesium to trace the activities of this mineral in the body.[49] It was observed that on a diet with an average amount of magnesium, 44 percent of the ingested radioactive magnesium was absorbed; on a low-magnesium diet, 76 percent was absorbed; and on a high-magnesium diet, only 24 percent was absorbed. These results indicate that there is no need to fear an overload of magnesium in the diet. Any excess will be excreted harmlessly, whereas a deficiency could have serious consequences.

Some researchers say that we don't absorb more magnesium because we evolved on a diet that was high in magnesium from sea vegetables and high-magnesium foods such as greens, nuts, seeds, and grains, and so we don't need mechanisms to conserve it. That could be one of the underlying reasons that we are so deficient—our diet has betrayed us. Dietary excess of magnesium is actually as rare as hen's teeth because of the deficiency of magnesium in the soil.

In the first edition of *The Magnesium Miracle* I listed a number of other conditions that also influence the degree of absorption, but those factors have shifted significantly because all the early research was based on the absorption of magnesium oxide. The absorption of ReMag does not depend on a healthy gut, protein transport molecules, or parathyroid hormone, and its assimilation is not inhibited by other minerals. The last block mentioned in the following list, about iron impeding magnesium absorption, is now referenced with a study showing that this is true of magnesium oxide but not of more absorbable forms of magnesium.

Blocks to Magnesium Absorption

- Intestinal condition (diseased intestines absorb less)
- Availability of the protein transport molecule for magnesium
- Availability of parathyroid hormone
- Poor hydration
- The rate of water absorption, because magnesium is soluble in water
- The amounts of calcium, phosphorus, potassium, sodium, and lactose (milk sugar) in the body, all of which can inhibit magnesium absorption
- Supplemental iron, which can impede magnesium oxide absorption and vice versa (if you take both, you should take them several hours apart)[50]

Whether your intestines are healthy or diseased is said to be the most important factor in nutrient absorption. Having written extensively on irritable bowel syndrome (IBS) and yeast overgrowth in *IBS for Dummies*[51] and *The Yeast Connection and Women's Health*,[52] I used to have great concern about magnesium absorption in people who have a leaky gut (micropunctures of the intestinal lining, caused by infection and injury, that allow absorption of toxins into the bloodstream).

A common cause of leaky gut is overgrowth of the yeast *Candida albicans,* which normally lives mostly unnoticed in the large intestine. When it moves into the small intestine, however, it sends out threadlike filaments that can poke microscopic holes in the intestinal tissue. Yeast grows beyond its normal environment in the large intestine under the influence of antibiotics, cortisone and other steroids, birth control pills, estrogen, stress, and a high-sugar diet. It produces 178 different by-products, most of which are toxins that can be absorbed through a leaky gut.

I say I *used* to have great concerns about magnesium absorption, because most people were taking magnesium oxide. As I've mentioned before, magnesium oxide is only 4 percent absorbed, and it has a strong laxative effect on most individuals, further irritating a leaky gut. However, picometer magnesium, ReMag, is fully absorbed at the cellular level, does not cause diarrhea, and does not irritate the intestines, and its absorption is not impeded by a leaky gut.

In the section above called "Magnesium and Yeast Overgrowth Syndrome" I talk about the yeast toxins that require magnesium in order to be detoxified. However, I'm not just advocating that you take magnesium to medicate the symptoms of yeast overgrowth. A full yeast treatment program should be implemented. (See #18 in the list "Dr. Dean's Personal Recommendations" in the Resources section.)

I've noticed a rise in the diagnosis of microscopic colitis, which causes intestinal distress and diarrhea. This condition appears to be a combination of leaky gut and the continuum of bowel disease that I wrote about in *IBS for Dummies.* In that book, I state that the intestinal distress of irritable bowel syndrome (IBS), with its many possible causes and triggers, can proceed to inflammatory bowel disease (IBD), Crohn's disease, and ulcerative colitis if not properly diagnosed and treated. Microscopic colitis has come to light because more people are undergoing biopsies as doctors look for structural damage to explain their intestinal distress.

We know that low magnesium levels can compromise cell membrane integrity by damaging the vital fatty layer in the cell membrane, which makes it more susceptible to destruction and allows leakage through the membrane.[53] Treatment with a non-laxative magnesium, ReMag, can help heal the leaky cell membranes of microscopic colitis and not worsen the condition by causing diarrhea like most other magnesium products.

MAGNESIUM BLOCKED BY CERTAIN FOODS

It's important to know which foods are high or low in magnesium, but you should also know that certain foods contain natural chemicals that block absorption of magnesium. For example, there is much evidence that a high-protein diet makes magnesium deficiency worse, and if you are following such a regimen, you should take at least 300 mg of supplemental magnesium for that reason alone.[54] Another potential source of problems is the tannin in tea, which binds and removes a portion of all minerals, including magnesium, from the body. If you suspect you are magnesium deficient, it's best to avoid both black and green tea, especially if they are strongly bitter. Less bitter teas do not contain such high amounts of tannins and may be less of a problem.

Oxalic acid, which is found in spinach and chard (among other foods), can form insoluble compounds (called oxalates) with magnesium and other minerals, causing these minerals to be eliminated rather than absorbed. Cooking vegetables removes most of the oxalic acid, so it's best to steam your spinach, chard, and other high-oxalic-acid vegetables instead of eating or juicing them raw.

The authors of a chapter on the treatment of kidney stones in a textbook called *The Kidney and Body Fluids in Health and Disease* wrote, "Some patients with intestinal hyperabsorption of oxalate and malabsorption also have magnesium deficiency. Replenishment of body magnesium stores increases urinary magnesium excretion, and magnesium oxalate is much more soluble than calcium oxalate."[55] What I take away from this is the possibility that by saturating yourself with magnesium you can bind up oxalates and remove them from the body through the urine. Magnesium oxalate is much more soluble than calcium oxalate; you never find magnesium oxalate kidney stones. Calcium oxalate is responsible for 80 percent of human kidney stones and will form as crystals when calcium levels in the blood are higher than magnesium levels. Kidney stones, gout, rheumatoid arthritis, and chronic vulvar pain (vulvodynia) can all be aggravated by oxalic acid. Instead of just avoiding oxalates, which is often an impossible task, I make sure people are saturated with magnesium.

Phytic acid, found in the hulls of seeds and the bran of grains, can form insoluble compounds called phytates with magnesium and other minerals, helping them to be eliminated rather than absorbed. In the process, those minerals are lost. Preventing the binding action of phytic acid in

grains and seeds is not so simple. Grains and seeds should be
soaked for eight to twelve hours to remove the phytic acid,
but few people make this effort. You can, however, purchase
sprouted sunflower seeds and pumpkin seeds. A diet high in
grains and non-sprouted seeds, while providing many valuable nutrients, is another reason to take magnesium supplements to replace the portion lost to phytic acid.

Soybeans, too, are full of phytic acid; they have one of
the highest levels of any legume. Unlike other foods, soy's
phytic acid is not destroyed with extended cooking time.
Only fermentation (as is done in the production of miso and
tempeh) will reduce soy's phytic acid levels. This explains
why I recommend only fermented soy and advise people to
stay away from soy powders and soy milk as well as tofu, especially when these foods are offered as a substitute for meat
and dairy.

As a cheap alternative to meat, soy (as soy protein isolate
and textured vegetable protein) has exploded on school
lunch menus and in the fast-food industry. This is unfortunate, as too much soy can cause mineral deficiencies in children, who really need their minerals to build strong bones
and teeth—their structural body.

Moreover, menopausal women may be overusing soy (for
its natural phytoestrogenic effects) and developing similar
mineral deficiencies. While the phytoestrogens in soy may
be helpful to older women, they are another reason to avoid
using unfermented soy in the diets of growing boys and girls.

JUNK FOOD LACKS MAGNESIUM

Even in a healthy diet with proper protein intake, studies
show that the addition of as little as 150 mg of elemental
magnesium a day can make dramatic changes in health.[56]
The lesson here is that if a good diet can leave you magne-

sium deficient, a poor diet can seriously undermine your health.

We live in strange times, when people avidly watch gourmet cooking shows while devouring junk food. As I mentioned earlier, junk food provides 25 percent of most people's daily calories; an astounding 70 percent of our food dollar is spent on processed foods. People who drink soda and soft drinks may be magnesium deficient because sugar uses up magnesium.[57, 58] Many carbonated beverages and processed foods (such as luncheon meats and hot dogs) contain phosphates, which bind with magnesium to make magnesium phosphate, an insoluble substance that is not absorbed by the body.

PART TWO

Magnesium Deficiency Conditions

Anxiety, Depression, Sleep

**THREE THINGS YOU NEED TO KNOW ABOUT
MAGNESIUM, ANXIETY, AND DEPRESSION**

---

1. Magnesium supports our adrenal glands, which are overworked by stress, leading to combined magnesium deficiency
symptoms and adrenal exhaustion symptoms of anxiety, depression, muscle weakness, fatigue, eye twitches, insomnia,
anorexia, apathy, apprehension, poor memory, confusion, anger,
nervousness, and rapid pulse.
2. Serotonin, the "feel-good" brain chemical that is artificially
boosted by Prozac, depends on magnesium for its production
and function.
3. Magnesium deficiency has been strongly linked to sleep disorders, which can either cause or increase anxiety.

ADRENALINE WASTES MAGNESIUM

Adrenaline is like an unstable accelerant that gets you all
revved up with no place to go! It's not just a theory that stress
causes magnesium deficiency and a lack of magnesium mag-
nifies stress. Experiments where adrenaline is given intrave-

nously show that it decreases magnesium as well as calcium, potassium, and sodium. This proves that when you are in a revved-up state and burning adrenaline, you are also burning off magnesium.

There are more than a dozen major metabolic processes that are affected by bursts of adrenaline, including heart rate, blood pressure, blood vessel constriction, and contraction of all muscles, including the heart. Each of these functions requires magnesium to bring them back into balance. When IV adrenaline is stopped in these experiments, the body recovers in about thirty minutes, showing a rise in potassium during that time. However, it takes much longer for magnesium to reach normal levels.

Darcy had driven across a mile-long bridge every day for years, so why one morning did she suddenly feel as though she would die if she didn't pull over? She was sweating and her heart was pounding; she felt sick to her stomach and couldn't get her breath. What was happening to her? Fortunately, she had her cell phone and called her best friend, Sara, who helped her calm herself and make her way across the bridge safely. Later, while talking with Sara to try to make sense of the episode, Darcy said she had been on a liquid protein diet for a few weeks. Sara pointed out that it could have thrown something out of balance, and she reminded Darcy that she had warned her of the dangers of this type of diet.

The two women reviewed the list of supplements that Darcy had been taking as part of the program and found that she had neglected to take the magnesium that had been suggested because it was causing the laxative effect. Sara grabbed a natural health encyclopedia and, sure enough, magnesium deficiency was listed as one of the possible causes of panic attacks. If Sara had read further, she would have found that the body demands more magnesium when on a liquid protein diet and that the dangers of such a diet have been documented for decades.[1] By eating only protein, Darcy had set herself up for a terrifying attack. Fortunately, she discovered she was probably magnesium deficient before pursuing a prescription for a tranquilizer to deal with the frightening symptoms of panic attack.

Lack of magnesium may not have been the only cause of Darcy's panic attack. As well as creating an extra demand for magnesium, her high-protein diet could have led to symptoms of hypoglycemia. When blood sugar (glucose) is low, the body reacts with a surge of adrenaline to bring glucose levels back to normal in order to keep this essential nutrient fueling the brain. Adrenaline acts to speed the heart and retrieve glucose from liver storage. Sometimes people perceive a normal adrenaline rush as a panic attack. Interestingly enough, magnesium is also a requirement for proper blood sugar control.

Women tend to pay attention to their feelings and interpret symptoms such as panic attacks as signs of emotional imbalance, for which they seek support. The support they get, however, is often in the form of a prescription for an antianxiety drug instead of sound advice to eat a balanced diet, exercise, and take the right balance of supplements.

Magnesium deficiency itself, even in the absence of erratic surges of adrenaline from the adrenal glands, can be an underlying cause of anxiety and depression, as determined in several clinical trials.[2] A 2016 review of the literature concluded that "the efficacy of Mg in the treatment of anxiety in the mildly anxious and those reporting premenstrual-syndrome-related anxiety is suggestive of a beneficial effect of Mg intake."[3]

Symptoms of chronic magnesium deficiency include anxious behavior, hyperemotionality, apathy, apprehensiveness, poor memory, confusion, anger, nervousness, muscle weakness, fatigue, headaches, insomnia, light-headedness, dizziness, nervous fits, the feeling of a lump in the throat, impaired breathing, muscle cramps (including leg cramps), a tingling or pricking or creeping feeling on the skin, rapid pulse, chest pain, palpitations, and abnormal heart rhythm.[4, 5] See the list "100 Factors Related to Magnesium Deficiency" in Chapter 1.

Even the hyperventilation that may accompany anxiety can further drop magnesium levels. Why is this? Hyperventilation makes the blood more alkaline than it should be, and that alkalinity must be neutralized with an intricate dance of sodium, potassium, calcium, and magnesium. It's much more unobtrusive, however, to take magnesium supplements for anxiety than to pull out a paper bag and breathe into it.

I think it's fairly safe to say that the flood of adrenaline that occurs in the body during periods of acute stress can cause you to experience anxiety and panic attacks. As the stress becomes chronic and your adrenal glands are depleted, you can fall into a state of depression.

CHRONIC STRESS

When the adrenals are stimulated to release adrenaline on a constant basis, due to long-term stress, they can become depleted and the release of adrenaline can become erratic. Some alternative medicine practitioners call this adrenal fatigue. However, according to allopathic medicine, the adrenals are either working just fine or collapsed, a condition called Addison's disease, which is treated with prednisone; there is no in-between place and no in-between treatment.

According to Hans Selye, the Canadian doctor famous for his work on stress, magnesium is depleted when the body shifts from a short-term fight-or-flight reaction to a chronic stress reaction. The adrenal glands produce stress hormones.

One is norepinephrine, which acts like adrenaline and is more a short-term stress hormone. Another is cortisol, a steroid hormone in the glucocorticoid class of hormones. Humans produce it in the middle or zona fasciculata of the adrenal cortex within the adrenal gland. It is released in response to chronic stress and low blood sugar. Elevated cortisol is an indication of chronic stress. Production of both norepinephrine and cortisol cause depletion of magnesium, and both can be active at the same time.

Chronic stress can come from feeling insecure and threatened, or from exposure to toxic chemicals, heavy metals, or even loud noise, all of which assault the nervous system and overwork the immune system. For example, in one study, constant loud noise in an industrial work setting induced a significant increase in serum magnesium (as magnesium was released from tissues) and significantly increased urinary excretion of magnesium (indicating magnesium deficiency), which lasted for forty-eight hours after exposure.[6]

MAGNESIUM DEFICIENCY ANXIETY

How do you go from being a calm person with your nervous system under control to being an anxious, fearful individual? I think it's due to a gradual but chronic decrease in magnesium reserves. When your body is stressed—which can happen for a dozen different reasons—your magnesium reserves dump this crucial mineral into your bloodstream, and you immediately become one of those people blessed with the ability to cope. You are both calm and alert. Your friends and relatives think it's just who you are, but it's really how much magnesium you have in reserve.

If the stress continues and you don't rest or replace your magnesium between episodes, your magnesium stores become depleted. Then when you are faced with the next stressor, your stress hormones (adrenaline and cortisol) cannot activate your magnesium reserves, with the consequent calming effect. Instead, adrenaline revs up your heart rate, elevates your blood pressure, and tenses your muscles in a fight-or-flight reaction.

Millions of people try unsuccessfully to cope with their problems by taking pharmaceuticals or through addictive behaviors such as overeating, cigarette smoking, alcohol abuse, or use of street drugs, among others. We are a nation suffering a 32 percent incidence of anxiety, depression, and drug problems. Instead of treating stress reactions properly with magnesium, each year millions of people are introduced to the merry-go-round of psychiatric drugs and psychological counseling for symptoms that may in fact be rooted in magnesium deficiency.

You're stressed out, not sleeping, tense, and irritable and you don't know that simply taking a good magnesium supplement could pull you out of that downward spiral. All these symptoms are interwoven, as you can see from the following cases of people who fortunately discovered that much of their suffering was due to magnesium deficiency.

A very special friend of ours was going through a very bad patch earlier this year. A relative, who she was extremely close to, was suffering with liver failure, and another relative, who has prostate cancer, had just had a test showing a rise in his PSA despite his good diet and supplement regime. My friend said she was suffering from dreadful stress and feeling constantly anxious with a tight pain constantly around her chest.

I suggested maybe it would be good to try some of the ReMag that her husband was taking. I think she thought it would be a waste as it wouldn't change the situation. Fortunately, she did try it, and literally a few days later she started feeling better. Her chest pains went away, as did her nightly cramps, and the constant feeling of tension lessened to such a degree she felt she could cope once more.

Sadly, her relative with liver failure died a few weeks later, but she said the ReMag really helped her through what was an incredibly stressful situation.

I have been using ReMag for about two weeks for my anxiety attacks and I already feel so much better. I am up to 1 tsp twice a day.

I've been sleeping very well, experiencing very little or no anxiety, hardly any or no heart palpitations—this is after having suffered atrial fibrillation and anxiety for almost ten years. I'm stronger in the evening hours than I used to be and can do many, many things throughout the day and night that I couldn't do before without some kind of a reaction. I do relax and rest and pace myself. I faithfully take my ReMag and ReMyte, ReAline and RnA Drops. Sometimes I don't always get all my salt water down, but I aim to reach my goal every day.

I am doing all your formulas now as well as a soil-based probiotic and feel fantastic! My night sweats have ceased and I've had no more issues with my Crohn's disease. Everything is moving along great. I have no more anxiety issues and I have increased energy. What more could I ask for!

I just want to thank you! Because of you, I have renewed hope in life! I have all the signs of magnesium deficiency—things I never thought about, like low blood pressure. I thought that was a good thing, but it's gotten so low in the past that I had severe vertigo. I saw a doctor the day after I literally could not get up, and she said she was surprised I was vertical! She gave me IV minerals. She said to drink Gatorade but I took sea salt water instead, like you recommend. I also have magnesium-deficiency muscle tension and anxiety that started in (early) menopause nineteen years ago, for which I was prescribed Xanax! I'm already able to taper off that. I have many other niggling symptoms, all due to magnesium deficiency! I love what you write about first replacing minerals, not hormones, and I love your minerals. It all rings true and feels true.

Is anxiety driven by brain hyperexcitability or adrenaline surges? It's likely to be both. Neurons in constant firing mode can't turn off because there is too little magnesium to repel calcium, which is the firing trigger. The neurons keep firing until the cell collapses.

An important study done in 1995 showed that even marginal magnesium deficiency could induce the brain to become hyperexcitable, as shown by EEG measurements.[7] The study lasted six months. During the first three months thirteen women ingested a very deficient 115 milligrams of magnesium daily. This amounts to only 30 percent of the RDA. During this time their EEGs showed hyperexcitability.

During the second three months, they received 315 mg daily—a little closer to the 360 mg RDA for women. On this dose of magnesium, it took six weeks for EEG readings to show significant improvement in brain function and decreased excitability. Studies such as this one convinced me to recommend twice the RDA for people with obvious magnesium deficiency symptoms.

Stress is so prevalent in our daily lives that we have become desensitized to it and the message it is trying to give us, which is to slow down. Anxiety is a chemical reaction created when the adrenal glands respond to a stressful event by releasing adrenaline. Adrenaline is very useful if you're trying to escape from a dangerous situation, because it stimulates the fight-or-flight response: your heart starts pumping faster; digestion slows down; energy stores are released from your liver and made available to the heart, lungs, and muscles; and the muscles of your arms and legs are activated. All of these responses require magnesium. So each time you experience any kind of stress, your magnesium stores are tapped to minimize stress reactions and to keep the body's thousands of enzyme processes active.

This magnesium depletion itself stresses the body, which can result in panic attacks, causing even more stress. Not only do your overworked adrenals cause magnesium depletion, but even more adrenaline is released under stress. If your magnesium levels are already low, you feel even more irritable, nervous, edgy, or ready to explode. It's the proverbial Catch-22.[8] To put an end to anxiety, you need to replenish your magnesium daily.

During stress reactions, calcium is also required to stimulate the release of adrenaline, but calcium excess can cause a flood of adrenaline. However, having sufficient magnesium will buffer excess calcium and keep it within normal levels, limiting the stress response. Magnesium is important because it naturally diminishes the excitability of the nervous system and lowers the level of calcium around nerve cells. This function of magnesium is also significant in heart disease and other stress-induced illness.[9, 10]

Magnesium regulates the hypothalamic-pituitary-adrenal axis, as shown in an animal study where magnesium restriction in mice enhanced anxiety-related behavior.[11] The chemical findings showed elevated plasma ACTH levels, which indicates a revved-up stress response. In the second arm of the study, anxiety symptoms were reversed with anxiolytic and antidepressant drug treatments. The obvious question is why on earth they didn't just give magnesium to the poor mice.

You can read more about this topic in my free ebook *Mineral Deficient Anxiety*, which you can access at http://bit.ly/mg-miracle-gift.

MAGNESIUM DEFICIENT DEPRESSION

Social epidemiologist Myrna Weissman at Columbia University reports that more and more Americans are becoming depressed, getting depressed at a younger age, and experiencing more severe and frequent periods of depression. Each generation born in the twentieth century has suffered more depression than the previous one, and since World War II the overall rate of depression has more than doubled.[12, 13] A study in the *Archives of General Psychiatry* showed a doubling of depression in women from 1970 to 1992, with the use of psychiatric drugs skyrocketing as a result.[14]

People do not develop anxiety, panic attacks, or depression because they have a deficiency of Valium or Prozac. Our bodies do not require these substances for essential metabolic processes. However, we can develop a myriad of psychological symptoms because of a deficiency of magnesium, a nutrient our bodies do require. Does it make any sense to merely switch our addictions from sugar, alcohol, drugs, and cigarettes to prescription medication without looking at the possible underlying metabolic causes? Psychiatrists all too often rely on prescription drugs for suffering patients and have no insight into the metabolic functioning of the mind and body and what happens when nutrients are deficient. Anxiety and depression are often nutrient deficiency diseases and chemical sensitivities, certainly not drug deficiency diseases.

A remarkable study of almost 500 depressed people by Drs. Cox and Shealy found that the majority of sufferers were magnesium deficient. The authors of the study advised clinicians that they should consider the distinct possibility of a therapeutic benefit from the use of magnesium therapy in chronic depression.[15]

When I went through menopause I had a glimpse of what depression must feel like. Just before a hot flash would strike, a feeling of impending doom would come over me. That horrific feeling would pass after only a few seconds, replaced by a hot flash. Each time it occurred I had no awareness that it was just notification of an upcoming hot flash; I was completely embedded in that moment. The feeling of doom and the hot flashes eventually subsided, but not the knowledge that depressive symptoms can be the result of highly charged biochemistry. That's why I truly believe magnesium can be extremely helpful in the prevention and treatment of depression.

However, I would never say that magnesium deficiency is the only factor in depression, and I often recommend a mega nutrient compound for the treatment of depression and manic depression. It is called EMPowerplus Advanced; I mention it below under "Supplements for Anxiety and Depression," and describe it in the Resources section.

A 2016 study, "Dietary Magnesium Intake and the Incidence of Depression: A 20-Year Follow-up Study," declared itself the first prospective study with twenty years of follow-up to report the association between magnesium intake and the incidence of depression in men.[16] I think it's worth looking up this study to see the impressive list of references. It seems that researchers have been proving the connection between depression and magnesium for a long time but the medical world hasn't been paying attention. An earlier study by the same group, published in 2009, found an association between magnesium intake and anxiety as well as depression.[17]

It may be the way that researchers report their results that prevents doctors from jumping on the magnesium bandwagon. In the 2016 twenty-year follow-up study, instead of shouting their conclusion from the rooftops that "magnesium intake may have an effect on the risk to develop depression," the researchers mildly say, "Further studies are needed to investigate whether sufficient magnesium intake could have implications for prevention or treatment of depression."

Lord suffering cats! Why on earth can't magnesium researchers come down from their ivory tower, make a definitive statement, and demand that clinicians listen to them? Lives are at stake! Instead, they just make their observations, never draw conclusions, and continue to demand funding for research that will never end while the public waits for science to tell them what to do!

Let me explain one of the ways magnesium functions to relieve the mind of anxiety and depression. You may be familiar with serotonin, the body's natural "feel-good" brain chemical. Magnesium is important in the serotonin story because it is a necessary element in its production as well as in the release and uptake of serotonin by brain and gut cells. With proper amounts of magnesium, nature makes sufficient serotonin and you experience emotional balance. But when stress depletes magnesium, a vicious cycle spins out of control, and depression can occur.

Authors of the October 2014 paper "Role of Dietary Factors in Psychiatry" made the following statement: "It was found that the individuals with low cerebrospinal fluid [CSF] levels of magnesium also have lower cerebrospinal fluid levels of 5-hydroxyindoleacetic acid which is a metabolite of serotonin, indicating serotonin deficiency."[18] CSF levels of magnesium were lower in patients with major depression as compared with controls, and low in people who attempted suicide. The authors concluded, "Deficiency of magnesium can cause depression, behaviour and personality changes, apathy, irritability and anxiety."

Instead of looking at dietary factors in psychiatric conditions, including magnesium deficiency, the pharmaceutical industry has focused its research for the treatment of depression on selective serotonin reuptake inhibitors, such as Prozac, to capitalize on serotonin's chemical effects instead of giving serotonin what it really needs—magnesium.

SSRIs create artificially elevated levels of serotonin in the body by preventing its breakdown and elimination; serotonin lingers longer in the brain and theoretically causes mood elevation. This is what is supposed to happen, on paper, but everyone has a different reaction to the manipulation of his or her brain chemicals. For some people, prolonged, rising levels of serotonin can liberate them from a long-term depression. For others, the drug can lead to anxiety and irritability. A small but significant group can feel released from their apathy just long enough to act on suicidal or homicidal thoughts. Another group of people tend to have flattened moods in which they can neither weep nor laugh, keeping them from the extremes of depression or mania but relegating them to a one-dimensional life.

This was my patient Maggie's situation. She was on Prozac and desperately trying to eliminate it because she was unable to cry or experience real emotions. Maggie was down to one-quarter of a 10 mg tablet but was afraid to stop in case her depression came back. She also had high blood pressure, high cholesterol, periodic muscle cramps, and constipation— all signs and symptoms of magnesium deficiency. I asked

Maggie to have her magnesium tested, and her cardiologist said it was normal. He said she didn't need magnesium but should continue to take her five prescription medications to control her symptoms.

Maggie called me when her primary care physician thought her worsening muscle cramps were actually a major blood clot in her leg. We didn't have time to ship a blood sample to the lab that performs magnesium RBC testing, so I encouraged her to take 300 mg of magnesium twice a day and go for a Doppler scan to rule out blood clots. Fortunately, the scan was negative, so Maggie was able to avoid several more medications to treat blood clots, and the magnesium was already working to relieve her symptoms. Within a few months Maggie was finally off the last small amount of Prozac and able to laugh and cry again.

I would not presume to tell a severely depressed person that taking magnesium is all he or she needs. I don't claim to treat depression, although I'm told often enough that my Completement Formula does help this condition. Instead I refer people to EMPowerplus Advanced from www.TrueHope .com. You can read more about it in the Resources section.

SLEEP AND MAGNESIUM

We take sleep for granted—until we start losing it! There are countless causes of insomnia, and many of them are either due to magnesium deficiency or treatable with magnesium supplements. The long list includes numerous medications, caffeine, alcohol, heart disease, pounding heartbeat, nighttime cortisol surges, restless legs, pain, hormone shifts, fear, stress, anxiety, heartburn, constipation, depression, dementia, OCD, ADHD, arthritis, and poor recovery from exercise. I'll talk more about these many conditions and explain their relationship to magnesium deficiency in this chapter.

Insomnia is actually one of the first symptoms to be alleviated with magnesium therapy. There is a saying in magnesium circles that the mineral is so effective that if a person complains that magnesium isn't helping them sleep, then they just haven't taken enough. Many people find that the laxative effect prevents them from reaching therapeutic levels of magnesium. Fortunately, the discovery of ReMag solves that problem.

There are many sleep studies that confirm the effectiveness of magnesium supplementation. However, I find it frustrating that magnesium sleep research is repeated over and over, yet doctors don't get the message to report this to their patients. If they do recommend magnesium, they reference magnesium oxide, which may partially work but usually causes an extreme laxative effect, and often the patient discontinues the treatment.

How does magnesium help us sleep? Twitchy, restless, tense muscles keep you from falling into a deep sleep. Tight muscles make you hyperalert and irritable, and in that condition any noise or even an active dream will wake you up. Magnesium relaxes tight, twitchy muscles so you can reach a deeper level of sleep. There are many other mechanisms, and I will briefly outline them.

- GABA is the main inhibitory neurotransmitter of the central nervous system, and so activation of GABA(A) receptors favors sleep.[19] Magnesium binds to GABA gates and increases their effects.[20]
- As mentioned above, one sleep study reported on magnesium-deficiency-induced, anxiety-like behavior in mice, which were then treated with sleep meds.[21]
- Research on magnesium and sleep shows that oral magnesium reverses age-related neuroendocrine and sleep EEG changes.[22]

- Magnesium supplementation improves magnesium deficiency symptoms and inflammatory stress in older adults (over age fifty-one) with poor sleep.[23]
- Magnesium reduces heart rate response to sympathetic nervous stimulation, to exercise, and to sleep problems.[24]
- Two studies showed that chronic sleep deprivation reduces intracellular magnesium, increases heart rate, and raises plasma catecholamines.[25, 26]
- A study found that dietary magnesium deficiency decreases plasma melatonin in rats.[27]

RESTLESS LEGS

Over the years I've received a tremendous number of reports from people whose restless leg syndrome (RLS) improved or even vanished when they took therapeutic levels of magnesium. Factors beyond magnesium deficiency that can cause or worsen restless legs include iron deficiency, Parkinson's disease, kidney failure, diabetes, peripheral neuropathy, pregnancy, extreme emotional stress, and various medications. Many commonly prescribed drugs induce RLS; they include antipsychotics used to treat manic-depression and schizophrenia, antidepressants (especially the selective serotonin reuptake inhibitors, or SSRIs), antiemetics (for nausea and vomiting), and antihistamines (found in many over-the-counter allergy and sleep aids).

Considering that 70 percent of the American population is taking one or more medications,[28] there is a very great likelihood of RLS being a drug side effect in a certain percentage of patients. The underlying reason that patients may develop drug-induced RLS could be because of the magnesium deficiency that is commonly caused by drugs.

A 2009 review of treatments for restless leg syndrome and periodic limb movement disorder made it clear that drug management is the allopathic medical standard of care for both conditions, and the investigators recommended behavioral therapy—not magnesium.[29] There were, however, two studies investigating magnesium. One, published in 1998, showed that magnesium treatment may be a useful alternative therapy in patients with mild or moderate RLS and periodic limb movement syndrome.[30] Another, published in 2006, found that magnesium sulfate may relieve restless legs syndrome in pregnancy.[31] IV magnesium was used in this study, which may not be a viable treatment option for most people. However, I've found that oral ReMag can match and even exceed the effectiveness of IV magnesium.

By 2012, it's as if magnesium for RLS never existed—a systemic review and meta-analysis in the journal *Sleep* made no mention of magnesium as a possible treatment for restless leg syndrome.[32] It did mention using iron supplements if the patient's ferritin levels were low. However, the number of drugs used to treat RLS had escalated. I find this of great concern because drug toxicity can cause RLS, so it makes no sense to treat possible drug side effects with more drugs unless someone is first given a proper trial of therapeutic magnesium.

The unfortunate fact in RLS research is that there is no funding to do proper studies on the possible effectiveness of magnesium. However, I think there is enough research and anecdotal confirmation of the effectiveness of magnesium that people can do their own personal clinical trials of magnesium and test it for themselves.

Magnesium is such a safe nutrient, with few to no side effects, that it should be the first step in the management of RLS. See Chapter 18 for a discussion about ReMag as the best-absorbed magnesium. First have blood tests run for magnesium RBC, iron, and potassium to determine deficiencies. If iron is low, try to increase your iron with foods—liver (from free-range animals), blackstrap molasses, deep green leafy vegetables (such as spinach). If potassium is low, eat more vegetables and make a rich Potassium Broth (see Appendix E.) And, of course, if your magnesium RBC level is less than 6.0 mg/dL, supplement with magnesium.

DIET ADVICE FOR ANXIETY AND DEPRESSION

My general diet recommendations are as follows:

- Eliminate alcohol, coffee, white sugar, white flour, gluten, fried foods, and trans fatty acids (found in margarine and in baked, fried, and processed foods made with partially hydrogenated fats).
- If you eat animal protein, choose organically raised grass-fed beef, free-range chicken and eggs, and fish (especially wild-caught salmon).
- For vegetarian protein, choose fermented dairy, lactose-free cheese, and ReStructure Meal Replacement (it has no casein, very-low-lactose whey protein, and pea and rice proteins).
- Vegan protein choices include legumes, gluten-free grains, nuts, and seeds.
- Eat healthy carbs such as a variety of raw, cooked, and fermented vegetables, two or three pieces of fruit a day, and gluten-free grains.
- Include magnesium-rich foods listed in Appendix A and calcium-rich foods listed in Appendix B.
- For fats and oils, choose butter, olive oil, flaxseed oil, sesame oil, and coconut oil.

SUPPLEMENTS FOR ANXIETY AND DEPRESSION

- **ReMag:** With picometer, stabilized ionic magnesium you can reach therapeutic amounts without laxative effects. Start with ¼ tsp (75 mg) and work up to 2–3 tsp (600–900 mg) per day. Add ReMag to a liter of water and sip all day to achieve full absorption.

- **ReMyte:** Picometer twelve-mineral solution. Take ½ tsp three times a day, or add 1½ tsp to a liter of water with ReMag and sip throughout the day.

- **ReCalcia:** Picometer, stabilized ionic calcium, boron, vanadium. Take 1–2 tsp per day (1 tsp provides 300 mg calcium) if you don't obtain enough calcium from your diet. It can be taken with ReMag and ReMyte.

- **ReAline:** B vitamin complex plus amino acids. Take 1 capsule twice per day. Contains food-based B_1 and four methylated B vitamins (B_2, B_6, B_{12}, and folate), plus L-methionine (precursor to glutathione) and L-taurine (which supports the heart and weight loss).

- **Tryptophan:** Take one or two 500 mg capsules at bedtime on an empty stomach. This amino acid is converted to serotonin. It acts like Prozac but has no side effects.

- **St. John's wort:** Taking 300 mg standardized extract three times a day is beneficial in mild to moderate depression.

- **EMPowerplus Advanced:** This high-potency vitamin, mineral, and amino acid formulation from www.TrueHope.com treats depression and bipolar disease, as proven in twenty-seven scientific clinical trials. (See Resources.)

SLEEP AIDS

- **ReMag:** Take an extra dose of ReMag at bedtime, ½–1 tsp (150–300 mg).

- **Melatonin:** 2–3 mg one hour before bedtime.
- **5-hydroxytryptamine (5-HTP):** 50–200 mg half an hour before bedtime, on an empty stomach.
- **Hops, valerian, and skullcap herbal combinations:** One or two 500 mg capsules before bedtime.

STRESS RELEASE

Exercise is excellent for alleviating both anxiety and depression. Try walking, biking, yoga, Pilates, T-Tapp, and swimming. Other forms of stress release include prayer, meditation, long baths, journal writing, and Emotional Freedom Technique (EFT).

Because depression can be so debilitating, even life-threatening, it's understandable that doctors feel strong measures are required to combat it, but these strong measures don't always work. The alternative that many doctors are missing is the nutrient connection. Magnesium deficiency is a potential cause for every type of depression. All treatment protocols should begin with adequate doses of this valuable mineral.[33]

MAGNESIUM AND MUSICIANS

One case of sound-induced magnesium deficiency became evident to a parent who heard me talking about this condition on a New York radio station. She called in to the program and said that a few months after her son began playing in a rock band, his left eyelid started to twitch uncontrollably. Listening to me on the radio show, she realized that it might be due to magnesium deficiency.

Her son's twitching was likely a result of magnesium being used to buffer against the stress of sounds at a decibel level that sets off alarm bells in the body. Loud sounds cause a reflexive fight-or-flight response, and constant loud sound is not something the body gets used to and ignores—it must continually adapt to the noise, all the while using up valuable nutrients such as magnesium to do that job.

Exposure to loud music can increase urinary excretion of magnesium, which lasts for days after exposure. If magnesium is not replaced through an excellent diet and supplements, magnesium deficiency symptoms may begin to appear. Although I do know some rock musicians who are vegetarians and don't smoke or drink alcohol, that may not be the norm. Smoking, coffee, alcohol, and the rock star lifestyle all contribute to magnesium deficiency.

Musicians have more than one reason to use magnesium. Nervousness, anticipation, and anxiety are all part of the buildup to a musical performance, whether it's classical, rock, punk, or rap. To deal with the anxiety and the resulting elevated heart rate that often accompanies it, musicians may feel they have to turn to drugs, alcohol, or even medication. Inderal (propranolol) is a beta-blocker that is normally prescribed to treat rapid heart rate, high blood pressure, and heart arrhythmias. It's called "the musicians' underground drug" because it is used for performance anxiety. It's underground because it's used off-label, which means that the FDA has not approved propranolol for anxiety. There have been some small studies reporting that musicians felt less anxious about their performance on beta-blockers, which block physical reactions to fear. When your heart begins to race, your palms sweat, and you just want to run as fast and as far as you can, you are experiencing the fight-or-flight response. Adrenaline is pumped from the adrenal glands to ready your muscles to run or fight. But musicians need to be calm so that their hands don't slip off their instrument due to shaking or sweating. They need their heart to stop thumping so loudly in their head that they can't hear their cue or be so distracted they can't even see the conductor or bandleader. And for bandleaders and conductors, the fear inherent in being responsible for the success of the band's performance elevates their heart rate and anxiety.

Beta-blockers are used to decrease heart rate, but some of them, including Inderal, also cause constriction of the bronchial tubes, which makes them dangerous to use if you have asthma. They can also worsen congestive heart failure, diabetes, allergic reactions, and Raynaud's syndrome. Some people may have no side effects using small doses only on rare occasions, but higher doses and becoming physically dependent on beta-blockers to calm you before every performance can take its toll.

Inderal is contraindicated in pregnancy and has the following side effects:

Most Frequent

Decreased sexual function, drowsiness, fatigue, general weakness, insomnia.

Less Frequent

Abdominal pain with cramps, anxiety, bronchospastic lung disease, chronic heart failure, constipation, depression, diarrhea, dizziness, nasal congestion, nausea, nervousness, sensation of cold, vomiting.

Rare

Agranulocytosis, allergic reactions, anaphylaxis, arthralgia, back pain, chest pain, conduction disorder of the heart, dry eye, dysgeusia (metallic taste), erythema, erythema multiforme, exfoliative dermatitis, hallucinations, impaired cognition, laryngeal spasms, leukopenia, nightmares, ocular irritation, orthostatic hypotension, pharyngitis, pruritus of skin, psoriasis, severe dyspnea, Stevens-Johnson syndrome, thrombocytopenic disorder, toxic epidermal necrolysis.

Most musicians may not think they have any side effects from taking Inderal; they take the medication because they need to, and they know lots of others who are doing the same. They may not realize that their sexual dysfunction, insomnia, and skin rash are due to the medication or that the medication removes the creative edge that adrenaline would normally give them. And for some, even if they do know, it's the price they pay in order to function in their profession.

What they don't know is how much more effective and safe magnesium is for treating and preventing anxiety and stress. It can also function to increase energy and performance levels that Inderal may actually block. The absolute irony of using Inderal for anxiety is that it is known to reduce levels of magnesium in the body, causing increased excretion through the urine. So if magnesium depletion is a cause of your anxiety, Inderal can actually make it worse. Another benefit of taking magnesium is reduction in the buildup of lactic acid that occurs after hours of playing. Repetitive motion injuries common to musicians can be eased by taking magnesium orally and using magnesium liquid on the injured neck, arm, or shoulder. See Chapter 18 for more on magnesium supplementation.

The best oral form of magnesium for musicians is ReMag, sipped through the day in your drinking water, to which you should add unrefined sea salt, pink Himalayan salt, or Celtic sea salt. Other enhancements to performance include a good balanced diet to overcome any symptoms of hypoglycemia, which also causes anxiety; meditation and relaxation therapies; and yoga, swimming, walking, and other forms of exercise to increase circulation and burn off excess adrenaline.

NOTE: It is inadvisable to suddenly stop using Inderal if you have been taking it regularly. Check with your doctor about weaning off the drug as you increase your doses of magnesium and see the benefits.

MAGNESIUM-DEFICIENT KIDS

It's not just adults who can get anxious because of a magnesium-deficient lifestyle. Our children are also susceptible when their favorite foods are magnesium-deficient hot dogs, pizza, and soda. The stress in their lives—from peer pressure, bullying, academic and athletic performance pressures, worries about body image, the changes and hormonal fluctuations of puberty, and exposure to negative events and violence through the media—all contribute to magnesium deficiency. As noted above, even burning off steam by playing in a band can be a risk factor.

Children are underdiagnosed when it comes to magnesium deficiency, but they develop magnesium deficiency for the same reasons as adults. Attention deficit hyperactivity disorder (ADHD), autism, juvenile delinquency, and childhood depression are associated with magnesium deficiency, and some say these conditions can be caused by it.[34]

Dr. Sharna Olfman, a professor of clinical and developmental psychology, expresses her concerns in her book *No Child Left Different*.[35] She warns that psychiatric illnesses in American children have soared from the early 1990s up to the time her book was published in 2008. She quotes the National Institute of Mental Health (NIMH), which estimates one in ten children and adolescents in the United States "suffers from mental illness severe enough to result in significant functional impairment." Also she notes that mood-altering drugs have become "the treatment of first choice rather than the treatment of last resort." The number of medications used in patients under twenty had increased threefold in the same period. In her research, she found that

"Over 10 million children and adolescents are currently on antidepressants, and about 5 million children are taking stimulant medications such as Ritalin."

In 2005, Columbia University initiated a program called Teen Screen throughout forty states, which screened teens and children for mental health problems. Unfortunately, such screening usually leads to more drug prescriptions. Instead of reaching for Ritalin or Prozac for kids, consider whether they're getting enough magnesium first. If these children were simply taken off sugar and put on magnesium, we would have much happier children and far fewer side effects from powerful drugs.

Dr. Leo Galland, author of *Superimmunity for Kids*, speculates that hyperactive children need extra magnesium due to their constantly high adrenaline levels. Dr. Galland recommends 6 mg per pound of weight per day (for example, 240 mg per day for a 40-lb child). I agree with this recommendation because it is more than twice the 6 mg/kg RDA of magnesium.

Because magnesium in pill form is difficult for young children to take, Galland suggests 1 tsp to 1 tbsp of magnesium citrate (mixed in water) a day.[36] Since there may be a concern about a laxative effect with this amount, I recommend the non-laxative picometer magnesium ReMag, ½ tsp twice a day hidden in juice or a smoothie. You can also put it in a spray bottle to use transdermally.

Migraines, Pain, Neuralgia, Issues for Athletes

THREE THINGS YOU NEED TO KNOW ABOUT MAGNESIUM AND MIGRAINES

1. Magnesium prevents platelet aggregation and the thickened blood and tiny clots that can cause blood vessel spasms and the pain of a migraine.
2. Magnesium relaxes the head and neck muscle tension that makes migraines worse.
3. Magnesium and vitamins B_2, B_6, and folate are important nutrients that treat and prevent migraine headaches.

Martha knew that a migraine was looming when the sparks and wavy lines appeared before her eyes and she became nauseous. Working became impossible, and she was looking at the loss of at least one day to a severe migraine attack. Medications such as codeine and ergotamine had not helped her over the years, instead making her feel drugged and tired after the headache finally passed. The fancy new drugs called triptans did nothing for her head pain, and neither did Imitrex, Depakote, or Midrin. Instead they caused chest pain and made her more nauseated. All Martha could do was lie in a darkened room with a cool cloth over her eyes. This time, however, instead of trying to keep hydrated with lots of diet soda, as she usually did, she was going to drink mineral water with lemon and natural fruit juice.

Martha's daughter Mary, a nurse, had told her that aspartame, the sweetener in diet soda, causes headaches. Even though Martha loved her diet soda—she suspected that she was addicted to it, drinking two liters a day on average—she knew she had to do something to stop these headaches, both the daily ones and the one or two massive migraines she got every week.

Over the next few days, Martha's skin itched and she was nauseated, dizzy, and depressed. She thought she was having a reaction to the medication she had taken for her migraine, but Mary told her she was going through aspartame withdrawal. She was also having strong cravings for her diet soda, but Mary insisted that she stay away from it. Mary did some more research on aspartame and how to cope with withdrawal and brought her mother a bottle of magnesium supplements. Martha took 150 mg three times a day, which seemed to help right away.

By the following week, Martha's head felt clearer; she was more alert and less achy. She hadn't even realized that her joints and muscles had been tight and sore until she no longer had those symptoms. To her great relief, two weeks after eliminating aspartame from her diet, she realized that she hadn't had any daily headaches or even one of those migraines that she used to get once or twice a week. After two months of strictly avoiding aspartame, she still had no more headaches or migraines, except once after she had eaten something she had not known contained artificial sweeteners. That convinced her even more that, for her, aspartame was poison, and avoiding it and taking magnesium were the solution.

ASPARTAME AND MSG: EXCITOTOXINS

Aspartame is an excitotoxin, one of a group of substances, usually acidic amino acids, that in high amounts react with specialized receptors in the brain, causing destruction of certain types of neurons.

A growing number of neurosurgeons and neurologists are convinced that excitotoxins play a critical role in the development of several neurological disorders, including migraines, seizures, learning disorders in children, and neurodegenerative disorders such as Alzheimer's disease, Parkinson's disease, Huntington's disease, and amyotrophic lateral sclerosis (ALS).[1]

Glutamate and aspartate are two powerful amino acids that act as natural neurotransmitters in the brain in very small concentrations, but they are also commonly used as food additives. Glutamate is in MSG, a flavor enhancer, and in hydrolyzed vegetable protein, found in hundreds of processed foods. Aspartate is one of three components of aspartame (NutraSweet, Equal), a sugar substitute. In the higher concentrations as food additives, and as single amino acids, these chemicals constantly stimulate brain cells and can cause them to undergo a process of cell death known as excitotoxicity—the cells are excited to death.

HYPOGLYCEMIA

I touched upon hypoglycemia in Chapter 3, but it deserves more attention because it can be responsible for many symptoms that can go undiagnosed and mistreated.

The brain becomes extremely vulnerable to excitotoxins during episodes of low blood sugar or hypoglycemia. Pound for pound, the brain uses more sugar (in the form of glucose) than any other part of the body. Low blood sugar occurs when you are malnourished or even when you skip meals. It also occurs in individuals whose adrenal glands are depleted and can't mount the necessary adrenaline response to raise blood sugar from glycogen stored in the liver.

Magnesium is responsible for balancing blood sugar. With sufficient magnesium and balanced mealtimes, you can protect yourself from headaches, attention deficit hyperactivity disorder, mood disorders, and even premenstrual tension, all of which are associated with hypoglycemia. Supporting the brain as much as possible with safe nutrients and a healthy lifestyle, you may never need the brain-altering medications that are prescribed for these disorders.

Hypoglycemia is recognized medically when blood sugar (glucose) drops to a low of 50 mg/dL (normal is about 80–110 mg/dL). If you eat a highly refined diet with lots of white sugar and white flour, foods whose carbohydrates are rapidly absorbed into the bloodstream, your blood sugar will quickly become elevated; when it reaches a certain point, insulin enters the bloodstream and quickly ushers the excess glucose into the cells of the body, causing your blood sugar to drop.

The more sugar you eat and absorb, the more insulin is released and the quicker and lower your blood sugar can fall. It is the abruptness of this drop, not just reaching 50 mg/dL, that causes adrenaline to be released from the adrenal glands to make sure that the blood sugar does not fall so low that you faint. When that adrenaline mobilizes the sugar stores in the liver to elevate your blood sugar, however, it also produces a fight-or-flight reaction, which may give you a sense of anxiety or impending doom. It may even feel like you're having a panic attack because you don't equate your symptoms with low blood sugar.

At this point, if you eat a confection containing food dyes or an aspartame-containing diet drink to pick you up or comfort you, or if you are exposed to other environmental toxins, your glucose-deprived, magnesium-deficient brain will be more vulnerable to the effects of the excitotoxins. Many diseases of the nervous system are associated with excitotoxin buildup in the brain, including migraines, seizures, strokes, and brain injury.

If you have magnesium deficiency and regularly use aspartame, the toxicity is magnified and can result in headaches and migraines. You can easily identify whether your headaches are caused by aspartame—eliminate aspartame for sixty days and judge for yourself. If you want to minimize the withdrawal effects, sip ReMag in sea-salted water throughout the day. See Chapter 18 for more on magnesium supplements.

Magnesium helps prevent the chain of events that causes cell death due to low blood sugar and exposure to other toxins besides excitotoxins. Magnesium is one of the most important neuroprotectants. It helps defend our cells against potential environmental neurotoxins such as pesticides, herbicides, food additives, solvents, and cleaning products.[2] I'll cover more about the effects of magnesium on aging, Alzheimer's, Parkinson's, and dementia in Chapter 15.

MIGRAINE MECHANISMS

Twenty-five million Americans suffer from migraines. Statistically, more women experience migraines than men, especially in the twenty-to-fifty-year-old age group. The following biochemical events involving low magnesium have been identified in migraine sufferers and may set the stage for a migraine attack.[3]

- In women who have not yet reached menopause, estrogen rises before the period, causing a shift of blood magnesium into bone and muscle. As a result, magnesium levels in the brain are lowered.

- When magnesium is low, it is unable to do its job to counteract the clotting action of calcium on the blood. Tiny blood clots are said to clog up brain blood vessels, leading to migraines. Several other substances that help create blood clots are increased when magnesium is too low.
- Similarly, magnesium inhibits excess platelet aggregation, preventing the formation of tiny clots that can block blood vessels and cause pain.
- Low brain magnesium promotes neurotransmitter hyperactivity and nerve excitation that can lead to headaches.
- Several conditions that trigger migraines are also associated with magnesium deficiency, including pregnancy, alcohol intake, diuretic drugs, stress, and menstruation.
- Magnesium relaxes blood vessels and allows them to dilate, reducing the spasms and constrictions that can cause migraines.
- Magnesium regulates the action of brain neurotransmitters and inflammatory substances, which may play a role in migraines when unbalanced.
- Magnesium relaxes muscles and prevents the buildup of lactic acid, which, along with muscle tension, can worsen head pain.

NOTE: You can do your own experiment to identify food allergies that may trigger migraines by following an elimination diet for three weeks and then testing foods individually, such as gluten, dairy, sugar, yeast, corn, citrus, and eggs.

A group of 3,000 patients given a low dose of 200 mg of magnesium daily had an 80 percent reduction in their migraine symptoms.[4] This 2001 study did not have a control group, so the results could be questioned, but it aroused a great deal of excitement and triggered a flurry of research on magnesium and migraines. Much of that research was done by Dr. Alexander Mauskop, director of the New York Headache Center, working with Drs. Bella and Burton Altura, who have been studying migraines and migraine treatments for many years. This research team consistently found that magnesium is deficient in people with migraine and many other types of headache and, even more important, that supplementing with magnesium alleviated headaches.

Dr. Mauskop with the Alturas undertook many research studies using sensitive magnesium ion electrodes.[5] During one of their first studies they found a deficiency in ionized magnesium but not serum magnesium in migraine patients.[6] This discrepancy highlighted the lack of correlation between magnesium-deficient states and serum magnesium. This is because only 1 percent of the magnesium in the body is found in the blood. A measurement of magnesium ions, the active form of magnesium, is much closer to the total amount of magnesium in the body and indicative of magnesium-deficiency disease.

When migraine sufferers with low magnesium ion levels were given intravenous magnesium, they experienced complete alleviation of their symptoms, including sensitivity to light and sound.[7] Subsequent studies of migraine patients established a common pattern and confirmed the role of magnesium deficiency in the development of headaches.[8] The researchers found that an infusion of magnesium resulted in rapid and sustained relief of acute migraine headaches. Because of an excellent safety profile and low cost, they recommend oral magnesium supplementation for migraine sufferers at a level of 6 mg/kg/day.[9]

In my clinical experience, migraine sufferers usually require double that amount. For a 150-pound patient, 6 mg/

kg is only 400 mg. The reason most doctors will not go much above the RDA is in order to avoid the laxative effect common to most magnesium products. Please read Chapter 18 about ReMag, the non-laxative form of magnesium, which allows migraine sufferers to take therapeutic levels of magnesium without experiencing diarrhea.

Another research team, using 300 mg of magnesium twice a day, treated eighty-one patients who suffered ongoing migraine headaches. The frequency of migraines was reduced by 41.6 percent in the magnesium group but by only 15.8 percent in a control group that received a placebo. The number of migraine days and drug consumption for pain also decreased significantly in the magnesium group. The researchers concluded that high-dose oral magnesium appears to be effective in migraine treatment and prevention.[10]

By 2012, Dr. Mauskop had sufficient clinical success and had published enough about treating migraine with magnesium to title his paper "Why All Migraine Patients Should Be Treated with Magnesium."[11] Dr. Mauskop enthused that "all migraine sufferers should receive a therapeutic trial of magnesium supplementation." As he explains, "A multitude of studies have proven the presence of magnesium deficiency in migraine patients." Double-blind, placebo-controlled trials have produced mixed results, but, as Dr. Mauskop writes, this is "most likely because both magnesium deficient and non-deficient patients were included in these trials." Clearly, if researchers wish to show that magnesium deficiency is a cause of migraine, it's important to test for magnesium deficiency using the ionized magnesium test beforehand; otherwise, the results will be seriously flawed.

Dr. Mauskop agrees with my statements in Chapter 16 that we do not have a readily available reliable test to determine magnesium deficiency. He is right when he states that serum magnesium levels are "entirely inaccurate." As he notes, the magnesium RBC test is more reliable. This test is available to the public at a very reasonable cost, $49. See Chapter 16 for more on magnesium testing and where to obtain the magnesium RBC test without a doctor's prescription.

Unlike other research papers that hem and haw when it comes to conclusions, Dr. Mauskop's paper makes a declarative statement: "Considering that up to 50% of patients with migraines could potentially benefit from this extremely safe and very inexpensive treatment, it should be recommended to all migraine patients."

Where Dr. Mauskop and I disagree is on the matter of magnesium supplement recommendations. He advises 400 mg of magnesium oxide daily. As I note throughout this book, absorption studies show that only 4 percent of a dose of magnesium oxide is absorbed; the remaining 96 percent acts as a strong laxative. Dr. Mauskop also recommends magnesium aspartate, but as I note in Chapter 18, neurosurgeon Dr. Russell Blaylock advises against magnesium aspartate because it has the potential to act as a neurotoxin and excitotoxin in the brain.

I asked Dr. Blaylock in 2016 for an update on this recommendation. He still suggests that people not use magnesium aspartate (or magnesium glutamate). He says that even though the concentration of aspartate may be low, there is some evidence that it "can be high enough to trigger excitotoxic effects—precipitating migraines in sensitive people. Those with neurological disorders certainly should avoid them." Dr. Blaylock cautions that even though some studies may indicate that magnesium aspartate offers neuroprotection, he thinks that is only because the magnesium component of the compound, which is in a much higher concentration, overrides the toxic effect of the aspartate.

Dr. Mauskop is so convinced of the efficacy of magnesium that he urges that if the initial dose is ineffective, patients should look for other magnesium deficiency symptoms. He suggests doubling the dose if a patient has cold extremities, premenstrual syndrome, or leg or foot cramps. He does note the limitation of diarrhea and abdominal distress due to magnesium's laxative effect; his option for patients who are unable to tolerate oral magnesium is frequent IV magnesium.

Since IV magnesium is very expensive and inconvenient, I recommend ReMag, the picometer, stabilized ionic form of magnesium. I've seen it perform even better than IV magnesium because it can be taken several times a day, it's fully absorbed at the cellular level, and it has no laxative effects. I also recommend that migraine sufferers get their magnesium RBC test done; the optimum level is 6.0–6.5 mg/dL. See Chapter 16 for more on magnesium testing.

A 2016 meta-analysis that aimed "to evaluate the effects of intravenous magnesium on acute migraine attacks and oral magnesium supplements on migraine prophylaxis" gleaned results from twenty-one clinical trials.[12] The investigators concluded, "Intravenous magnesium reduces acute migraine attacks within 15–45 minutes, 120 minutes, and 24 hours after the initial infusion and oral magnesium alleviates the frequency and intensity of migraine. Intravenous and oral magnesium should be adopted as parts of a multimodal approach to reduce migraine." The pain of migraines is excruciating, and you would think that this magnesium cure would draw headlines or at least be common knowledge among doctors. A study in late 2016 found that the likelihood of migraine attacks is increased thirty-five times in sufferers with low serum magnesium levels.[13]

In Dr. Mauskop's book *What Your Doctor May Not Tell You About Migraines* he outlines his "triple therapy" for migraines.[14] His triple therapy includes magnesium aspartate, vitamin B$_2$

(riboflavin), and a well-known migraine herb, feverfew. Dr. Mauskop has apparently given up on magnesium oxide but still recommends magnesium aspartate. As I mention above, Dr. Russell Blaylock recommends that we avoid magnesium aspartate because it can break down into aspartic acid and act as a brain excitotoxin.

Several B vitamins have helped people with migraines; however, I don't recommend these as first-line therapies until you have saturated yourself with magnesium. If people can't take therapeutic amounts of magnesium because of the laxative effect, they often switch to other remedies, making them popular. However, taking ReMag allows you to achieve therapeutic levels without getting diarrhea and is effective for most migraines.

In a journal article in *BioMed Research International* discussing the B vitamins and why they help treat migraines, the investigators reported that "deficits in mitochondrial energy reserves can cause migraine because they allow an increase in homocysteine levels, which can lead to migraine attacks; therefore, vitamins could play a vital role in migraine prevention." They say that (1) vitamin B_2 influences mitochondrial dysfunction and prevents migraines, (2) the C677T variant of the methylfolate enzyme is associated with elevated plasma levels of homocysteine and migraine with aura, and (3) homocysteine breakdown requires vitamins B_6, B_{12}, and folic acid, which can decrease the severity of migraine with aura.[15]

I'd like to remind these researchers that deficits in mitochondrial energy reserves are a direct consequence of magnesium deficiency, since magnesium is a necessary cofactor in six of the eight steps in the Krebs cycle. Regarding elevation of homocysteine as a cause of migraines, please read the section on homocysteinemia in Chapter 6, where I describe how important magnesium is for balancing homocysteine levels in the body. However, since nutrients do work synergistically, along with ReMag I do recommend my ReAline product, with its four methylated B vitamins, for treating migraine headaches.

Does allopathic medicine have anything new or better to offer migraine sufferers? Unfortunately not—a new class of migraine drugs, triptans, is now suspected of doing more harm than good. The triptans comprise about sixteen tryptamine-based drugs approved by the FDA in the 1990s. They manipulate serotonin, but their mechanism of action is still not known. Millions of prescriptions for triptans have been written, but a study presented at the 2013 International Headache Congress on the American Migraine Prevalence and Prevention (AMPP) Study found that there is a heart disease contraindication to taking triptans for at least five million Americans.[16] The study's principal investigator, Dr. Richard Lipton, noted, "These data highlight an area of unmet need for acute migraine treatment that does not have cardiovascular risk and contraindications."

I would add that we also need a migraine drug that works in more than 20 percent of migraine patients, which is the "success rate" for triptans. The triptans that cause heart disease are probably doing so by depleting magnesium. The heart contains the highest amount of magnesium in the body, so the more magnesium deficient you are, the more your heart will suffer. Any painkiller—any medication at all—will deplete the body's magnesium stores, because magnesium plays a role in breaking down all medications that are delivered to the liver through the bloodstream. Such a deficiency will only cause more migraine symptoms and magnesium deficiency symptoms, the worst being cardiovascular side effects.

CLUSTER HEADACHES

Patients with cluster headaches, a very severe form of recurrent headache, have also been reported to have low magnesium ion levels. Some people suffer up to twenty bouts of head pain daily in a siege that can last for months. Another study from the Alturas and Dr. Mauskop examined the possibility that patients with cluster headaches and low magnesium ion levels may respond to an intravenous infusion of magnesium sulfate. Within fifteen minutes of an intravenous dose of magnesium, nine patients with cluster headaches had their acute headache aborted.[17] Blood ionized magnesium testing is useful in elucidating the cause of cluster headaches and in identifying patients who may benefit from treatment with magnesium, much as it does for migraines.[18]

SUPPLEMENTS FOR MIGRAINE

- **ReMag:** With picometer, stabilized ionic magnesium you can reach therapeutic amounts without laxative effects. Start with ¼ tsp (75 mg) and work up to 2–3 tsp (600–900 mg) per day. Add ReMag to a liter of water and sip all day to achieve full absorption.
- **ReCalcia:** Picometer, stabilized ionic calcium, boron, vanadium. Take 1–2 tsp per day (1 tsp provides 300 mg calcium) if you don't obtain enough calcium from your diet. It can be taken with ReMag and ReMyte.
- **ReAline:** B vitamin complex plus amino acids. Take 1 capsule twice per day. Contains food-based B_1 and four methylated B vitamins (B_2, B_6, methylfolate, and B_{12}, which help lower homocysteine levels in migraine sufferers), plus L-methionine (precursor to glutathione) and L-taurine (which supports the heart and weight loss).
- **Feverfew** (*Tanacetum parthenium*): 100 mg per day.

ADDITIONAL THERAPIES FOR MIGRAINE

- **Anti-stress therapies:** Breathing exercises, meditation, prayer, singing, and yoga.
- **Regular exercise:** Walking, swimming, T-Tapp, Egoscue Method.

Aspirin has been used to treat headaches for decades. Heavy users, however, prefer magnesium-buffered aspirin. I think magnesium could be responsible for some of aspirin's beneficial effects. The same applies to magnesium-buffered aspirin used in heart disease.

MUSCLE PAIN AND SPASMS

A patient came for a consultation and wanted a total body CT scan because she was having such severe episodes of pain—her whole body would go into spasm—that she thought she must have cancer. I asked her to try taking 300 mg of magnesium three times a day. Within three days she no longer had the spasms, and after three weeks she was free of pain.

THREE THINGS YOU NEED TO KNOW ABOUT MAGNESIUM AND MUSCLE PAIN

1. Magnesium helps muscles and nerves relax.
2. Magnesium eliminates spasms.
3. Magnesium relaxes the smooth muscles in blood vessels in the fingers to treat Raynaud's syndrome; relaxes artery walls, which lowers blood pressure; and relaxes fallopian tubes, which enhances fertility.

Although this patient did not have cancer, research has shown that even the pain of cancer can respond to magnesium. Cancer sometimes metastasizes into nerve bundles located in the neck or lower back and may not respond to even the strongest analgesics such as morphine. There is a special receptor site called NMDA that is responsible for creating this type of nerve pain. Magnesium helps block this receptor. In cases of severe pain, intravenous magnesium has shown very powerful analgesic effects.[19]

ReMag has the same potential to help eliminate severe pain since it is even better absorbed than IV magnesium. A fifty-seven-year-old woman with a twenty-five-year history of ankylosing spondylitis and two hip replacements reported that on ReMag she experienced immediate relief of her severe muscle pain. Her neck region pain also subsided and her mobility improved.

Muscle twitches, tics, and spasms may seem like minor irritations to the onlooker, but to the person suffering, it's like water torture—only instead of water slowly dripping on your forehead, your eye or lip or a small muscle in your leg may constantly jump and writhe. Muscle twitches are a sure sign of magnesium deficiency. The nervous system is hyperexcitable and fires off small muscle groups to try to release some tension. But the only way to eliminate muscle spasms and twitches is by relaxing the nervous system with the proper amounts of magnesium.

LOW BACK PAIN

While I was working on this 2017 edition, a woman whose low back pain was greatly relieved when using magnesium commented on Facebook that in the earlier edition of *The Magnesium Miracle* I didn't emphasize the importance of magnesium for this condition, yet she had had incredible relief when she used magnesium supplementation. I immediately searched the book for "back pain" and only found it described in two case histories and mentioned in my list of conditions associated with magnesium deficiency. I'll remedy this oversight, but first let's find out how many people are affected by low back pain.

In a 2015 review of twenty-eight studies involving low back pain, the authors found that "chronic low back pain prevalence was 4.2% in individuals aged between 24 and 39 years old and 19.6% in those aged between 20 and 59. Of nine studies with individuals aged 18 and above, six reported chronic low back pain between 3.9% and 10.2% and three, prevalence between 13.1% and 20.3%."[20] WebMD says that 80 percent of the population at some point in their lives will experience low back pain, and it lists the main causes as slipped discs, spinal stenosis, and scoliosis. These seem to be very extreme causes of low back pain, and doctors will offer muscle relaxants, saying that muscles will be in spasm around an area of low back injury. They may recommend physical therapy as well. However, if the medications and therapy don't work, you're referred to an orthopedic surgeon and may be told you need to have back surgery.

I have a very different way of looking at low back pain. What if magnesium deficiency causes muscles that are irritated and overworked to go into spasm and that's the cause of many cases of chronic low back pain? I've talked about my heart palpitations and leg cramps as my main magnesium deficiency symptoms. However, during the six months I was writing this edition, I began experimenting with reducing my ReMag intake. On less than 300 mg a day I developed occasional leg cramps and heart palpitations, and I saw the resurgence of some low back pain that I had been plagued with many years ago. I even had to go to conferences wearing a brace to support my lower back. Now I realize I was suffering from low back muscle spasms that came and went and I didn't even associate them with my magnesium deficiency or their disappearance with my magnesium intake!

In 2013, the journal *Anaesthesia* reported on a study using sequential IV and oral magnesium therapy for chronic low back pain.[21] This study reported that "persistent mechanical irritation of the nerve root sets up a series of events mediating sensitization of the dorsal roots and dorsal horns in the spinal cord. Current evidence supports the role of magnesium in blocking central sensitization through its effect on N-methyl-d-aspartate receptors." In the study all patients were already being treated with anticonvulsants, antidepressants, and simple analgesics. Additionally, forty patients in the control group received a placebo for six weeks, while another forty patients in the experimental group received IV magnesium for two weeks followed by oral magnesium capsules for another four weeks. The researchers found that in a six-month period, a rotating schedule of two weeks of IV magnesium followed by four weeks of oral magnesium reduced pain intensity and improved lumbar spine mobility in this group of patients with intractable low back pain and associated nerve involvement.

When I go over my case histories of people who report benefits from magnesium, low back pain comes up very often, and magnesium should be the first line of treatment for this condition. You can take oral magnesium, soak in Epsom salts baths, and spray magnesium locally on the painful areas. ReMag is the most therapeutic magnesium that you can use, and it also works well when sprayed directly on painful areas.

Of course, you should have your back examined by your doctor, including X-rays if necessary, to make sure there is no anatomical damage that might require surgery. However, most low back pain is muscular and worsened by stress, including the stress of being concerned that you might have a chronic condition. To learn more about the stress and emotional component of back pain, read rehabilitation specialist Dr. John Sarno's book *Healing Back Pain*.[22]

RAYNAUD'S SYNDROME

Sally had terrible leg cramps. During the night, her legs felt jumpy and twitchy and kept her awake. If she did fall asleep, muscle cramps in her calves would wake her up. In addition, her fingers began turning white, blue, or red at different times. A young internist diagnosed her as having Raynaud's syndrome, a circulatory condition caused by spasms in tiny arteries, especially in the hands and feet.

Raynaud's syndrome may occur suddenly or as a result of chronic illnesses such as connective tissue disease, trauma, or pulmonary hypertension, in which case it is called Raynaud's phenomenon. Raynaud's syndrome is seen mostly in young women and rarely leads to damage of the extremities. Cold is often the only stimulus that initiates the blood vessel spasms, which may last from minutes to hours. Emotional stress can also play a role in bringing on an attack. Besides the noted color changes, there can be agonizing pain, especially when the fingers are rewarming. Symptoms of tingling, numbness, and burning are common. Many people who have this condition just put up with it. Even if they consult their doctors for a diagnosis, there is no safe, effective drug treatment for it. Sometimes calcium channel blockers are used, which is ironic, because magnesium is a natural calcium channel blocker.

Fortunately, Sally's internist knew that magnesium is the most effective treatment for muscle cramps. He put her on magnesium, 300 mg twice a day, a food-based multiple vitamin and mineral supplement, and dietary calcium. They were both surprised that her Raynaud's also responded.

Magnesium improved Sally's peripheral circulation, stopped the smooth muscle spasms in the small arteries of her fingers, and cut down her stress reactions. Sally couldn't believe how much better she felt all over. Her muscle cramps improved within a week, and symptoms that she had thought were just part of getting old dramatically improved. Her energy increased, as she was able to sleep better. Her bowel movements were also more regular, and she was much calmer than she had been in a long time.

Nutritional recommendations for Raynaud's include liver-cleansing foods such as beets, dandelion greens, burdock root, and lemons, and foods rich in magnesium, including nuts, seeds, green vegetables, and whole grains. Foods to avoid or reduce to lessen the symptoms of Raynaud's syndrome include meat, alcohol, spices, and fatty, rich, fried, or salty foods.

SUPPLEMENTS FOR RAYNAUD'S

- **ReMag:** With picometer, stabilized ionic magnesium you can reach therapeutic amounts without laxative effects. Start with ¼ tsp (75 mg) and work up to 2–3 tsp (600–900 mg) per day. Add ReMag to a liter of water and sip all day to achieve full absorption.
- **ReMyte:** Picometer twelve-mineral solution. Take ½ tsp three times a day, or add 1½ tsp to a liter of water with ReMag and sip throughout the day.
- **ReCalcia:** Picometer, stabilized ionic calcium, boron, vanadium. Take 1–2 tsp per day (1 tsp provides 300 mg calcium) if you don't obtain enough calcium from your diet. It can be taken with ReMag and ReMyte.
- **ReAline:** B vitamin complex plus amino acids. Take 1 capsule twice per day. Contains food-based B_1 and four

methylated B vitamins (B_2, B_6, methylfolate, and B_{12}), plus L-methionine (precursor to glutathione) and L-taurine (which supports the heart and weight loss).

- **Vitamin E, as mixed tocopherols:** 800 IU per day, preferably Grown by Nature brand.
- **Evening primrose oil:** 6 capsules per day.
- **Quercetin:** 500 mg per day of this bioflavonoid.

TOURETTE SYNDROME

Tourette syndrome was first defined in 1885 by a French physician whose name was—you guessed it—Tourette. This syndrome is characterized by violent muscle contortions called motor tics in most sufferers. Fewer patients, 5–15 percent, also experience vocal disruptions, which sometimes involve outbursts of obscenities. Tourette syndrome itself was thought to be a rare condition; however, the National Institutes of Health reports that the prevalence of Tourette syndrome is substantially higher than previously estimated.[23] Tourette syndrome is also associated with obsessive-compulsive disorder, ADHD, and learning problems in children. The muscle contortions that characterize Tourette syndrome are increased by stress and associated with anxiety, depression, and sleep disorders. Since all these associated conditions are affected by magnesium, it only makes sense to look at magnesium deficiency as a possible cause. In fact, researchers have identified a central role of magnesium deficiency in Tourette syndrome, and this bears further investigation.[24]

I recommend magnesium for Tourette because it is extremely safe and often very effective. In Chapter 16 you will find Dr. Mildred Seelig's recommendation that athletic adolescent boys and girls may need 7–10 mg/kg/day (3.2–

4.5 mg/lb). It would only seem logical that if a child had magnesium deficiency symptoms, he or she would need at least that amount in supplemental form.

NEURALGIA, NEURITIS

Neuralgia is a stabbing, shocking, burning, and often quite severe pain that occurs along a damaged or irritated nerve. It's a catchall diagnosis that makes people think there's more going on than inflammation, and it invites the use of pain medication that can become addictive. The irritated nerves may be anywhere in the body, but they are most common in the face and neck because there are so many nerves and muscles in that region. Sitting at computers all day, poor posture, holding a phone to your ear with your shoulder, poor sleep position—these are a few of the many things that can build inflammation in the neck, scalp, and face.

Trigeminal neuralgia is inflammation of the fifth cranial nerve, which innervates the face. Trigeminal neuralgia occurs mostly in people over age fifty. Doctors find that up to 95 percent of cases are caused by an artery pressing on the trigeminal nerve, where the brain stem meets the spinal cord. The current treatment is surgical.

All sources admit that they do not know why trigeminal neuralgia happens. But I have an idea. What if there is vascular calcification in that particular artery? Most arteries do become calcified as we age, especially if there is magnesium deficiency causing a relative excess of calcium. The pressure would have to come from a rigid artery that irritates the trigeminal nerve. If this is the case and the calcified artery is exerting pressure on the trigeminal nerve, the nonsurgical treatment would be to take therapeutic levels of magnesium in order to dissolve the buildup of calcium.

Neuritis and *neuropathy* are general terms for inflammation of a nerve or the general inflammation of the peripheral nervous system. Peripheral neuropathy is inflammation or degeneration of the nerves in areas outside the brain or spinal cord. Diabetes causes peripheral neuropathy that affects 50 percent of the older diabetic population.

I mentioned earlier that patients with neuralgia are given pain pills. They are also prescribed medications such as gabapentin, which is FDA-approved for the lingering pain of shingles. However, it's also being given to people who have undiagnosed magnesium-deficiency-related nerve pain. Perhaps it works for some people, but I receive emails and calls from people for whom the drugs aren't working; they want to get off these drugs and find something that does work for their pain.

LIVING WITH NEURITIS

Neuritis is an inflammation of any nerve in the body (for example, optic neuritis, or inflammation of the optic nerve) or the general inflammation of the peripheral nervous system (which is any nerve in the body excluding the brain and spinal column). Below is Susan's story about her experience with occipital neuritis, or inflammation of the back of her head.

Susan, a forty-year-old mother of four, emailed me about a strange tingling sensation she was having on the back of her head—it had already lasted for three years. From her history I realized it was a combination of magnesium deficiency and yeast overgrowth caused by several recent courses of antibiotics. But instead of treating these conditions, doctors had initially told her she had anxiety and gave her Ativan.

A year of taking Ativan did not help Susan's scalp symptoms, and when she stopped it suddenly, she went into severe withdrawal symptoms—heart palpitations, exhaustion, insomnia, dissociative feelings, and panic attacks. She was admitted to a rehab clinic and was put on Neurontin for the withdrawal symptoms.

Susan found this book and began taking ReMag to help her wean off Neurontin and get rid of the zombie-like feelings that it gave her. After two months on ReMag, she was 75 percent better with her scalp tingling and Ativan withdrawal symptoms, and much improved with her sleep and muscle pains.

But, desperate and impatient to be 100 percent better, she found a doctor online who described her symptoms exactly and called it occipital neuralgia—which simply describes the location of her nerve problem, which I said was still due to magnesium deficiency. He said Susan needed to fly to his clinic for what seems to be craniosacral therapy—gentle manipulation of the cranial bones to release pressure. However, if your scalp muscles are in spasm because of magnesium deficiency, it's magnesium that will release those muscle spasms. Another doctor was offering Botox injections, to relax the muscles. I don't recommend Botox injections because they don't address the underlying problem and can have dangerous side effects. Another doctor, a neurologist, told her she might have a herpes infection in her occipital nerves and should take an antiviral drug, acyclovir.

The lesson from this case is that you do have to be patient when recovering from long-term magnesium deficiency. It took you quite a while to develop magnesium deficiency, often decades, and you can't build up your magnesium stores overnight. Susan needed to keep sipping her ReMag, along with a multimineral supplement (ReMyte), in sea-salted water throughout the day. She also needed to buckle down and do a yeast-free diet, probiotics, and natural antifungals to eliminate yeast toxins that could be continuing to aggravate her symptoms. Fortunately, Susan did all these things and continued to improve. I also asked her to mark her daily improvements in a journal and say the following affirmation, "Every day in every way I am getting better and better!"

MAGNESIUM AND ATHLETES

THREE THINGS YOU NEED TO KNOW ABOUT MAGNESIUM AND EXERCISE

---

1. Magnesium is lost during exercise through increased metabolism and sweat.

2. Lactic acid, which causes postexercise pain, is decreased by magnesium.

3. Magnesium deficiency may cause sudden cardiac death in healthy athletes.

When your muscles are engaged in the rapid-fire contraction and relaxation of physical exercise, if there is too much calcium (the initiator of contractions) and too little magnesium (the initiator of relaxation), muscle cramps and a buildup of lactic acid can result.

Too little magnesium is very common in athletes because so much is lost through sweating, and instead of replacing with proper mineral electrolytes, including magnesium, athletes tend to chug down sodium- and sugar-loaded concoctions that cause brain swelling in the short term and diabetes in the long term.

Even though most athletes and coaches don't know it, magnesium is one of the most important nutrients athletes can possibly take. As noted earlier, mitochondria in our cells make energy molecules called adenosine triphosphate (ATP), and magnesium is necessary for this process to occur.

Some of the first studies investigating the relationship between magnesium and physical performance were done on animals and showed that decreased exercise capacity can be an early sign of magnesium deficiency. When the animals were given magnesium dissolved in water, their endurance was restored. Most human studies also confirm that both brief and extended exercise deplete magnesium.

When I talk to college or professional athletes about their magnesium losses and how to avoid them, I'm often asked if drinking alcohol is okay. I've noted before that alcohol is a diuretic, so it is going to deplete magnesium. Alcohol will also stimulate yeast overgrowth and can lead to all kinds of intestinal distress and body-wide symptoms. Yeast produces toxins, so the body has to use up even more magnesium in order to help eliminate them from the body. I think alcohol, especially the binge drinking often seen among college students and during tailgate parties, may be the root cause of magnesium-deficiency induced panic attacks and depression, which seem to be epidemic in these circles. What could be worse for a six-foot, 300-pound college or pro football player than to suffer frightening atrial fibrillation and humiliating panic attacks and have to give up his $10 million contract, when all he had to do was drink sea-salted water along with magnesium and multiple minerals?

A study in the journal *Magnesium Research* notes that magnesium works so well for the athlete because it directly affects muscle function, which includes oxygen uptake, energy production, and electrolyte balance.[25] One of the benefits of exercise, they emphasize, is that it encourages magnesium redistribution to accommodate metabolic needs. They report on studies showing that marginal magnesium deficiency impairs exercise performance and exacerbates the oxidative stress that comes with strenuous exercise. The researchers comment that strenuous exercise causes sweat and urinary losses of magnesium that may increase magnesium requirements by 10–20 percent. They say that taking in less than 260 mg of magnesium a day for males and 220 mg/day for females can result in magnesium deficiency. They conclude, "Magnesium supplementation or increased dietary intake of magnesium will have beneficial effects on exercise performance in magnesium-deficient individuals."

One of the most amazing effects of magnesium on the neuromuscular system is that it produces energy (via the production of ATP), even though the mineral generally acts as a relaxant and not a stimulant. If you are magnesium deficient, your energy level will be low because you aren't producing the necessary ATP to run your body. When you start taking magnesium, your energy level goes up because you are making more ATP.

Magnesium's interactions with calcium help keep calcium from causing excessive muscle contraction. Too much calcium causes tension and tightness in all the muscles of the body, but when you have a balancing amount of magnesium, this tension releases within weeks, days, or even hours, depending on the underlying level of magnesium deficiency in your body.

Exercise is often prescribed therapeutically for anxiety and depression—to burn off steam, to increase the circulation, and to get your adrenaline pumping. Magnesium allows the body to burn fuel and create energy in an efficient cycle during exercise that does not lead to lactic acid production and buildup. For some individuals who exercise excessively or suffer from chronic fatigue syndrome, painful amounts of lactic acid build up in their muscles, making exercise an unpleasant experience. Exercise itself places stress on your body, to which your adrenal glands respond by pumping out adrenaline.

Heavy exercisers, especially long-distance runners, can

build up lactic acid and suffer shin splints and painful muscles, but they keep on running because they may be addicted to the adrenaline rush they get when they reach "the wall" in their workout. The wall feels like something you just can't break through, but you keep on pushing, and suddenly you get a burst of adrenaline and you're flying. That's the power of your adrenal glands when pushed to the max. Yet that stress-induced high will be followed by a crash if you don't repair the damage to your adrenal glands with good nutrition, hydration with sea-salted water, and the magnesium and other minerals that are lost during exercise.

Many studies have shown that magnesium supplementation enhances the performance and endurance of long-distance runners, cross-country skiers, cyclists, and swimmers. It also reduces lactic acid buildup and postexercise cramps and pain. Since athletes experience severe physical stress as well as the psychological drive to win, and most ingest suboptimal amounts of magnesium, they are vulnerable to magnesium deficiency.[26]

Years ago the coach of a Florida high school football team was concerned about his players' frequent complaints of leg cramps, so he gave them a calcium supplement on a very hot day before a rigorous game. Early in the second half, eleven players became disoriented and had difficulty walking. Their speech was slurred, they complained of muscle spasms, and they were breathing very deeply. Within an hour, eight of the boys collapsed into full-blown seizures; two had repeated seizures. Those having the worst symptoms had been playing the hardest. Thirteen more players reported headaches, blurred vision, muscle twitching, nausea, and weakness.[27]

Eventually all the boys recovered, but what happened to create such a frightening scene in this group of healthy young men? With the increased magnesium loss from excessive sweating plus the calcium supplement, their magnesium stores had been driven dangerously low.[28]

Magnesium deficiency may also play a role in sudden cardiac death syndrome, which can affect athletes.[29] Another study concluded that the sudden death of athletes and other individuals during extreme exertion is triggered by the detrimental effects of persistent magnesium deficiency on the cardiovascular system.[30] In a study of young, healthy, well-conditioned men, strenuous exercise was reported to give rise to persistent magnesium deficiency and a related long-term increase in cholesterol, triglycerides, and blood sugar.[31]

MAGNESIUM SUPPLEMENTS FOR EXERCISERS AND ATHLETES

Dr. Seelig, an internationally recognized magnesium expert, recommends that athletes in training obtain at least 6–10 mg/kg/day (or 2.7–4.5 mg/lb/day) of magnesium to help replace the losses from exertion, sweating, and stress. For a 220-pound man that would be 600–1,000 mg per day. For a 150-pound woman that would be 400–680 mg per day. In my clinical experience, athletes and people with magnesium deficiency conditions may require 10–15 mg/kg per day. These doses can be cut by 150 mg for people who exercise moderately (one to two hours a day).

However, as I've indicated previously, you must go by your clinical symptoms and your magnesium RBC blood test to define your magnesium requirements—and be aware they can shift according to the many variables I outline throughout the book.

The CNS, Stroke, Head Injury, Brain Surgery

**THREE THINGS YOU NEED TO KNOW
ABOUT MAGNESIUM AND THE BRAIN**

---

1. Magnesium protects the brain from the toxic effects of chemicals such as food additives.
2. Magnesium keeps excess calcium out of cells. When magnesium is low, calcium rushes in, causing cell death.
3. When blood sugar and magnesium are both low, excitotoxins such as glutamate (in MSG) and aspartic acid (in aspartame) can more easily enter brain cells, causing cell death.

Magnesium does much more than any drug to protect the blood circulation and the brain:

- It's a vasodilator, opening up blood vessels.
- It protects the endothelium, or innermost layer of blood vessel walls.
- It closes the calcium channel to excessive calcium influx.

MAGNESIUM-DEFICIENT BRAINS

With most of the U.S. population deficient in magnesium,[1] many Americans are at greater risk for a host of serious problems, including stroke with severe poststroke complications. Depending on the degree of magnesium deficiency, there can be poor recovery from head injury and escalating neurological damage. Lack of magnesium can enhance neurotoxin damage from vast numbers of chemicals in our air, food, and water, stimulating seizure disorders. The complexity of the mechanisms of central nervous system (CNS) hyperexcitability due to magnesium deficiency is only now being appreciated.[2]

In the Introduction, I mentioned a free online book from the University of Adelaide called *Magnesium in the Central Nervous System* (2011).[3] I recently did an interview where I went into some detail about the various chapters in that book, referencing content from *The Magnesium Miracle* to explain the importance of magnesium in the brain. I'll include a listing of the chapters here to inspire you to look for the whole book online. Several of the chapter topics are covered in other parts of this book.

Chapters in *Magnesium in the Central Nervous System*

1. Free Magnesium Concentration in the Human Brain
2. Intracellular Magnesium Homeostasis
3. Magnesium Transport Across the Blood-Brain Barriers
4. Intracellular Free Mg^{2+} and $MgATP^{2-}$ in Coordinate Control of Protein Synthesis and Cell Proliferation
5. Magnesium and the Ying-Yang Interplay in Apoptosis
6. Brain Magnesium Homeostasis as a Target for Reducing Cognitive Ageing

7. The Role of Magnesium Therapy in Learning and Memory
8. The Role of Magnesium in Headache and Migraine
9. Magnesium in Edema and Blood-Brain Barrier Disruption
10. Magnesium and Hearing Loss
11. The Role of Magnesium in Pain
12. The Role of Magnesium in Traumatic CNS Injury
13. The Use of Magnesium in Experimental Cerebral Ischaemia
14. Magnesium in Subarachnoid Hemorrhage
15. Magnesium in Clinical Stroke
16. Magnesium in Cancer: More Questions than Answers
17. Magnesium in Parkinson's Disease: An Update in Clinical and Basic Aspects
18. Magnesium and Alzheimer's Disease
19. Magnesium and Stress
20. Magnesium in Neuroses
21. Magnesium, Hyperactivity and Autism in Children
22. Magnesium in Psychoses (Schizophrenia, Bipolar Disorder)
23. Magnesium and Major Depression
24. Magnesium in Drug Abuse and Addiction

CHARCOT-MARIE-TOOTH DISEASE

Here's a testimonial about the effects of ReMag and ReMyte on a hereditary neurological disease:

> A friend of mine, who is forty-two, was diagnosed with the genetic condition called Charcot-Marie-Tooth disease. She was told that it was all downhill from here and that she would keep losing feeling in her limbs until she could no longer walk without foot and leg braces, and

would eventually end up in a wheelchair. The doctor said she should just enjoy her life while she can! Thankfully she had the good sense to talk to me and we immediately ordered ReMag, ReMyte, and Blue Ice Royal [a supplement made from fermented cod liver oil and butter oil that contains vitamins A, D, and K_2]! I'm so happy to report that she is walking properly again! She feels amazing and all her symptoms are gone. She says she feels like all her body parts are now connected!

Charcot-Marie-Tooth disease (CMT) is one of the most common inherited neurological disorders, affecting approximately 1 in 2,500 people in the United States. The neuropathy of CMT affects both motor and sensory nerves. Motor nerves that control voluntary muscle activity such as speaking, walking, breathing, and swallowing will deteriorate. Damage to the sensory nerves causes pain that can range from mild to severe.

HEAD INJURY AND MAGNESIUM

Traumatic brain injury (TBI) is a major public health problem throughout the world. There are more than 400,000 patients with TBI in the United States alone. From animal studies, we know that brain magnesium levels fall dramatically at the site of a head injury, as this mineral is depleted in a nonstop cascade of acute events.[4]

In sixty-six human subjects with acute blunt head trauma, the greater the degree of injury, the greater the calcium-ion-to-magnesium-ion ratio. More calcium than magnesium in brain neurons is never a good thing—excess calcium causes ceaseless neuron stimulation, leading to cell death.

Measuring magnesium ion levels in the blood after TBI

can be of both diagnostic and prognostic value in treating brain injury.[5] Studies of animal and human brain trauma victims indicate that higher magnesium levels are associated with a better recovery.[6] Also, giving sufficient magnesium will create a better healing outcome. Intravenous magnesium sulfate significantly reduces brain edema following brain injury and is used without adverse effects to treat patients with severe TBI.[7] This is crucial information to give your doctor if your child suffers a head injury or any family member is involved in a motor vehicle accident.

Ionized magnesium testing, used in research studies, makes the diagnosis of posttraumatic headaches much easier. Abnormalities in magnesium ion concentration and the calcium-ion-to-magnesium-ion ratio were found in children with posttraumatic headaches even though serum magnesium levels were normal.[8] Obviously, studies using only the serum magnesium test would miss the diagnosis and doctors would fail to properly treat these patients. See Chapter 16 for more on magnesium testing.

Magnesium depletion created by a head injury is slow to reverse. According to neurosurgeon Dr. Russell Blaylock, magnesium takes thirty minutes to get into the spinal fluid, three hours to reach the cortical area directly under the skull, and a full four to six hours for sufficient amounts of magnesium to reach the deep brain tissues.[9] Experiments with Navy SEALs and marathon runners show that after a month of intensive training they experience magnesium deficiency, and if no supplements are taken, the deficiency is still present three to six months later. It only makes sense that if your diet is deficient and you're under stress, physical or emotional, you need to replace your magnesium stores daily.

BRAIN INJURY, ALCOHOL, AND MAGNESIUM

Drs. Bella and Burton Altura discuss the direct cause-and-effect relationship between alcohol-induced headache and risk of brain injury and stroke in one of their numerous papers.[10] They note that binge alcohol drinking is associated with an ever-growing number of strokes and cases of sudden death, with alcohol causing spasm and rupture of magnesium-deficient cerebral arteries.[11] In animal studies, high doses of alcohol instigate a rapid fall in levels of magnesium ions in the brain and an elevation of calcium, followed by cerebral vessel spasm and rupture of cerebral blood vessels (stroke).[12, 13] People who consume more than three alcoholic drinks a day can be deficient because alcohol blocks magnesium absorption as well as acting like a diuretic.[14]

In human studies, people with mild head injury have been found to exhibit early deficits in magnesium ions; the greater the degree of head injury, the greater and more profound the deficit in magnesium ions, and the greater the level of calcium ions compared to magnesium ions. Patients with a history of alcohol abuse or ingestion of alcohol prior to head injury exhibited greater deficits in magnesium ions (and higher calcium-ion-to-magnesium-ion ratios) and, unlike the subjects without alcohol, remained in the hospital at least several days longer. Data on 105 men and women with different types of stroke indicate that, on average, a 20 percent deficit in magnesium ions is seen using the ionized magnesium test, even though serum magnesium levels are usually normal.[15]

As pointed out many times in this book and discussed in detail in Chapter 16, serum magnesium is a highly inaccurate measurement of the body's magnesium because only 1 percent of the magnesium in the body resides in the blood. The Alturas report that in many human studies, migraines, headaches, dizziness, and hangover that accompany alcohol ingestion are associated with rapid depletion of ionized magnesium levels but not of serum magnesium. The diagnosis is missed if only serum magnesium is measured. Since magnesium is necessary to regulate calcium, when magnesium is deficient, it's the excess calcium that creates vascular spasms and pathology.[16]

Alcohol-associated headaches can be treated with intravenous magnesium sulfate.[17] Premenstrual tension headache and its exacerbation by alcohol in women is also accompanied by deficits in magnesium ions and elevation in the calcium-ion-to-magnesium-ion ratio, and can also be corrected by intravenous magnesium sulfate. Don't be concerned that you must find someone to give you IV magnesium therapy to alleviate your symptoms. Clinical experience shows that oral ReMag is even more effective than IV magnesium. See Chapter 18 for more on magnesium supplementation.

STROKE

A burst or blocked blood vessel in the brain is all it takes to cause a stroke. The damage in so confined a space destroys critical brain functions. Stroke is initiated by hypertension, atherosclerosis, and diabetic complications—all of which are associated with low magnesium. Keeping blood vessels strong, preventing blood from clotting inappropriately, and healing stroke-damaged areas are all within the scope of the miracle of magnesium.

Stroke has devastated the lives of more than 6.5 million people in the United States. Each year, 15 million people worldwide suffer a stroke. The CDC's Stroke Facts, updated in 2015, paint a very scary picture.[18] Every year, almost 800,000 people in the United States have a stroke. Almost one quarter, 185,000 people, have had a previous stroke. Stroke kills almost 130,000 Americans each year; many of the rest are left disabled. Stroke is a leading cause of serious, long-term disability.

What evidence is there of the importance of magnesium in stroke? All deaths due to stroke among Taiwan residents (17,133 cases) from 1989 through 1993 were compared with deaths from other causes (17,133 controls). It was determined that the higher the magnesium levels in drinking water used by the Taiwanese residents, the lower the incidence of stroke.[19] Also, in a study of 4,443 men and women ages forty to seventy-five, lower dietary magnesium intake was associated with higher blood pressure and stroke risk. The investigators said such results "may have implications for primary prevention."[20]

Decades of research show that withdrawal of magnesium from cerebral arteries causes them to spasm, whereas elevated magnesium produces relaxation.[21, 22, 23] Animal studies show that when there is normal or elevated magnesium in the brain, the damage caused by stroke is reduced and the neurological deficit is lessened. This is because magnesium blocks calcium from flooding the cells and causing injury. Research also indicates that the area of the brain damaged by stroke contains injured neurons that can remain hyperactive (if they don't have enough magnesium) for several hours after the stroke has occurred.[24]

Damaged neurons are frantically struggling to survive and need even more oxygen, glucose, and magnesium than normal. In addition, when these vital nutrients are deficient, those neurons become especially vulnerable to the damaging effects of excitotoxins that rush in to fill the void left by depleted nutrients. Hospitalized patients commonly have low magnesium levels, which means that neurons are even less likely to survive. According to one researcher, a state of severe magnesium deficiency alone is enough for rats to develop widespread brain injury, affecting key brain functions.[25]

A study of stroke patients in New York highlights the absolute requirement for magnesium intervention in the ER. Ninety-eight patients admitted to the emergency rooms of three hospitals with a diagnosis of stroke exhibited early and significant deficits in magnesium ions as measured with a sensitive ion-selective electrode. The stroke patients also demonstrated a high calcium-ion-to-magnesium-ion ratio, signs of increased vascular tone, and abnormal cerebral vessel spasm.[26]

Animal experiments show that intravenous magnesium can prevent alcohol-induced hemorrhagic stroke and the subsequent fall in brain magnesium ion levels as well as other metabolic factors.[27] Recent data indicate that alcohol-induced cellular loss of magnesium ions is associated with cellular calcium overload and the generation of free radicals.[28]

What about humans? Can they benefit from IV magnesium to reverse the symptoms and the damage caused by stroke? I interviewed Dan Haley, a former New York assemblyman, on this topic. Dan spent over a decade researching alternative healing modalities and wrote a book called *Politics in Healing*.[29] When Dan suffered a stroke that paralyzed his entire left side in August 2004, one of his many friends advised him to see a doctor in Washington, D.C., who offers IV magnesium and oxygen for stroke recovery. Dan had already seen some improvement with several acupuncture treatments and could move his left hand, but his doctor had to go to China, so Dan went to Washington. Within ten days of receiving daily treatments as an outpatient, Dan was walking and had full use of his left arm again.[30]

Dr. Bruce Rind is Dan's Washington doctor. He and Dr. Sean Dalton developed the RELOX procedure for stroke, which consists of an intravenous vitamin-mineral solution, with a heavy emphasis on magnesium, and the simultaneous application of oxygen by mask. In Dan's case, Dr. Rind added hour-long sessions in a hyperbaric oxygen chamber to further enhance the delivery of oxygen to the brain.

Drs. Dalton and Rind presented their RELOX protocol at the Neuroscience 2005 Conference in Washington. The conference was attended by 30,000 people and honored with a keynote address by the Dalai Lama. In their talk, "Stroke Rehabilitation: An Investigation of Clinical and Neurological Recovery with a Nutrient-Oxygen Intervention," the doctors pointed out that there has been little research focused on the potential of cost-effective nutraceutical-biologic interventions to improve/restore clinical and neurological function in subacute-chronic stroke patients who are functioning with paralysis and no hope of cure. They told the audience that the RELOX procedure has been administered to a patient population of more than 200 who have suffered the aftereffects of stroke from periods ranging from a few days to twenty-plus years.

Their results have been nothing less than miraculous. Patients with mild to moderate impairment experienced "moderate to significant, relatively sustained clinical recovery of cognitive, motor, and sensory functions after three 40-minute treatments with no significant adverse effects." SPECT scans of these patients suggested "cerebral functional volume recovery correlated with CBF [cerebral blood flow] and metabolic increases."

Contrary to most medical opinion, Drs. Rind and Dalton are proving that the area of stroke damage "may represent relatively viable, functionally depressed, albeit potentially salvageable regions for a more extended period following stroke or other cerebral insult than heretofore estimated."

The good doctors know this to be a real possibility because their procedure has helped the majority of patients that have been treated. They advise that, "given the potentially remarkable personal, social, and economic benefits for patients and society, further investigation of the RELOX Procedure's clinical and neurological efficacy, safety, and mechanisms of action is warranted." Dr. Rind, as of 2016, is practicing in Gaithersburg, Maryland, and has RELOX listed as one of his many modalities.

In the meantime, I've had some success with using ReMag in place of IV magnesium therapy. In Chapter 18, Lynn writes about her husband, Dana, and how he was able to replace his thrice-weekly IV magnesium drips with ReMag and improve his magnesium blood test results and his health. So I was not too surprised when I received the following email about ReMag's effect on stroke symptoms.

> My wife had a stroke four years ago. While researching brain damage repair after stroke I discovered that brain glial cells have a collagen structure and need magnesium and vitamin C, so she's been taking both according to your blog recommendations. Apparently Einstein's brain was overly abundant in glial cells, which made me decide to try and increase my wife's. Guess what? She has made big strides in speech recovery and organizational activities at home in just three months of ReMag. I don't think this is placebo not at 77 years of age. Also, since I've been using ReMag, it's reduced my AFib [atrial fibrillation].

THREE THINGS YOU NEED TO KNOW ABOUT MAGNESIUM AND BRAIN SURGERY

1. Good neurosurgeons give IV magnesium to all their surgical patients.
2. Magnesium helps the brain recover from brain surgery.
3. Magnesium can prevent postsurgical strokes or make them less damaging.

BRAIN SURGERY AND MAGNESIUM

During and after brain surgery, magnesium's many attributes come into play by preventing stroke, keeping calcium from entering damaged cells, reducing neuron excitability, and decreasing the incidence of seizure and spasm. These favorable effects have all been proven unequivocally in animal studies, but clinical experience in the neurosurgical operating room also proves its efficacy as lives are being saved. Many surgeons make it standard procedure to administer intravenous magnesium to all their surgical patients before, during, and after an operation.

Dr. Bernard Horn, a general surgeon in California, has given intravenous magnesium sulfate to more than 8,000 patients over a fifteen-year period. Dr. Horn reports that blood pressures as high as 200/150 would normalize before surgery.[31]

Intravenous magnesium sulfate enhances the effects of general anesthetic, so during surgery the dose of chemical anesthetics can be safely reduced. Using intravenous magnesium also results in lower postoperative pain scores, less pain medication is needed in the twenty-four hours after surgery, and there is less postoperative nausea and vomiting. Magnesium sulfate is therefore a safe and cost-effective addition to such general anesthetics as propofol, remifentanil, and miva-curium.[32]

I have a concern about one inhaled anesthetic, desflu-rane, which has six fluorine atoms embedded in its structure. You can read about the potential dangers of fluoride drugs in Chapter 2 and their potential to irreversibly bind magne-sium. The admitted side effects of desflurane include hyper-tension, arrhythmia, and tachycardia—all magnesium deficiency symptoms.

MAGNESIUM AND SEIZURES

The brain is in a state of constant electrical activity. Brain cells are either stimulated or suppressed in a delicate push-and-pull balance of activity. Switches control these cells; some switches are turned on and some are turned off by neu-rotransmitters. The action of these neurotransmitters could not take place without calcium, magnesium, and zinc, which play various roles in the response of the nerve cells to electri-cal stimulation. Brain cells altered by trauma, chemicals, or severe stress can be permanently switched on and fire exces-sively due to excess calcium in the damaged cells. Repeated firing in groups of nerve cells can result in seizures.

Chapter 7 of *Magnesium: The Nutrient That Could Change Your Life,* by J. I. Rodale, is about the treatment of epilepsy using magnesium.[33] The book was written in 1963 and my reference gives you access to it online.

Rodale writes about the evidence he found showing that seizures could be successfully treated with magnesium. Dr. Lewis B. Barnett, head of the Hereford Clinic and Deaf Smith Research Foundation, in Hereford, Texas, learned that magnesium is deficient in people with epilepsy. In the 1950s he presented evidence on thirty cases of childhood sei-zures that responded exceptionally well to high oral doses of magnesium. Barnett found that as his patients' blood magnesium reached normal levels, their seizure activity diminished. He also reported that the treatment was entirely harmless. As a result of his research, Barnett speculated that the main cause for the 3 million clinical and 10–15 million subclinical cases of epilepsy in the population at that time was a deficiency of magnesium.

Even as late as 2012, sixty years after Dr. Barnett proved the importance of magnesium in seizures, there is still only speculation about its use. One paper asked the question, "Can magnesium supplementation reduce seizures in people with epilepsy?"[34] The authors reviewed the literature, saying that animal models of epilepsy show that magnesium deficiency decreases seizure thresholds and low magnesium solutions can generate spontaneous epileptiform discharges from rat hippocampal (brain) slices. They confirm that "magnesium is a potential modulator of seizure activity because of its ability to antagonize excitation through the N-methyl-d-aspartate receptor." They report that "some studies have shown that people with epilepsy have lower magnesium levels than people without epilepsy." There are also "case reports of seizures being controlled with magnesium supplementation in people with specific conditions, and recently in an open randomized trial, children with infantile spasms responded better to adrenocorticotropic hormone (ACTH) plus magnesium than to ACTH alone." The authors "hypothesize that magnesium supplementation can reduce seizures in people with epilepsy." Of course they recommend more studies and suggest that, if proven, "supplementation needs to be considered in the overall management of people with refractory epilepsy."

Intravenous magnesium sulfate for the treatment of seizures and hypertension in pregnancy is safe and effective and universally accepted. Even though large clinical trials using magnesium for other types of seizures and epilepsy have not been forthcoming, many practitioners use oral magnesium as an adjunct to antiepileptic medication, so at least a number of those dealing with seizures are benefiting.

MAGNESIUM AND ELECTROMAGNETIC FIELDS

Some people insist that they are negatively affected by electromagnetic fields (EMFs) in the low- and microwave-frequency range. But until now, science has stayed neutral on EMFs, saying that the only effects from EMFs are due to heat.

EMFs can have positive effects, such as stimulating bone growth. However, a study focusing on negative effects showed that EMFs caused single-strand breaks in DNA. In fact, many people feel that EMFs can cause many side effects in the body. This condition has been labeled electromagnetic hypersensitivity (EHS), which unfortunately implies that only "sensitive" people feel these effects.

According to Wikipedia: "The reported symptoms of EHS include headache, fatigue, stress, sleep disturbances, skin symptoms like prickling, burning sensations and rashes, pain and ache in muscles and many other health problems. Whatever their cause, EHS symptoms are a real and sometimes a disabling problem for the affected persons." You will notice that the symptoms of EHS are also symptoms of magnesium deficiency. EMFs are stressors; therefore, they deplete magnesium, adding to our magnesium burn rate.

A paper by Dr. Martin Pall reviewing twenty-three EMF studies found that the production of EMF side effects has to do with voltage-gated calcium channels (VGCCs).[35] The wide range of actions caused by EMFs are thought to be due to two different pathways for VGCCs. Scientists don't know the cause of EHS, but when I see that voltage-gated calcium channels are possibly involved, I nominate magnesium deficiency as a probable cause.

In Chapter 1, I discuss calcium channels and how they are jealously guarded by magnesium. Magnesium, at a concentration 10,000 times greater than that of calcium inside the cells, allows only a certain amount of calcium to enter to create the necessary electrical transmission, and then immediately helps to eject the calcium once the job is done. Otherwise, if calcium accumulates in the cell it triggers hyperexcitability and disrupts cell function. Too much calcium entering cells can cause symptoms of heart disease (such as angina, high blood pressure, and arrhythmia), asthma, and headaches. Magnesium is nature's calcium channel blocker.

What are the main symptoms of magnesium deficiency and calcium excess? Headaches, fatigue, insomnia, muscle pain—just like EHS symptoms. My theory is that the negative effects of EMFs occur in people who are magnesium deficient, and their hypersensitivity to EMFs is because they don't have enough magnesium to block the calcium channels stimulated by EMFs. Maybe my theory will be validated in a decade or two; in the meantime, get your magnesium RBC test and begin taking magnesium to prevent upward of a hundred symptoms, including damage from EMFs. See Chapter 16 for information on magnesium testing and Chapter 18 for my magnesium supplement recommendations.

Obviously more studies are called for, but Dr. Pall's paper does help vindicate people who are concerned that EMFs are operating at more than just a heat-producing level.

Cholesterol, Hypertension

High cholesterol and high blood pressure are two conditions that plague Americans in epidemic proportions, and they appear to be the initial symptoms that lead to chronic heart problems. But not surprisingly, the real story behind both conditions could be a lack of magnesium.

CHOLESTEROL

Most of our cholesterol, 85 percent, is made in the body—the liver, to be exact. The rest comes from our diet. There are several types of cholesterol with different functions; some of these types we label "good" and some "bad." High-density lipoprotein, HDL, is generally considered to be beneficial to the body; it helps remove cholesterol from blood vessel walls and the blood itself, bringing it to the liver for processing and excretion. Low-density lipoprotein, LDL, is harmful to the body because it carries cholesterol into the bloodstream, promoting the buildup of cholesterol plaque on the arterial walls. Very-low-density lipoproteins, VLDLs, are made into LDLs and therefore are harmful.

All of these cholesterols are normally found in the body. What is not normal is the high amounts of oxidized cholesterol (cholesterol abnormally bound with oxygen) that we eat in processed foods, fast foods, and fried foods. In addition, chlorine, fluoride in water, pesticides, and other environmental pollutants can oxidize cholesterol in the body. It is this oxidized cholesterol that researchers are concerned about when it comes to heart disease.[1] What is most interesting about oxidized cholesterol is that it means cholesterol is an antioxidant. Cholesterol is sweeping up toxins in the body and trying to eliminate them and in the process becomes oxidized. So cholesterol is not the problem; toxicity from chlorine, fluoride, pesticides, and other environmental pollutants is the real problem.

Regular use of antioxidants such as magnesium, vitamin E, vitamin A, and vitamin C can lower oxidized cholesterol levels because they deal with the toxins that overload the body and spill into the cholesterol pool. Magnesium is likely the most powerful antioxidant in the body, and there is compelling evidence that magnesium therapy reduces cholesterol levels,[2, 3, 4] even when there is a genetic risk factor present for hypercholesterolemia.[5] Another important mineral in the cholesterol story is copper. Copper deficiency contributes to elevated cholesterol and a well-absorbed copper supplement, such as found in ReMyte, can help lower cholesterol, among many other positive things.

Unfortunately, there are no visible physical symptoms of high cholesterol beyond the associated signs of a bad diet, sedentary lifestyle, smoking, alcohol intake, and stress. You have to find it on a blood test. A poor diet with a high intake of saturated and polyunsaturated fats, hydrogenated oils, fried foods, meat, sugar, coffee, and alcohol will elevate cholesterol levels, especially when a person lacks fiber from whole grains and vegetables. Add a sedentary lifestyle with weight gain, and cholesterol increases. The very diet that promotes elevated cholesterol also causes magnesium deficiency.

Most doctors do not have the knowledge, time, or inclination to educate patients about correct eating habits that could reduce their cholesterol; instead they rely on medication to treat the problem. To be fair, many patients don't have the inclination to comply even if their doctor recommends dietary change, exercise, or weight loss. Adding magnesium supplementation to lifestyle changes, however, gives patients more dramatic improvement and the incentive to embrace change.

Many of us have been conditioned to believe that elevated cholesterol is the only cause of heart disease; that is why marketers have been so successful in getting us to replace saturated fat such as butter with hydrogenated vegetable oils. Yet epidemiologists and dental anthropologists proved long ago that various world cultures that ate high-cholesterol diets for thousands of years (meat, lard, cream, butter, and eggs) suffered very little, if any, heart disease.[6] Almost all the long-lived, healthy communities where degenerative disease and heart disease were unknown included significant amounts of natural, unprocessed meat or dairy in their diets. And it is also clear that once a population is exposed to refined and processed food, or "altered" meat and "altered" dairy, health declines in a number of ways.[7, 8, 9]

Hydrogenated oils are made from unsaturated oils and for that reason were thought to be healthier than saturated fats such as butter. But the processing of liquid vegetable oil by heat, pressure, and chemicals to change it into a solid fat creates an unhealthy synthetic product called a trans fatty acid (as opposed to the natural cis fatty acid).

Only in the late 1990s did research show that these

highly refined hydrogenated oils themselves promote atherosclerotic plaque much more than butter. In fact, some scientists say that the rise of heart attacks, and heart disease in
general, can be traced back to the late 1930s, when hydrogenated oils were first introduced. We now know that trans
fatty acids cause arterial damage as well as cancer. Be sure
to read labels to avoid this substance.

Let's follow those fats into the bakery. A major disadvan-
tage of low-fat products is that they often contain extra sugar
in order to capture the taste buds. Even worse is aspartame,
a synthetic sweetener with a daunting list of side effects to its
name. To maintain your health, avoid both.

WHAT CHOLESTEROL DOES

Not just adults but every schoolchild has been conditioned to
believe that cholesterol is the bad guy in heart disease. But
did you know that without cholesterol we wouldn't be able to
have sex, couldn't procreate, and would become extinct?
That's simply because sex hormones and stress hormones are
made from cholesterol. It's also necessary to create cell membranes and coat nerves with a protective fatty insulation that
makes up about 60–80 percent of our brain tissue. Cholesterol is also essential for proper food digestion and fat absorption because it produces bile salts. Moreover, if you
didn't have cholesterol, your bones would turn to mush because you couldn't make vitamin D from sunlight and
wouldn't be able to absorb calcium.

If cholesterol is so crucial to life, why are we trying so
desperately to get rid of it? Our body thinks cholesterol is so
important that the liver makes about 1,000 mg of cholesterol
a day; if we try to lower our cholesterol too much with drugs,
the liver merely gears up production. As I mentioned above,

normally the liver produces about 85 percent of the cholesterol measured on a blood test. The other 15 percent comes
from our diet.

WHEN CHOLESTEROL BECAME THE BAD GUY

In 1913 two Russian researchers fed large amounts of cholesterol to a group of hungry rabbits. When they saw yellow
gunk clogging the rabbits' arteries, they leapt to the conclusion that cholesterol must be responsible for coronary artery
disease.[10]

Robert Ford, as long ago as 1969, called the cholesterol
theory of heart disease a tragic blunder.[11] In his book called
Stale Food vs. Fresh Food, Ford gave us some very important
information about the Russian experiment that had been
overlooked for decades. He wrote, "Their finding was one of
those unfortunate half-truths which only served to mislead."
In his commonsense way of looking at the cholesterol theory
of heart disease, Ford said, "It is absurd to say that something we are largely made of would be harmful for us to eat."

Ford explained that dietary cholesterol is harmful only if
it is stale or rancid. When he read the original article by the
Russians he was amazed to discover that they had fed their
rabbits "pure crystalline cholesterol dissolved in vegetable
oil" to produce the cholesterol buildup in arteries. They
didn't stop to think that crystalline cholesterol is not something the body can use but is "an unnatural stale substance
now known as oxycholesterol, which is not found in fresh
food or in the healthy human body." Ford said the cholesterol theory of heart disease was untrue in 1913, is still untrue, and has served to deceive us by delaying discovery of
the real causes and cures.

Udo Erasmus wrote an enlightening book about fats and
oils called *Fats That Heal, Fats That Kill.*[12] From his decades-

long research he concludes, "The cholesterol scare is big business for doctors, laboratories, and drug companies. It is also a powerful marketing gimmick for vegetable oil and margarine manufacturers. In the end, cholesterol will be exonerated from its role as primary villain in cardiovascular disease. The accusing finger points at 'experts' who concocted the cholesterol theory to drum up business by spreading fear."

THE DRUG TREATMENT OF CHOLESTEROL

Statins are a group of powerful drugs that block a specific enzyme in the liver that helps make cholesterol. When that enzyme is blocked, cholesterol levels are lowered. That enzyme, however, does much more in the body than just make cholesterol, so when it is suppressed by statins there are far-ranging consequences.

One major side effect that medicine acknowledges is elevated liver enzymes and disrupted liver function. If you take statins, you must have regular blood tests to look for liver damage. Stopping statins if your liver is damaged usually reverses the problem.

Another acknowledged side effect, statin myopathy, is an iatrogenic (doctor-induced) condition that damages muscles and is entirely related to statin intake. Up to 20 percent of statin users can suffer muscle pain, tenderness, and weakness. But drug companies only report a 0.1 percent incidence of a type of muscle damage, called rhabdomyolysis, that is caused by statins, and therefore they can say muscle symptoms are rare. They ignore the one in five people who suffer their way through statin therapy, usually receiving other medications so that they can tolerate the statins' side effects.

Rhabdomyolysis is a severe form of toxic myopathy (muscle damage), which destroys striated muscles. Myoglobin is a muscle protein that is released into the bloodstream when the muscles break down and can be measured as a sign of statin myopathy. Interestingly, about 40 percent of the magnesium in the body is found in muscles. So when muscle is destroyed, magnesium is lost from this storage site, increasing muscle pain and spasm. Magnesium is also an indispensable mineral activator of many types of myosin (a large protein that forms muscle), including the myosin in skeletal muscle, smooth muscle, and cardiac muscle.[13] The myosin paper helps explain how magnesium deficiency can greatly disturb muscle function throughout the body.

Unfortunately, several statins are potentially toxic fluoride compounds that may release fluorine ions that can irreversibly bind to magnesium, contributing to muscle pain. For a larger discussion about fluoride drugs, see Chapter 1. Another side effect is the inhibition of coenzyme Q10 production, as the statins block pathways that help produce both CoQ10 and cholesterol. CoQ10 is a fat-soluble antioxidant found in the mitochondria. Mitochondria are the principle powerhouses of cells, producing energy for the whole body in a process called the Krebs cycle. CoQ10 is found in one of the eight steps of the Krebs cycle; magnesium is found in six of the eight steps. Lowered levels of coenzyme Q10 along with magnesium deficiency contribute to myopathy and also produce neuropathy (nerve damage); memory decline, including global amnesia; and cardiomyopathy (destruction of heart muscle).

Many alternative doctors prescribe high doses of expensive coenzyme Q10 supplements if you are on statin drugs but forget to give magnesium. If you are not a vegetarian, you should be able to get enough CoQ10 from fish, beef, pork, chicken heart, and chicken liver. Parsley and the minty herb perilla also provide CoQ10. If you also take magnesium, your CoQ10 levels should normalize. However, what might work even better is to use magnesium as your first line of treatment for elevated cholesterol so you don't have to touch statin drugs at all.

MAGNESIUM IS A NATURAL STATIN

A well-known magnesium expert, Mildred Seelig, M.D., just before she died in 2004, wrote a fascinating paper with Andrea Rosanoff, Ph.D., showing that magnesium acts by the same mechanisms as statin drugs to lower cholesterol.[14]

Every metabolic activity in the body depends on enzymes. Making cholesterol, for example, requires a specific enzyme called HMG-CoA reductase. As it turns out, magnesium slows down this enzymatic reaction when cholesterol is present in sufficient quantities and speeds it up when we need more. HMG-CoA reductase is the same enzyme that statin drugs target and inhibit. The mechanisms are nearly the same; however, magnesium is the natural way that the body has evolved to control and balance cholesterol, whereas statin drugs are used to destroy the whole process.

If sufficient magnesium is present in the body, cholesterol will be limited to its necessary functions—the production of hormones and the maintenance of membranes—and will not be produced in excess. Remember, most of the cholesterol in the body is produced in the liver, so if it's not needed, the body won't produce it—but this mechanism depends on having sufficient magnesium.

It's only in our present-day circumstances of magnesium-deficient soil, little magnesium in processed foods, and excessive intake of calcium and calcium-rich foods without supplementation of magnesium that cholesterol has become elevated in the population. If there is not enough magnesium to limit the activity of the cholesterol-converting enzyme, we are bound to make more cholesterol than is needed.

The magnesium/cholesterol story gets even better. Magnesium is responsible for several other lipid-altering functions that are not even shared by statin drugs. Magnesium is necessary for the activity of an enzyme that lowers LDL, the "bad" cholesterol; it also lowers triglycerides and raises the "good" cholesterol, HDL. Another magnesium-dependent enzyme converts omega-3 and omega-6 essential fatty acids into prostaglandins, which are necessary for heart and overall health. Seelig and Rosanoff conclude their paper by saying that it is well accepted that magnesium is a natural calcium channel blocker, and now we know it also acts like a natural statin.

In their book *The Magnesium Factor*,[15] Seelig and Rosanoff reported that eighteen human studies verified that magnesium supplements can have an extremely beneficial effect on lipids. In these studies, total cholesterol levels were reduced by 6 to 23 percent, LDL (bad) cholesterol was lowered by 10 to 18 percent, triglycerides fell by 10 to 42 percent, and HDL (good) cholesterol rose by 4 to 11 percent. Furthermore, the studies showed that low magnesium levels are associated with higher levels of "bad" cholesterol and high magnesium levels indicate an increase in "good" cholesterol.

NORMAL LIPID VALUES

Total cholesterol: 180–220 mg/dL
HDL cholesterol: greater than 45 mg/dL
LDL cholesterol: less than 130 mg/dL
VLDL cholesterol: less than 35 mg/dL
Ratio of total cholesterol to HDL: in men the optimal
ratio is less than 3.43 (average 4.97); in women the optimal
ratio is less than 3.27 (average 4.44)

When I went to medical school, the average total cholesterol level was 245 mg/dL. It wasn't until cholesterol-lowering drugs came on the market that doctors and drug companies began promoting much lower levels of cholesterol in a misguided attempt to prevent heart disease. For a protocol of supplements for high cholesterol, see "Supplements for Heart Disease" at the end of Chapter 7.

CORONARY CALCIUM SCAN

Since I wrote the first edition of *The Magnesium Miracle*, cholesterol has begun to fall out of favor in some circles as the primary cause of heart disease. Statin drugs have been around for about thirty years, so if cholesterol is the cause of heart disease and statins are the cure, why is heart disease still the leading cause of death? Drug industry papers say statins lower cholesterol, but independent studies say they do not prolong life. In the midst of this battle, cardiologists are now pointing the finger at calcium and measuring the levels of coronary artery calcium to assess heart disease risk.

Coronary calcium scans assess the degree of calcification in the cholesterol plaque of the coronary arteries using CT scanning. The coronary calcium scan has not caught on as a screening tool, probably because there are no drugs to dissolve the calcium in coronary arteries. Allopathic medicine continues to use ineffective calcium channel blockers, statin drugs, and stents (which then require lifelong blood thinners) as their treatments of choice. In my world, when there's excess calcium deposited in arteries, it means a relative lack of magnesium, and magnesium is a treatment for calcium buildup in the body. Here is a report about reversal of carotid artery calcification with ReMag:

> My wife had open-heart surgery 2½ years ago due mostly to hypertension and obstruction of the coronary arteries. After being on ReMag and ReMyte for several months her blood pressure had dropped from 180/95 to 110/60. Her last echocardiogram showed a healthy and

strong heart with an ejection fraction of 60 percent. The last ultrasound of her carotid artery showed a 30–40 percent lessening of calcified occlusions. This is all amazingly good news.

A recent study says that the higher the degree of calcification found on a coronary calcium scan, the greater the risk for atrial fibrillation. I'll write more about these scans in Chapter 7, in the "Arrhythmia" section.

MAGNESIUM AND HYPERHOMOCYSTEINEMIA

Researchers have identified various causes of damage to the inner lining of the arteries. They include high homocysteine, chlamydia infection, distorted blood flow around fat deposits, free radicals, high blood sugar, high blood pressure, and lack of oxygen. The damaged tissue of the artery wall initiates an inflammatory process. The inflammation then attracts "bad" cholesterol (LDL) and calcium, which build up into a solid scar to try to "heal" the inflammation. Magnesium has a role to play every step of the way by reducing homocysteine levels, naturally thinning the blood, preventing free radicals, balancing blood sugar, reducing high blood pressure, eliminating inflammation, and dissolving calcium.

When Russian researchers showed that oxidized cholesterol causes blocked arteries, instead of learning from that message that oxidized cholesterol might be the problem, everyone assumed all cholesterol was bad. A process that produces oxidized cholesterol from elevated homocysteine is described by Dr. Kilmer McCully. In 1969, Dr. McCully was the first researcher to identify increased levels of the amino acid homocysteine in the urine of patients with heart disease. He also found that those increased levels could be reversed with certain nutrients, not drugs.[16, 17]

Homocysteine is a normal by-product of protein digestion. If you don't have the specific nutrient cofactors (magnesium and B vitamins) to digest protein optimally, homocysteine
can build up. Elevated amounts of homocysteine can cause
the oxidization of cholesterol—and it is oxidized cholesterol
that damages blood vessels.

An optimal level of homocysteine is between 10 and 12
μmol/L. When homocysteine is elevated in the cells, it depletes cellular magnesium because magnesium is needed to
break it down. That's why a high-protein diet requires more
magnesium in order to metabolize the extra homocysteine
that is produced.

Twenty to 40 percent of the general population have
high levels of homocysteine in the blood called hyperhomocysteinemia. Individuals with high levels have almost four
times the risk of suffering a heart attack compared to people
with normal levels.[18]

Hyperhomocysteinemia is high on the list of risk factors
for heart disease and serves as an even stronger marker than
high cholesterol for heart disease and blood clotting disorders.[19, 20] However, it is not on a standard blood test panel for
heart disease—likely because there is no drug treatment to
lower homocysteine.

I say an even more relevant marker may be low magnesium since the major enzymes involved in homocysteine metabolism are magnesium dependent.[21] Dr. McCully blames
too much protein in the diet for hyperhomocysteinemia.
However, when magnesium, vitamin B_6, vitamin B_{12}, and
folate are deficient, the body is not able to properly digest
dietary protein. Magnesium and the B vitamins were readily
available in the typical diet a hundred years ago; now that
they are absent, homocysteine becomes elevated, resulting in
heart disease.

When these metabolic nutrients are reintroduced

through diet and supplements, the high homocysteine levels are reversed and the symptoms of heart disease diminish. Ongoing research confirms that B_6, B_{12}, and folate together with magnesium are necessary to prevent blood vessel damage induced by high levels of homocysteine in the blood.[22] It is clear that the successful treatment of hyperhomocystein-emia relies on dietary changes that include B vitamins and magnesium.[23, 24, 25] However, magnesium is often left out of the prescription for hyperhomocysteinemia in favor of the B vitamins—a common but serious error on the part of conventional medicine. The most effective B vitamins are in methylated form. The source I recommend is ReAline, which has four methylated B vitamins and also contains taurine—another nutrient that helps metabolize homocysteine. (See the Resources section.)

Researchers have found that high homocysteine is also a marker for all causes of mortality, which underscores that a deficiency in essential nutrients has far-reaching effects on the body beyond heart disease.[26]

HYPERTENSION

Hypertension is an elevation of blood pressure suffered by more than 50 million Americans. Most often, hypertension is diagnosed during a routine physical exam. It presents no distinguishing signs or symptoms unless the condition is very advanced, in which case headache, dizziness, and blurred vision can occur.

Normal blood pressure is a range: 100–140 over 60–90. Systolic pressure is the first number and relates to the pump pressure that the heart muscle creates to push blood into the arteries. Diastolic pressure is the second number and is the pressure that the arteries maintain when the heart is relaxed, between heartbeats, to keep the arteries open.

Hypertension is either primary or secondary. Primary hypertension is said to have no single cause and occurs in 90 percent of all hypertensive patients. Secondary hypertension is due to another disease. Causes of primary hypertension include high cholesterol, family history, obesity, diet, smoking, stress, and excessive table salt intake—but one major cause that is overlooked is magnesium deficiency.

The necessity to keep blood pressure as low as possible may be another myth of modern medicine, just like cholesterol. In the past decade the so-called normal value for high blood pressure has been lowered to the point that a majority of Americans fall into what's now called a prehypertensive category. When people are told they are prehypertensive, they don't hear the "pre-" part; they just hear "hypertensive," and it scares them—sometimes enough to elevate their blood pressure. This is known as "white-coat syndrome."

White-coat syndrome has your heart beating faster and your blood pressure rising when anyone in a white coat comes at you wielding a blood pressure cuff. Your blood pressure automatically rises in a fight-or-flight reaction because you are afraid your doctor will tell you that your blood pressure is elevated. Blood pressure that is normal at home but high in the doctor's office is white-coat syndrome, not hypertension. It's not a life-threatening medical condition that needs to be treated; it's a normal reaction to acute stress. It's another iatrogenic (doctor-induced) condition that often results in your taking medications unnecessarily.

Certainly high blood pressure is to be avoided, but these new values for normal blood pressure make it appear that almost everyone is susceptible to high blood pressure and should be on drugs. With the elderly and their slightly rigid blood vessels, a somewhat elevated blood pressure may be necessary to keep blood pumping to their head and extremities—and attempting to achieve a lower blood pressure in such individuals may cause dizziness and falls, resulting in dangerous fractures that could otherwise be prevented. A much more expedient solution is weight loss, exercise, stress reduction, and magnesium to treat and prevent hypertension.

DIURETICS AND DEHYDRATION

Diuretics are the first drugs allopathic medical providers resort to in order to treat high blood pressure. These drugs, in combination with salt restriction, help flush fluids from the body according to the theory that if there is less salt and water in your bloodstream, then there is less pressure on your blood vessels. But how is a doctor supposed to know if a patient has too much water in the bloodstream without doing complicated tests? And if you get rid of too much water, doesn't that make you dehydrated, thicken your blood, and make you susceptible to clotting-related conditions such as stroke and deep vein thrombosis?

Dr. Fereydoon Batmanghelidj, in his book *Your Body's Many Cries for Water,* says that dehydration causes high blood pressure.[27] When the body is even slightly dehydrated, it attempts to hold on to whatever water it can by constricting blood vessels throughout the body. You sweat less and lose less moisture when you breathe—but constricted blood vessels mean increased blood pressure!

Dehydration is very common; most people don't drink enough water anyway, so why squeeze out more with a diuretic? When patients are prescribed diuretics, they are warned that the most common side effect is a deficiency of potassium, which spills out in the urine. To prevent it, they are advised to eat bananas and oranges or take potassium pills. What they are not told is that magnesium is drained out along with potassium.

Recall that magnesium deficiency leads to blood vessels that are less relaxed and more susceptible to spasm and tension, a precursor to hypertension; thus the very treatment for hypertension worsens the problem.[28] Ironically, replacing potassium doesn't help patients who are also magnesium deficient, because the body is unable to deliver potassium to the cells without sufficient magnesium. Even the so-called potassium-sparing diuretics still commonly deplete other minerals, including magnesium.[29] The common side effects of diuretics include weakness, muscle cramps, joint pain, and irregular heartbeat; these are all symptoms of magnesium deficiency. Proper testing for magnesium RBC should be a routine procedure when you are taking diuretics, but it currently is not. See Chapter 16 for more on magnesium testing.

Another side effect that I see with diuretics is the elevation of cholesterol and blood sugar, a result of the chronic magnesium deficiency caused by diuretics. When patients are given statin drugs for their cholesterol and drugs for their diabetes, magnesium deficiency can become so severe that they develop atrial fibrillation or have a heart attack. One of the reasons doctors want patients to take medications for life is because they don't see their heart patients getting better. Little do they realize that their drugs may be causing incurable heart disease and heart failure!

EDEMA AND MAGNESIUM DEFICIENCY

I received the following email from one of my blog readers describing his experience using magnesium for his edema, or swelling.

> I have always had a problem with edema and have been on a potassium-sparing diuretic for many years to keep it under control. A few months ago the problem intensified and my legs were so badly swollen that I could hardly walk. My MD prescribed a leg massage for me

but I couldn't get an appointment for six weeks. In the meantime I decided to do some research on the web. In the many articles that came up, I found one that mentioned magnesium deficiency as being a possible cause. I picked up some 200 mg magnesium tablets and took one in the a.m. and another in the p.m., for a total of 400 mg per day.

Nothing happened at first, but after about five or six days, I started to urinate profusely and continued for more than a week. I started feeling better in general, was more alert, and most importantly, I could walk normally. The scale showed that I had lost about 40 pounds during that couple of weeks. I actually saw my ankles, which had gone missing years ago. I cancelled the massage appointment. I now feel and act like I did years ago.

One woman wrote and said that she has edema and her sodium levels were low but her doctor told her to avoid salt and lower her water intake to only 4 cups per day (32 ounces). I have many issues with the medical approach to edema. Doctors will limit water, prescribe diuretics, and withhold salt—all of which can prevent recovery and even create more edema.

In general, to treat edema, you need to drink more than 4 cups of water a day and you need to spike the water with sea salt, magnesium (ReMag), and a multimineral supplement (ReMyte). I recommend drinking half your body weight (in pounds) in ounces of water. If you weigh 150 pounds, drink 75 ounces of water a day. In each quart of water (32 oz) put ¼ tsp of unrefined sea salt, pink Himalayan salt, or Celtic sea salt. If that seems too strong at first, simply begin with a pinch of salt in a glass of water and work up. (Note: If sea salt seems to be causing fluid retention—

a rare occurrence—then stop it and have your sodium levels checked.)

It's a sad misconception that table salt and sea salt are the same. Nothing could be further from the truth. Sea salt is replete with seventy-two different minerals, and table salt is just plain sodium chloride. You could call sodium chloride a drug because of the damage it does to the body. Sea salt was a valued commodity in the past, so valued that it was at one time used as currency. Proper cell hydration, sea salt, and well-absorbed minerals are the keys to efficient and effective cellular function. When you have the proper amount of minerals in the cell, the cell automatically pulls in water to create the perfect electrolyte balance, allowing the cell to function efficiently.

If you don't take enough minerals, water can't find its way to your cells and begins to collect in extracellular tissues, especially feet, legs, and hands. You can develop "sausage fingers" and swollen ankles. If you have edema and symptoms of heart disease, such as chest pain and an irregular pulse, your doctor may diagnose you with heart failure. It's probably why they are so aggressive about treating edema with diuretics. But if they could only review basic fluid dynamics and cellular function, they might learn the truth.

DIURETICS DRY OUT THE BRAIN

A journal case study reported that an elderly woman's serum magnesium level became depleted because of a diuretic she was taking for hypertension.[30] She was admitted to the hospital with severe weakness and developed an overt psychosis with paranoid delusions. Fortunately, her magnesium deficiency was identified, and following large intravenous doses of magnesium, her symptoms disappeared within twenty-four hours. However, her symptoms returned as long as she was taking the diuretic. No other abnormalities were found to explain her condition. People who are prescribed diuretics should check with their doctor about taking at least 600 mg a day of supplemental magnesium in divided doses. In that way, many of the side effects of diuretics can be avoided.

THE BLOOD PRESSURE DRUG RECIPE

If blood pressure is not controlled with diuretics, the next choice may be ACE inhibitors, calcium channel blockers, antiadrenergic drugs, or vasodilators. The treatment of high blood pressure by an internist provides a good example of "recipe medicine." I arrived early for an interview with my doctor friend and he invited me to sit in on an appointment with a very stressed, overweight newspaper reporter who was suffering from intractable high blood pressure in spite of being on a total of four different blood pressure medications.

The patient said he was becoming depressed and was very concerned about his blood pressure. I recognized that the medications he was on could cause depression, as could the stress of having a case of high blood pressure that does not respond to treatment. I asked about impotence, suspecting this side effect of his drugs as a possible cause of his depression. He said he had been suffering impotence since going on the medications but had attributed it to stress.

As I noted earlier, the patient was overweight. When I asked about diet, the doctor admitted that he hadn't offered specific diet advice to the patient but had told him to try to lose weight. I also mentioned the usefulness of magnesium as a mineral that excels as a natural antihypertensive, muscle relaxant, antianxiety remedy, and sleep aid. The doctor said that if the four different types of antihypertensive drugs don't help a patient, he will add magnesium, and it always works. Only professional courtesy kept me from shouting, "Why not prescribe the magnesium first, before all the other drugs with their nasty side effects?"

Fortunately, a growing number of naturopaths, chiropractors, nutritionists, primary care doctors, internists, and cardiologists know that magnesium is a physiological necessity and a pharmacological treasure, and are willing to use it before drug intervention. They call magnesium the ideal drug: it is safe, cheap, and simple to use, with a wide therapeutic range, a short half-life, and little or no tendency toward drug interactions.

WEIGHT LOSS DROPS BLOOD PRESSURE

Long before drugs are even discussed, diet should be the first treatment of choice for hypertension. Research shows a direct relationship between the amount of magnesium in the diet and the ability to avoid high blood pressure.[31] The Alturas first demonstrated that diets deficient in magnesium will produce hypertension in experimental animals.[32] However, I've mentioned many times that the soil and the food we eat are woefully deficient in magnesium. Also, people eat larger quantities of food in an unconscious attempt to get the nutrients they require. When those nutrients are provided, insatiable hunger disappears.

Diet may lower the blood pressure through a combination of weight loss and increased intake of the vitamin and mineral cofactors necessary in blood pressure control. For example, increased levels of minerals such as potassium and magnesium in the diet have a suppressive effect on calcium-regulating hormones, which influence blood pressure.[33] The arterial blood pressure appears to go up as the levels of ionized magnesium and serum magnesium go down.[34]

Weight loss is given only a passing mention in most clinical textbooks on blood pressure. The authors in these texts admit that if you can get a person to lose weight, then his or her blood pressure will usually go down. Every study that's been done on this subject reports this association. However, most doctors say that because they have little success with helping their patients lose weight, they usually offer medications as the first line of treatment. Doctors have two strikes against them when it comes to weight loss: they receive no training in weight loss management in medical school, and a typical doctor's copay does not cover nutritional counseling or prevention of disease. It pays only when the doctor can produce a disease code for a patient visit.

For a protocol of supplements for high cholesterol, see "Supplements for Heart Disease" at the end of Chapter 7.

NOTE: Some forms of severe high blood pressure are hereditary or a result of kidney disease and do require medication. Also, if the arteries in the body are damaged from long-term atherosclerotic injury and scarring, unfortunately they may no longer respond to therapeutic magnesium alone and you may require additional medications to keep your blood pressure under control. If you have been cautioned to avoid magnesium because you have kidney disease, please read the section called "Kidneys Need Magnesium" in Chapter 11.

Heart Disease

**THREE THINGS YOU NEED TO KNOW ABOUT
MAGNESIUM AND HEART DISEASE**

---

1. Magnesium prevents muscle spasms of the blood vessels in the heart, which can lead to heart attack.
2. Magnesium prevents muscle spasms of the peripheral blood vessels, which can lead to high blood pressure.
3. Magnesium prevents calcium buildup in cholesterol plaque in arteries, which leads to clogged arteries, atherosclerosis, and stroke.

Annette was tired of people's shocked reaction when they learned that she was recovering from a heart attack. She knew that the common image of heart disease is that it afflicts aggressive, overweight men who smoke and eat too much. Annette, on the other hand, was slim, reserved, and a vegetarian who ate a low-fat diet. She groaned when friends tried to tell her about the Dr. Dean Ornish vegetarian diet for reversing heart disease, because she'd lived according to that diet.

She was only fifty-six, a nonsmoker, with exemplary cholesterol levels, but she did have elevated blood pressure, her only risk factor. And, as her doctor told her, she'd had a mild heart attack because of her blood pressure. Now she suffered from daily palpitations and was on several medications that seemed to drain her energy more with every passing day. She was also simply too afraid to exert herself for fear of bringing on another heart attack.

Annette was becoming a cardiac invalid, and at her next appointment her cardiologist was shocked at her worn-out appearance. He decided to run some blood tests and was urged by a student doctor to order a magnesium RBC test. The results of that test were so low that a nurse immediately called Annette to come in, saying the doctor had found something that would help her feel better.

Her doctor told her the causes of magnesium deficiency and wondered why Annette's levels were so low. She told him she used to run marathons and still worked out at every opportunity. She realized she had been sweating out her magnesium for years and not actively replacing it. Annette was recommended a magnesium citrate preparation that she mixed with water. It began to work within twenty-four hours, and she was amazed that her muscle aches, insomnia, palpitations, and fatigue all but disappeared. She was even able to cut back on her other medications. Her doctor vowed to test all his patients' magnesium red blood cell levels from then on, and wondered aloud if it had been low magnesium in the first place that had led to Annette's heart attack.

TAKING MAGNESIUM
WITH PRESCRIPTION DRUGS

You may experience a decreased need for your drugs as magnesium deficiency is corrected or as magnesium treats your symptoms or reverses your condition. In other words, the symptoms for which the drug was prescribed may clear up because of the magnesium, making the drug unnecessary or even toxic and causing side effects. Patients and doctors should be on the alert for a shift in symptoms. Be sure to work with your doctor to lower your medication safely, because your goal should be to take as few drugs as possible.

A 2003 study gives doctors all the evidence they need to include magnesium in their protocol for women suffering heart disease.[1] The findings from this study show that "dietary magnesium depletion can be induced in otherwise healthy women; it results in increased energy needs and adversely affects cardiovascular function during submaximal work."

As we will learn in Chapter 10, obstetricians are quite familiar with the use of magnesium for hypertension in women about to deliver. Unfortunately, they aren't talking to cardiologists or even to family doctors about the importance of magnesium in treating general hypertension or using magnesium to prevent heart problems.

The American Heart Association Heart Disease and Stroke Statistic Report from 2015 finds that:

- Heart disease is the number one cause of death in the United States, killing over 375,000 people a year.
- Heart disease is the number one killer of women, taking more lives than all forms of cancer combined.
- Cardiovascular operations and procedures increased about 28 percent from 2000 to 2010, according to federal data, totaling about 7.6 million in 2010.
- About 735,000 people in the United States have heart attacks each year. Of those, about 120,000 die.

Hypertension statistics are just as depressing. Almost 80 million U.S. adults have high blood pressure. That's about 33 percent of the population. About 77 percent of those are using antihypertensive medication, but only 54 percent of people taking drugs have their condition controlled.

When I first researched these statistics in the late 1990s, the number of Americans suffering hypertension was 50 million, with an estimated 29.3 million office visits a year to conventional medical doctors.[2] Prescriptions for antihypertensive drugs are given at most of these appointments, even though magnesium has been used with much more success for over half a century by a small group of medical doctors, osteopaths, and naturopathic doctors.[3, 4] I'm mentioning hypertension here, even though I covered it in Chapter 6, because medicating hypertension can lead to heart disease.

WOMEN AND HEART DISEASE

The Centers for Disease Control's *Morbidity and Mortality Weekly Report* notes that heart disease has been the leading cause of death in the United States since 1921.[5] Yet it's taken nearly a century for the American Heart Association (founded in 1924) to release its "First Scientific Statement on Acute Myocardial Infarction in Women."[6]

The report acknowledges that coronary artery disease affects 6.6 million American women each year, but doctors say the disease "remains understudied, underdiagnosed, and undertreated" in this group. "More than 53,000 women die each year from an MI [myocardial infarction] and approximately 262,000 are hospitalized for acute MI and/or unstable angina. In addition, 26% of women vs. 19% of men die within a year following their first MI; 47% vs. 36%, respectively, die within the 5 years after the event."

Investigators found that "coronary angiography is used less often in women, largely because their risk is underestimated, yet women have significantly higher mortality rates than men regardless of age." They say that the public and medical perception of heart attacks is that they occur mostly in middle-aged and elderly men. Doctors want to change that misperception so they can diagnose and treat women earlier. I suggest women take more magnesium to prevent heart attacks.

According to the investigators on this study, the literature shows that women who suffer a heart attack are more likely than men to have diabetes mellitus, heart failure, hypertension, depression, and renal dysfunction, and more women present with non-ST-segment elevation, myocardial infarction, or coronary artery spasm. They also have more bleeding complications, longer hospitalizations, and higher in-hospital mortality after undergoing coronary revascularization.

Investigators admit that the reasons for risk in young women remain unclear. For older women, it's been suggested that increased endothelial dysfunction and lipid deposition caused by menopause-related lack of estrogen could influence the risk of coronary heart disease (CHD). However, "studies evaluating exogenous estrogen hormone therapy for the primary prevention of CHD in postmenopausal women have been convincingly negative."

Diagnosis is often impaired because instead of chest pain, women experience tightness, pressure, or squeezing in the chest accompanied by nausea. The amount of arterial plaque is also different. In men, 76 percent of fatal heart attacks were caused by plaque rupture, compared to 55 percent in women. And women often present with less severe artery blockages than men, which can mean misdiagnosis and ineffective treatment.

The bottom line is that doctors don't know why women have more heart attacks and more complications than men.

So, of course, I look at all this through the lens of magnesium. We know that women require more magnesium than men—it's probably got to do with women's extra hormones, which means more biochemical pathways utilizing more magnesium. Women also take far more calcium supplements than men. There are over a half dozen studies by Bolland and his group that found an increased heart disease risk in women who simply take calcium supplements and do not balance them with enough magnesium. Those studies were not even mentioned in this report.

While investigators look at endothelial dysfunction and suggest an estrogen connection, I see the endothelium affected by lack of nitric oxide due to magnesium deficiency, mitochondrial dysfunction due to magnesium deficiency, and calcium-triggered endothelium dysfunction due to magnesium deficiency.

The complications that occur at higher rates in women are a complete list of magnesium deficiency symptoms: diabetes mellitus, heart failure, hypertension, depression, renal dysfunction, non-ST-segment elevation MI, and coronary artery spasm. I also find that the magnesium burn rate in women is higher than in men. In my opinion, women are more likely to work harder, worry more, and take more calcium and more medications than men and therefore burn off more magnesium.

Then I look at the fact that women suffer more adverse drug reactions than men. According to one study, 5 percent of all hospital admissions are due to drug side effects, and female patients have a 1.5- to 1.7-fold greater risk of developing an adverse drug reaction compared with male patients.[7] Of course, doctors also don't know why women have more drug side effects. This study noted that women are at increased risk for QT prolongation with certain anti-arrhythmic drugs compared with men. Again, they say the mechanisms are unknown. While the researchers speculate about the cause of these adverse events, I speculate that drug therapy in women, who are already magnesium-depleted, will lower their levels even more and cause more magnesium-deficiency-induced drug side effects.

Magnesium deficiency causes muscles to go into spasm. When the heart muscle goes into spasm, that is diagnosed as angina or a heart attack. I think magnesium deficiency should be the first area of investigation to solve the problem of higher incidence of heart attack in women. But doctors won't go there because medical schools don't teach about the clinical, therapeutic application of magnesium. So it's up to you, the reader, to do your homework and look for your own solutions.

THE SLIPPERY ROAD TO HEART ATTACK

STEP ONE: LOSS OF ARTERIAL ELASTICITY

The coronary arteries bringing oxygen-filled blood from inside the heart through the aorta to the heart muscle are very, very small, only about 3 mm across (a nickel is 2 mm thick). It doesn't take much to plug them up with a tiny blood clot or to cause them to collapse when in spasm. Magnesium prevents blood clot formation and artery spasm. These blood vessels get even smaller as they split into two, then four, then eight, and so on as they descend toward the bottom of the heart; some of the tiniest capillaries are only the width of a red blood cell. Each of these splits is called a bifurcation. According to cardiologists, about 85 percent of sclerotic plaques initially form near bifurcations. It is widely believed that the development of these plaques is a response to injury. This means that something, such as an infection, may be damaging the arteries, initiating the buildup of fat and calcium around the inflammation.

Endothelial cells are a single layer of specialized cells that form the inside membrane of an artery. The subendothelial layer (the next layer in) is a very thin connective tissue that contains elastin. As its name implies, this is the layer responsible for providing much of the elasticity in your arteries. It is important to note that your body requires magnesium to maintain healthy elastin. One of the earliest signs of magnesium deficiency is degeneration of elastin in the subendothelium. Seelig and Rosanoff discuss the deposition of calcium in elastin and replacement with fibrous tissue in animals suffering from magnesium deficiency.[8]

Smooth muscle cells are the next layer. Smooth muscle cells provide integrity and control the dilation of the arterial cavity, which is triggered by the calcium/magnesium ratio in the body. Calcium causes contraction and magnesium causes relaxation, which together control the blood pressure and flow in the artery. A final messenger for the dilation response is nitric oxide, which is dependent on magnesium. Animals on low-magnesium diets lose the elasticity of their arterial system. Coronary arteries require even more elasticity than other arteries because they must stretch and flex as the heart expands and contracts. Loss of elasticity results in inflammation of the endothelial and subendothelial layers at the points that are most mechanically challenged by stretching: the bifurcations. Imagine a small rubber-band-like tube shaped like a Y. In your mind's eye grasp the two legs of the Y in one hand. With your other hand, grip the single leg. Begin pulling them apart just as though they were stretching on the surface of the heart. Stretch it as far as you can. Where is the shape weakest? If we left the rubber tube out in the sun for a week or so, what would happen if you slowly stretched it again? Where might you expect the first crack to appear? Most of the time it would happen at or near where one tube becomes two—

at the bifurcation. If your artery loses elasticity, it makes sense that the problem might show up at or near the bifurcation.

STEP TWO: THE INFLAMMATORY RESPONSE

Inflammation begins with injury of the artery wall, leading to white blood cells and cholesterol hovering around trying to heal the damage. At this stage in the process, if there is too much calcium and not enough magnesium in the bloodstream, excess calcium precipitates around the area of inflammation in the artery wall. The area becomes rigid and interferes with blood flow. This calcification is now being measured by coronary artery scans.

STEP THREE: HEART ATTACK

Over time, the above steps weaken and plug the coronary arteries and slowly destroy small areas of the heart muscle. The final result is severe chest pain, damage to a larger portion of the heart muscle, and heart attack.

Some of the first evidence for the use of magnesium against heart disease came from epidemiological studies in Wales, Taiwan, Sweden, Finland, and Japan showing that death rates from coronary heart disease are higher in communities with magnesium-deficient water and magnesium-deficient diets.[9] Areas where calcium in the water is much higher than magnesium or where dietary intake of calcium is higher than magnesium showed even more coronary heart disease. A U.S. study done over a seven-year period followed 14,000 men and women and concluded that low magnesium in the diet may contribute to coronary atherosclerosis and acute heart attack.[10]

The Centers for Disease Control and Prevention in Atlanta followed 12,000 people for nineteen years, at the end of which 4,282 people had died, 1,005 from heart disease. Risk of dying from heart disease was highest in those with magnesium deficiency. Researchers made a conservative estimate that 11 percent of the half million deaths related to heart disease in 1993 could have been directly related to magnesium deficiency.[11] If more accurate measurements for magnesium deficiency were used, such as ionized magnesium testing, we would find the numbers to be even higher and the need for magnesium even greater.

The evidence has been mounting for decades that magnesium plays a crucial role in the prevention of both atherosclerosis and arteriosclerosis.[12, 13] Magnesium maintains the elasticity of the artery wall, dilates blood vessels, prevents calcium deposits, and is necessary for the maintenance of healthy muscles, including the heart muscle itself. For all these reasons, magnesium is critical to the maintenance of a healthy heart.[14] One of the pivotal metabolic chemicals in the body is nitric oxide. It is a very simple compound made from nitrogen and oxygen, but it packs a powerful punch. Nitric oxide controls vasodilation, but this activity is under the direction of magnesium.[15]

C-REACTIVE PROTEIN

A December 2005 study confirmed that C-reactive protein (CRP) had emerged as a powerful predictor of heart disease.[16] An optimal level of CRP is less than 6 mg/l. As more research is done, CRP could supplant cholesterol as the most significant heart disease predictor. Why is this important? Because CRP is a measure of inflammation—and, as previously noted, it's the injury and inflammation of heart blood vessels that underlie heart disease.

This 2005 study also examined uric acid, which is a product of incomplete purine breakdown. Purine-rich foods include anchovies, herring, kidney, liver, mackerel, meat extracts, mincemeat, mussels, and sardines. High uric acid is associated with inflammation, hypertension, heart disease, and damaged blood vessel walls. Uric acid is broken down by nitric oxide, thus depleting this anti-inflammatory substance, which increases inflammation in the body and elevates CRP.

Although the researchers say nothing about magnesium, it is important in the treatment of elevated CRP because it is such a powerful anti-inflammatory agent. Sufficient magnesium can calm inflammation at every stage, whereas the only other option, anti-inflammatory prescription drugs, are ineffective and can cause dangerous side effects. I discuss nonsteroidal anti-inflammatory drugs (NSAIDs) in Chapter 11.

A 2015 review article on CRP, inflammation, and coronary heart disease gives an excellent overview of CRP and shows that it is an important diagnostic tool.[17] You can search this article online, where the abstract alone gives you vital information about the role of inflammation in chronic disease. In summary, high-sensitivity CRP tests are being used increasingly as a "clinical guide to diagnosis, management, and prognosis of CHD."

A 2013 meta-analysis included a total of 532,979 participants from nineteen studies and concluded that there is a statistically significant association between lower dietary magnesium intake and increased risk of cardiovascular disease events.[18] Even more compelling evidence is that lower serum magnesium concentrations are associated with a higher risk of total cardiovascular disease events. I only wish they could have used the much more accurate ionized magnesium test or even the magnesium RBC test.

An April 2014 study in the *European Journal of Clinical Nutrition* concluded, "This meta-analysis and systematic review indicates that dietary Mg intake is significantly and inversely associated with serum CRP levels. The potential beneficial effect of Mg intake on chronic diseases may be, at least in part, explained by inhibiting inflammation."[19]

A U.S. study, reported in the July 2006 issue of the journal *Nutrition Research*, found that a daily magnesium supplement could reduce the levels of inflammation, as measured by C-reactive protein.[20] This is very encouraging news. It's also encouraging that researchers are investigating magnesium supplementation and not just dietary magnesium. In this study of more than 10,000 people, only 21 percent were getting the RDA for magnesium in their diet. Another 26 percent were taking magnesium supplements, and that group exhibited lower levels of C-reactive protein than the magnesium-deficient group.

ATHEROSCLEROSIS

It is easy to confuse the terms *arteriosclerosis* and *atherosclerosis*; in fact, many people use them interchangeably. *Arteriosclerosis* is the overall term for scarring of the arteries. *Atherosclerosis* is scarring or thickening specifically due to fatty plaques. When fatty deposits already narrow the diameter of an artery, a blood clot or an arterial spasm can be the final straw that results in angina, heart attack, or stroke. Complications of atherosclerosis, a preventable condition, cause over a third of all deaths in the United States. Don't forget that calcium deposits in the arteriosclerotic scarring and in the atherosclerotic fatty plaques are the real culprits, and that they will be dissolved with therapeutic amounts of magnesium.

ANGINA

Angina describes an episodic pain in the region of the chest and/or down the left arm due to lack of oxygen to the heart muscle and a buildup of carbon dioxide and other metabolites. Usually the pain, which can be a mild ache, a feeling of pressure, a sense of fullness, or a crushing pain, comes on with exercise (especially in the cold), emotional stress, a heavy meal, or even a vivid dream, and is relieved (usually within five minutes) by rest and nitroglycerine.

The lack of sufficient blood flow carrying life-giving oxygen and nutrients can be due to blocked coronary arteries or spasms in these tiny vessels. Angina is labeled "unstable" when symptoms become more severe; unstable angina implies a greater risk for heart attack. Another type of angina is called Prinzmetal's, which is angina that occurs at rest, rather than following some sort of physical stress.

James B. Pierce, Ph.D., believes he has identified the cause of Prinzmetal's, which occurs most commonly at two specific times in the day, early morning and late afternoon, coincidentally when magnesium levels are at their lowest.[21] Dr. Pierce estimates that up to 50 percent of sudden heart attacks may be due to magnesium deficiency. He has found that magnesium works better than nitroglycerine for his own stress-induced chest pains. In fact, Dr. Pierce knew that he would get chest pain after a stressful day, a long drive, or an emotional upset and would increase his intake of magnesium to forestall symptoms.

Risk factors for angina include magnesium deficiency, smoking, diabetes, hyperlipidemia, type A personality, sedentary lifestyle, poor diet, and family history of coronary artery disease. Diagnosis of angina, to differentiate it from myocardial infarction and unstable angina, includes an EKG (electrocardiogram) taken during an angina attack; an exercise tolerance test, which is an EKG taken while on a treadmill; and a coronary angiogram (an X-ray of dye in the coronary arteries) to assess whether the coronary arteries are open or blocked.

Once angina is diagnosed, the recommendations are universally known: stop smoking, lose weight, get blood pressure under control (with or without drugs), and in extreme cases of arterial blockages undergo placement of stents to open arteries or have bypass surgery to circumvent blocked arteries.

The best treatment for angina, however, is prevention. Eliminate sugar, alcohol, and junk food from your diet to help prevent heart disease; these foods are lacking in magnesium and serve only to create magnesium deficiency. When you eat a more balanced diet without processed foods, you have a better chance of increasing your magnesium intake. With supplemental magnesium, a few other heart-healthy supplements, a good diet, and an exercise regimen, you have a fighting chance of not becoming a statistic in this epidemic.

HEART ATTACKS

Myocardial infarction (MI), or heart attack, is now called acute coronary syndrome (ACS). It can cause permanent damage to the heart muscle and requires immediate hospitalization. ACS is the result of coronary artery disease due to atherosclerosis or due to spasms caused or aggravated by magnesium deficiency. The artery may be damaged gradually by plaque or become blocked by a blood clot, or both, and suddenly goes into spasm; either of these processes can be accelerated by excessive emotion. The calcified atherosclerotic plaque, the blood clot, and the arterial spasm can all be caused or worsened by magnesium deficiency.

Laboratory findings distinguish a heart attack from an episode of angina on the basis of heart muscle damage shown on an EKG and the elevation of certain heart enzymes on blood testing. After a heart attack, these enzymes remain elevated for several days. The immediate treatment for an acute heart attack usually includes anticoagulant drugs in an intravenous drip. Intravenous magnesium given as soon as possible after a heart attack, however, may provide the best protection for the heart. Oral magnesium treatment also inhibits blood clots in patients with coronary artery disease whether the patient is on aspirin therapy or not.[22] As more doctors read the considerable research on magnesium they are incorporating magnesium into their intravenous and oral protocols for heart patients.

Magnesium has been studied for its effects on the heart since the 1930s and used by injection for the treatment of heart conditions since the 1940s.[23, 24] Magnesium's lifesaving effects have been confirmed and reconfirmed in many clinics and laboratories. For example, in an analysis of seven major clinical studies, researchers concluded that magnesium (in doses of 5–10 g by IV injection) reduced the odds of death by an astounding 55 percent in acute MI.[25, 26] Over the past decade, several large clinical trials using magnesium have shown its beneficial effects. If intravenous magnesium is given (1) before any other drugs and (2) immediately after onset of a heart attack, the incidence of high blood pressure, congestive heart failure, arrhythmia, or a subsequent heart attack is vastly reduced.

One such study, called LIMIT-2, provided powerful evidence that early magnesium administration protects the heart muscle, prevents arrhythmia, and improves long-term survival.[27, 28, 29] Magnesium can improve the aftermath of an acute heart attack by preventing rhythm problems, increasing blood flow to the heart by dilating blood vessels, protecting the damaged heart muscle against calcium overload, improving heart muscle function, breaking down any blood clots blocking the arteries, and reducing free radical damage. Magnesium may also help the heart drug digoxin to be more effective in the treatment of cardiac arrhythmia;[30] without enough magnesium, digoxin can become toxic.[31]

The suggested criteria for magnesium intervention were not followed in a very large trial called ISIS-4 and the outcome did not show the same results as the LIMIT-2 trial.[32] In the ISIS-4 trial, magnesium was given many hours after the onset of symptoms, after blood-clotting had begun—and after clot-dissolving drugs had been administered. The two trials were as dissimilar as apples and oranges. Since the LIMIT-2 and ISIS-4 studies, several smaller trials have shown even greater recovery from heart attacks using intravenous magnesium, including a trial of 200 people with a 74 percent lower death rate.[33]

However, in the literature, researchers are using the large ISIS-4 trial to say that IV magnesium "cannot be recommended in patients with myocardial infarction today."[34] Unfortunately, that flawed trial will hold back widespread clinical application of magnesium for decades.

Dr. Michael Shechter is a committed magnesium researcher who in his numerous clinical trials has proven the benefits of magnesium in treating heart disease. His clinical trials began in 2000 and continued for several years, all maintaining that magnesium is a viable and necessary treatment for people with heart disease in spite of the ISIS-4 trial and another trial called MAGIC suggesting that it has no benefit.[35, 36, 37, 38, 39, 40]

Pharmaceutical companies, who want to promote their own drug therapies, cite the ISIS-4 trial as proof that magnesium sulfate doesn't work; supporters of magnesium cite the LIMIT-2 trial as proof that it does. Your doctor may be influenced by the ISIS-4 trial and think magnesium is not an important option in your care. But cardiologists who are looking for alternatives to the side effects of drug therapy and who read the magnesium studies thoroughly are using magnesium successfully.

I wish I could help you find these cardiologists. In the Resources section in the back of this book, I name several alternative medicine associations that you can contact for local practitioners. Unfortunately, I see a greater regimentation in the current HMO system that prevents doctors from doing anything outside the standard practice of drugs and surgery. Most doctors who practice alternative medicine are not covered by insurance. That's why books like *The Magnesium Miracle* are so important to help educate you about alternatives to drugs and surgery that you can implement as you take charge of your own health.

One of the major side effects of heart medications, especially diuretics, is magnesium deficiency. I've already spoken about diuretics depleting magnesium in Chapter 2. You will know you are deficient by your symptoms of leg cramps, heart palpitations, insomnia, irritability, and more. You can also have your magnesium levels tested with a magnesium RBC test. If your levels are below 6.0 mg/dL, be sure to take 6 to 10 mg/kg/day of magnesium. At 1,000 mg of elemental magnesium per day, most magnesium products will have a laxative effect, but not ReMag. See Chapter 16 for more on magnesium testing. See Chapter 18 for more information on ReMag, a non-laxative magnesium product.

HEART FAILURE

There appears to be an epidemic of heart failure in the Western world. But, in my opinion, hearts aren't failing; it's doctors who are failing to treat magnesium deficiency, which is an underlying cause of heart disease and subsequent heart failure. The problem begins with the very name that doctors use for this disease. They don't seem to realize that a declaration that the patient's heart is failing sets the patient up for just that!

Investigators in a paper published in the July 2013 issue of *Circulation: Cardiovascular Quality and Outcomes* comment on the high hospital readmission rate of heart failure patients.

They report: "A million people are hospitalized with heart failure each year, and about 250,000 will be back in the hospital within a month. If we could keep even 2% of them from coming back to the hospital, that could equal a saving of more than $100 million a year." If we could give everyone magnesium and prevent them from ever having to enter a hospital for heart failure, we would save billions.

High on the list of signs and symptoms of heart failure is an enlarged heart—especially left ventricle hypertrophy (LVH). In fact, LVH is a significant predictor of adverse cardiovascular events up to and including heart failure. An important study found that low serum magnesium is one of the strongest predictors of increased left ventricular mass over a five-year period.[41] Why aren't doctors using that measurement and improving patients' magnesium levels to prevent heart failure?

Heart failure is more routinely diagnosed by a combination of cardiac catheterization, CT scan or MRI, and ultrasound to measure the ejection fraction of the heart. The ejection fraction gauges the strength of the heart muscle, specifically the ventricles, and their ability to pump blood through the vast network of arteries and capillaries in the body. There's a good reason the highest amount of magnesium in the body is found in the heart ventricles. Those muscle cells depend on the proper balance of magnesium and calcium for proper function. If the ventricles are not ejecting blood properly, I would first look to magnesium deficiency, as identified in the above study.

Instead of reading the scientific literature and incorporating magnesium into their diagnostic and treatment plan, doctors have a standardized treatment for heart disease of about six drugs—often sold together in blister packs so you don't miss a dose. The drugs are to control blood pressure, cholesterol, blood sugar, and fluid retention, and to push the heart to beat stronger—and, ironically, they all contribute to magnesium deficiency!

Even worse, people tell me their doctors warn them not to take magnesium in case it interferes with their medication! How has it come to the point where patients are being warned not to take something that's as important as air, food, and water because it will lessen their need for drugs? What has occurred to cause doctors to distrust necessary nutrients and prescribe drugs for life?

Cardiologists are convinced that the natural progression of heart disease is to develop into heart failure. That's why they put all their patients on "preventive" doses of blood pressure drugs, statins, and diabetic drugs because they think that high blood pressure, high cholesterol, and high blood sugar are inevitable consequences of heart disease. But what they fail to recognize is that the very drugs they are prescribing cause more magnesium deficiency and more heart disease and bring on symptoms of high blood pressure, high cholesterol, and high blood sugar.

Here's a common scenario that I've heard from countless patients. You've been under even more stress than usual, but it's time for your annual physical. When the new physician's assistant takes your blood pressure, it's high. You explain it's always a bit high when you go to the doctor. However, the physician's assistant looks at your chart and insists that it's time you took medication because your hypertension is only going to get worse with age. You are scared by what you hear, so you take the prescription for a diuretic (which depletes magnesium) and go back for a follow-up visit in a month. Your blood pressure is even higher, and the physician's assistant says, "Look, we caught it just in time, but now you need two more drugs," both of which cause magnesium deficiency. After another two months you go back for blood tests to make sure your liver can handle the drugs, and—seemingly out of the blue—your cholesterol and blood sugar are both high for the first time. The PA says it's just part of the disease progression and puts you on another two or three drugs. It's the downward spiral of magnesium-deficiency-induced heart disease, and it will keep spinning out of control unless you begin taking therapeutic amounts of magnesium and work with your doctor to slowly wean off those unnecessary medications.

SPASTIC HEART

Between 40 and 60 percent of people who suffer sudden heart attacks may actually have no arterial blockage.[42] Two suspected causes are spasms in the coronary arteries and the occurrence of a severe heart rhythm disturbance, such as atrial fibrillation. Both of these conditions can be caused by a deficiency of magnesium. Low magnesium makes the heart muscle hyperirritable, leading to the development of a rhythm disturbance that can't be stopped without emergency medical intervention. An astute physician recognizes the possibility of magnesium deficiency and immediately gives magnesium intravenously, as in the LIMIT-2 trial. Rapid heartbeat (atrial tachycardia), premature beats, atrial fibrillation, and ventricular tachycardia have all responded to treatment with IV magnesium.[43, 44, 45, 46]

The most common time for the onset of heart attacks is around 9:00 a.m. on Monday as people gird their loins for another long workweek.[47] As mentioned earlier, people who suffer from spasm-induced angina attacks most often experience them at the same time each day, usually in the morning and late afternoon, when magnesium levels are at their lowest. The morning deficiency is likely the result of overnight fasting and the loss of magnesium through the urine when you empty your bladder in the morning. Deficiency in the afternoon may be caused by depletion of magnesium induced by the stress of the day and not yet replenished by the evening meal. In view of this, it seems reasonable that people with angina, heart spasms, hypertension, or heart disease should consult with their doctors and take a magnesium RBC test; if it is below optimal (less than 6.0 mg/dL), they should go on magnesium supplementation. See Chapter 16 for more on magnesium testing and Chapter 18 for my magnesium product recommendations.

BROKEN HEART SYNDROME

Broken heart syndrome is another missed diagnosis, and a missed opportunity for modern medicine to truly help patients. I think part of medicine is very pleased with itself for even acknowledging this condition's existence. Although another part wants to be much more scientific about this condition. Thus, there is a recent move to drop the name Broken Heart Syndrome and call it Takotsubo cardiomyopathy. Researchers are also trying to find the pathology that goes with this condition. They think it might be microscopic coronary artery disease but they really don't know what causes it or how to treat it.

Experts say that broken heart syndrome, which most often affects women in their sixties or older, is brought on by strong emotions, such as grief, anger, and anxiety, or by physical stress or even intense joy or excitement. A common trigger is a loved one's illness or death, thus the name. The symptoms mimic a heart attack but without any evidence of coronary artery disease.

Researchers suspect these patients suffer from an impaired parasympathetic nervous system—the calming part of the nervous system is just not making you calm anymore. Of course, I see it as another obvious symptom of magnesium deficiency and taking this one mineral, magnesium, can help a person cope with severe stressors.

Doctors, always looking for a drug solution, have prescribed beta-blockers to prevent symptoms, but a recent study found these drugs are ineffective. This study recommends that relaxation techniques such as breath therapy, yoga, and meditation should be investigated to prevent broken heart syndrome, while other branches of medicine still want to medicate the problem with drugs.

In Chapter 15, I talk about magnesium deficiency in the elderly, in whom deficiency causes "autonomic nervous system disturbances that involve both the sympathetic and parasympathetic nervous systems, causing hypotension on rising quickly or borderline hypertension. In elderly patients, excessive emotionality, tremor, weakness, sleep disorders, amnesia and cognitive disturbances are particularly important aspects of magnesium deficiency."[48]

If a person who is already magnesium deficient is overwhelmed with grief and shock, the magnesium burn rate soars, and the person can experience a coronary event. Although breathing exercises, yoga, and meditation may be beneficial to calm your parasympathetic nervous system, the best treatment is magnesium, and the most therapeutic magnesium is ReMag.

How is it that I can unearth the research showing that magnesium deficiency compromises the parasympathetic nervous system but these doctors cannot? Why is a drug solution the only route that doctors will travel, and why are nutrients considered useless at best or quackery at worst? There is a formidable anti-nutrient lobby at work that is threatening our health and our lives. Our only recourse is to take responsibility for our own health and protect it. Please know that magnesium is important for all stress and all types of grief and trauma.

In Chapter 3 I mentioned a case where someone was "suffering from dreadful stress and feeling continually anxious with a tight pain constantly around her chest." She took ReMag and "her chest pains went away, as did her nightly cramps, and the constant feeling of tension lessened to such a degree she felt she could cope once more." She said the magnesium "really helped her through what was an incredibly stressful situation."

After I wrote a blog post about broken heart syndrome, I received several emails from women who thanked me for finally putting a label on what they had suffered after a traumatic emotional experience. They were also grateful to learn that they could use magnesium to help alleviate their physical as well as their emotional symptoms.

ARRHYTHMIA

Magnesium's ability to neutralize the heart-damaging effects of catecholamines and prevent many of the sequelae of acute heart attack, such as arrhythmia, was reported decades ago in 1994.[49] *Catecholamines* is the name given to the grouping of epinephrine, norepinephrine, and dopamine, which function both as neurotransmitters and as hormones in the body. Release of epinephrine and norepinephrine from the adrenal glands is part of the fight-or-flight response to stress.

Catecholamines have contradictory effects on the heart depending on their concentration. These effects were studied in a 2009 paper called "Role of the Excessive Amounts of Circulating Catecholamines and Glucocorticoids in Stress-Induced Heart Disease."[50] According to this paper, at low concentrations catecholamines stimulate the heart by promoting calcium entry into heart muscle cells. However, excessive amounts of catecholamines create cardiac dysfunction by overloading heart cells with too much calcium, leading to heart spasms.

The authors further note that under stressful conditions, high concentrations of catecholamines become oxidized and generate free radicals. These oxidation products and high intracellular calcium levels produce coronary spasm, arrhythmias, and cardiac dysfunction as well as defects in energy production by cellular mitochondria and myocardial cell damage.

To my way of thinking, cellular overload of calcium is best treated with magnesium. Magnesium deficiency contributes to abnormal heart rhythms because magnesium is responsible for maintaining normal concentrations of electrolytes inside heart muscle cells. A balance of potassium, sodium, calcium, and magnesium allows for normal heart muscle contraction and maintains normal heartbeat. A central pacemaker within the heart muscle creates a normal pumping action that travels across the heart.

Cardiac arrhythmia occurs when other, less suitable areas of the heart are forced to assume the role of the central pacemaker when it becomes damaged or irritated by lack of oxygen due to blocked blood vessels, drugs (including caffeine), hormonal imbalance, or deficiency of magnesium. These new pacemakers are even more sensitive to magnesium deficiency but are responsive to magnesium therapy, which has been successfully used since 1943.[51]

Magnesium is also an accepted treatment for ventricular arrhythmias,[52, 53] congestive heart failure (where the heart is weak and unable to empty after each heartbeat),[54, 55] and before and after heart surgery, including coronary bypass grafting.[56, 57, 58] All these studies indicate that the frequency of ventricular arrhythmias is reduced by administration of intravenous magnesium, and they support an early high-dose administration of intravenous magnesium in the wake of myocardial infarction.

I have not expanded the above entry about arrhythmias since 1999, but in the meantime, arrhythmia—especially atrial fibrillation, or AFib—has become epidemic. A 2007 meta-analysis gathered data about the efficacy of administering IV magnesium compared to placebo and medications in the acute treatment of rapid atrial fibrillation.[59] Data were pooled from twelve trials with a total of 779 patients. Magnesium was effective in achieving rate control and rhythm control. A positive response was achieved in 86 percent of the magnesium group versus 56 percent of the control groups. And the magnesium group responded much more quickly to treatment. The investigators concluded that intravenous magnesium is an effective and safe strategy for the acute management of rapid AFib. Also, it has no side effects compared to drug management. And doctors should also consider that magnesium may "cure" the condition in individuals whose AFib is caused by magnesium deficiency.

In 2013, investigators with the Framingham Heart Study acknowledged that low serum magnesium is linked to increased risk of atrial fibrillation following cardiac surgery. They wanted to investigate whether magnesium deficiency predisposes to AFib among the Framingham study participants. Of 3,530 participants, they found that those with the lowest levels of serum magnesium were approximately 50 percent more likely to develop AFib.[60] The results would probably have been even higher if a more accurate measurement of magnesium was done using ionized magnesium testing.

In 2015 I wrote a book called *Atrial Fibrillation: Remineralize Your Heart*. The book arose from my experience with recommending magnesium for arrhythmia, for which I was recognized when the Heart Rhythm Society in the United

Kingdom presented me with an award for Outstanding Medical Contribution to Cardiac Rhythm Management, 2012. Even with mounting evidence of the importance of magnesium in treating arrhythmias, I do not see it being implemented in the doctor's office. Or if doctors do recommend magnesium, they will prescribe the ineffective and laxative-effect-producing magnesium oxide. The advice in *Atrial Fibrillation: Remineralize Your Heart* has helped countless people regain their health. Below I'll excerpt from the book so the information can reach a wider audience. The book in its entirety is available for free under the "Books" link on my RnA ReSet website.[61]

ATRIAL FIBRILLATION: REMINERALIZE YOUR HEART

Most clients who have consulted with me about their symptoms of atrial fibrillation are very distressed about their condition. Additionally, most patients have also been traumatized by their interaction with the medical community. Doctors give AFib patients no natural or alternative options; they immediately prescribe several medications and recommend cardioversion or catheter ablation of the fibrillating area in the heart. They provide no reassurance, instead assuring patients that their condition is lifelong and incurable and will only get worse with time. If a patient doesn't seem compliant with the standard treatment for AFib, doctors scare them into taking their drugs by warning them that they otherwise risk having a stroke or heart attack.

Since doctors do not look closely at the role that magnesium plays in AFib, they miss the opportunity to give their patients a treatment that can help the heart's electrical disharmony. If doctors do acknowledge and prescribe magnesium, it's usually magnesium oxide, a form that's very poorly

absorbed, causing an overwhelming laxative effect and rein-
forcing to doctors the notion that magnesium is ineffective!
On top of that, diarrhea can flush out even more magnesium, further upsetting the electrolyte balance. Doctors focus
on magnesium oxide because it's the form that has been used
in the majority of magnesium studies and they assume diarrhea is a normal side effect of taking magnesium.

A reader of my blog sent me the following story of how
she developed her AFib but the doctors would never admit
the cause.

> In 2014, on June 30, I developed abdominal pain, nau-
> sea, and vomiting. Within several hours the pain local-
> ized in the right lower quadrant, so I went to the hospital
> ER, and after several more hours I was diagnosed with
> acute appendicitis.
>
> Since this was a major teaching hospital and it was
> now July 1, there were additional problems and delays
> due to changing over to the new rotation of interns! So
> I didn't get to surgery until eighteen hours after I had
> presented to the ER and twenty-four hours after the
> onset of symptoms. By this time, my appendix had per-
> forated.
>
> When I woke up, I was on two IV antibiotics—
> Flagyl and Levaquin—in addition to IV narcotic pain
> meds and nausea meds. I continued to have severe nau-
> sea and vomiting—now due to the narcotics, which also
> had me so sedated that I was barely aware of what was
> going on around me. After three more days of constant
> vomiting, I began refusing the narcotics and my symp-
> toms improved quite quickly.
>
> On my fourth hospital day, I developed AFib with a
> rapid ventricular response and was admitted to the
> ICU. At that point I also refused the Levaquin, although

the cardiologist assured me that it had nothing to do with my arrhythmia. From reading your material, I now know Levaquin is a fluoride drug that binds magnesium!

They finally checked my electrolytes. Serum magnesium and potassium were both low—apparently they had not been checking them postop despite the fact that I had been vomiting constantly for four days!

I converted to normal sinus rhythm fairly quickly after discontinuing Levaquin and taking magnesium and potassium and a short course of the antiarrhythmia drug amiodarone. A couple of days later I was able to go home, I discontinued all meds and have been happily taking ReMag and ReMyte ever since with no further problems.

I likely had low magnesium prior to the hospitalization, which was exacerbated by vomiting and Levaquin. I had never had a problem with low potassium prior to this.

It is truly shocking how unaware conventional medicine is of basic biochemistry and also of the dangerous side effects of the medications they prescribe. I am very fortunate that they didn't kill me.

I receive many unsolicited testimonials each week like the following:

Your products have increased my family's health tremendously. Before ReMag, ReMyte, and RnA Drops, I was dealing with undiagnosed atrial fibrillation or heart arrhythmias/palpitations. Sometimes it would go on for hours and sometimes into the next day, draining every ounce of energy in my body. I no longer have any episodes of this kind anymore.

EPIDEMIC OF ATRIAL FIBRILLATION

Why are so many hearts suddenly beating erratically and mystifying doctors?

1. Because 80 percent of the population is magnesium-deficient.
2. Because doctors don't even measure magnesium when they investigate atrial fibrillation.
3. Because doctors don't ask their patients if they are drinking enough water.
4. Because doctors don't make sure their patients are taking enough magnesium and other minerals, including sea salt in their water.

I think there is more focus on AFib currently because there are newer drugs to treat some of the symptoms. Specifically, drug companies are marketing new blood thinners. Blood thinners are the primary treatment for AFib's potential to produce clots—a rapidly fibrillating heart may not empty completely, leaving some blood behind that could clot if it doesn't keep moving. Blood thinners don't heal the condition; they just prevent blood clot formation. But the side effects of the newer drugs can be devastating, causing irreversible bleeding.

WHAT IS ATRIAL FIBRILLATION?

Atrial fibrillation is the most commonly diagnosed heart arrhythmia, reaching epidemic proportions. In the United States, AFib hospitalizations increased by 23 percent between 2000 and 2010.[62] The number of people in 2010 with AFib was about 5.2 million, and this is predicted to increase to about 12.1 million cases in 2030.[63] I believe the increase in AFib parallels the increase in magnesium deficiency in the population.

Doctors believe that most cases of AFib are secondary to heart disease, so the treatment is to medicate those symptoms to try to alter the course of the disease. At one time doctors described adrenal stimulation and vagus nerve relaxation as factors in AFib. But doctors no longer discuss these causes of AFib with their patients, leaving them to worry endlessly. That happened to a client of mine who experienced arrhythmia, anxiety, and shortness of breath from drinking cold water. When I explained what could be happening, she was quite relieved and said the doctors made her feel like she was crazy. I personally used to get a burst of coughing when my heart kicked out extra beats. Of course, all that is gone now because I drink enough salted water and take my own ReMag and ReMyte formulas, which I will discuss in Chapter 18 and in the Resources section.

Adrenal Stimulation

Certain activities can stress the adrenal glands, causing them to pump out excess adrenaline: stress, exercise, exertion, and stimulants (coffee, alcohol, tobacco). Over time this type of reaction can cause an increase in blood pressure (by constricting blood vessels) and lead to structural damage to the heart, which may involve the pacemaker areas and thus interfere with the heart rate and rhythm.

Vagus Nerve Relaxation

This type of AFib occurs at night, after a meal, or when resting after exercising, or is associated with digestive problems. The vagus nerve controls peristalsis and stomach secretions and is part of the parasympathetic nervous system, which tends to slow the heart and dilate blood vessels.

Doctors say that if you have AFib, you are at increased risk for heart failure, clots, and strokes. But that's only if you already have heart disease. Most people I speak with do not have a heart problem; they have a magnesium deficiency problem.

Unfortunately, the medications that are used to treat AFib can themselves cause heart disease, which may just increase the likelihood of maintaining an AFib condition. And those patients with heart disease, high blood pressure, and high cholesterol are on medications that cause more heart disease because those meds cause magnesium deficiency. That's probably why doctors say that AFib is incurable. They don't know that magnesium deficiency may be the cause and magnesium supplementation may be the cure for many people. AFib is more common in people age sixty and older, possibly because we become more magnesium-deficient as we age.

The heart has four chambers; the top two are atria and the bottom two are ventricles. What causes the atria to fibrillate? In a healthy heart, the electrical impulses in the atria are coordinated by the proper balance and interaction of several minerals that function as electrolytes: magnesium, calcium, sodium, and potassium. It seems logical that an imbalance of these minerals is the cause and balancing them is the cure. But doctors skirt around that issue—probably because they don't even measure magnesium in a routine electrolyte panel. Just look at your most recent blood tests and you'll see that I'm right. They test for sodium, potassium, calcium, and chloride but not magnesium.

The electrical firing that occurs to make the heart beat regularly begins in the atria. So that's the first place where things can go wrong. The sinoatrial node is a cluster of cells in the right atrium that has the ability to create an electrical impulse on its own and trigger adjacent cells to carry the current, like a Pac-Man progression. The electrical impulse runs to the atrioventricular node and down into the ventricles.

However, a huge factor in the realm of heart electrical activity is the little-discussed fact that the heart has multiple backup pacemakers. There are several areas along the conduction pathway where clusters of cells can start an electrical impulse from scratch.

The body is a genius operation, and having backup pacemakers is pretty smart. But what happens when one of those backup pacemakers gets caught up in a magnesium deficiency spasm? It will fire erratically, potentially causing increased heart rate and abnormal heart rhythm.

WHAT CAUSES OR TRIGGERS ATRIAL FIBRILLATION

Cardiologists say that damage to the structure of the heart is the most common cause of AFib. I found a list of AFib causes on the Mayo Clinic website, and I expanded and embellished it, below. But remember, it is the disorganization of the electrical activity of the cells of the heart that causes the heart to beat erratically. So instead of just listing off the causes, why aren't they able to say why each one can potentially cause AFib?

I've discovered that each one of these causes may be due to magnesium deficiency, which can lead to structural changes in the heart by causing normal muscle cells to go into dangerous spasm. As will be made quite clear, there is no single cause of AFib for everyone, and several causes may be in play for some.

Read this long list of thirty-three AFib triggers and you will find the ones that most apply to your case. But please don't panic; it's very important to know what triggers your AFib, and you will soon realize that magnesium can eliminate most if not all of these triggers.

ATRIAL FIBRILLATION TRIGGERS

1. **Air pollution.** Data mining from patients with implanted defibrillators shows that during times of air pollution there are more episodes of fibrillation. It's the very fine particles of pollution from cars and power plants that travel deep into the lungs and trigger bronchial irritation, coughing, and atrial fibrillation. You can stay indoors during times of high air pollution. However, magnesium can help prevent bronchial spasm and help clear pollution from the lungs. The ingredients in Re-Aline can help the liver detoxify pollutants, even heavy metals.

2. **Alcohol.** Drinking alcohol releases catecholamines from the adrenal glands—especially noradrenaline. Additionally, alcohol causes the release of adrenaline stored in the heart. Plasma acetaldehyde, the main metabolite of ethanol, raises catecholamine concentrations systemically and in the heart muscle. Withdrawal of alcohol also results in increased release of catecholamines. Alcohol directly, and the above metabolites, stress the heart, with prolonged PR, QRS, and QT times, facilitating atrial arrhythmias.

   Alcohol excess is associated with hypertension. The residues of sulfites, pesticides, and fungicides can be found in some wines and trigger reactions in susceptible people. Alcohol depletes magnesium, and the breakdown products of alcohol, such as acetaldehyde (a heart stimulant), require magnesium in order to break them down and eliminate them from the body.

   Alcohol also feeds intestinal yeast, resulting in yeast overgrowth and production of 178 yeast toxins, including acetaldehyde.

3. **Calcium.** Taking calcium supplements or eating a diet high in dairy products can overwhelm your magnesium stores and lead to a relative magnesium deficiency state. When you reduce your calcium intake you may find that your AFib attacks diminish.

4. **Coronary artery disease.** CAD affects more than 15 million Americans, making it the most common form of heart disease causing arrhythmia, angina, and heart attack. CAD is mostly attributed to atherosclerosis, which happens when a waxy plaque made of cholesterol, fatty compounds, calcium, and a blood-clotting material called fibrin forms inside the arteries. However, coronary artery calcium is being investigated as a much more important cause of CAD. You can read about cholesterol and its treatment with statin drugs in Chapter 6.

   Magnesium is able to dissolve calcium, but when you don't have enough magnesium or when you take calcium supplements, eat a lot of dairy, or take high-dose vitamin D, you build up calcium deposits in the body, including in your arteries, creating CAD.

   Unabsorbed calcium precipitates in tissues, causing kidney stones, gallstones, heel spurs, and breast tissue calcification as well as coronary artery disease. On the other hand, if you take too much magnesium, it has a laxative effect, which aids in its elimination, so it does not build up in the body.

5. **Dehydration.** Adequate hydration with pure water is essential for proper blood circulation and heart function. However, when we purify water these days, we eliminate most of the good minerals along with the bad chemicals. So water and remineralization go together. I recommend drinking half your body weight (in pounds) in ounces of water and adding salt (unrefined sea salt, pink Himala-

yan salt, or Celtic sea salt—¼ teaspoon per quart), as well as ReMag and ReMyte for the best effect.

Alcohol, coffee, and heavy exercise (including hot yoga) are all dehydrating, and they all cause magnesium deficiency. Attacks of vomiting and diarrhea can also be dehydrating and deplete your minerals. Always carry a water bottle with salted water, ReMag, and ReMyte.

6. **Dental infections, fillings, crowns, and cavitations.** Biological dentists agree with Chinese medicine that each tooth corresponds to an acupuncture meridian. They will check to see if there is a problem with the teeth that are on the same meridian that flows through the heart. The testing instrument they use is called EAV. But you will have to do your research to find a reliable holistic physician or dentist who can do EAV.

7. **Diabetes.** This disease increases the risk of high blood pressure and heart disease. Blood sugar levels also influence heart rates.

8. **Electrolyte imbalance.** An imbalance of minerals such as sodium, potassium, magnesium, and calcium can alter the way the heart conducts electricity. Magnesium, at a concentration 10,000 times greater than that of calcium inside the cells, allows only a certain amount of calcium to enter to create the necessary electrical transmission, and then immediately helps to eject the calcium once the job is done. If magnesium is deficient, calcium accumulates in the cell, causing hyperexcitability, calcification and cell death. Because doctors don't regularly test for magnesium with an accurate blood test, they miss the importance of magnesium and focus on potassium and sodium instead.

9. **Gas, bloating, and hiatal hernia.** Mechanical pressure from the stomach and intestines pushing up on the

diaphragm, which is directly below the heart, can trigger an AFib attack. The pressure can come from a hiatal hernia or gas pressing on the heart and great vessels or irritating the vagus nerve. Avoiding sugar, alcohol, and gluten and treating yeast overgrowth can all help reduce gas and bloating. A chiropractor or naturopath trained in the technique of hiatal hernia adjustment can "pull down" a hiatal hernia using an external massage technique.

10. **Gluten and glutamate sensitivity.** This trigger for AFib may surprise you, but it's important to include it since more people seem to be reacting to this group of natural chemicals. I've written about this topic in an article, "Solving the MSG Problem with Magnesium," and include an edited excerpt here.[64]

MSG, gluten, glutamine, and glutamic acid are all in the same family and are all placing a strain on our magnesium stores. Wheat has been hybridized, which increases the gluten content. Glutamates such as MSG are used in most processed foods. But few people realize that the main reason we are becoming more gluten-sensitive and glutamate-sensitive is because we are all very magnesium-deficient.

MSG is difficult to avoid if you eat processed foods. Glutamate and glutamic acid are often considered substitutes for salt; the FDA categorizes them as "generally recognized as safe," or GRAS. Glutamic acid and glutamate in food can be metabolized into the equivalent of MSG and reach the brain and the heart—it just takes longer and makes it harder to track the cause of your brain rush or heart palpitations.

Glutamine is the most abundant amino acid in the body. Most glutamine is made and stored in muscles and lung tissue, and it helps protect the lining of the gastrointestinal tract. For that reason, some researchers have suggested that people who have inflammatory bowel disease (ulcerative colitis, Crohn's disease) may not have enough glutamine. This finding led to the widespread use of glutamine for leaky gut and all manner of intestinal imbalance. However, two clinical trials found that taking glutamine supplements did not improve symptoms of Crohn's disease.

And, as my friend Dr. Russell Blaylock wrote in his book *Excitotoxins: The Taste That Kills,* "high doses of the single amino acid glutamine will be converted into glutamate." A person who is low in magnesium will be unable to prevent glutamate from flooding into unprotected brain and heart cells.

Psychology Today published an article called "Magnesium: The Original Chill Pill."[65] The author discusses the relationship between magnesium and glutamate in brain neurons, saying that magnesium is found in the junction between two nerve cells along with calcium and glutamate. Magnesium is calming but calcium and glutamate are excitatory in their actions, and if they are in excess, they are toxic. Calcium and glutamate activate the NMDA receptor, whereas magnesium guards the receptor to keep out excess calcium and glutamate. If magnesium is deficient, there is no guard, no protection against too much calcium and glutamate. The author concludes, "Calcium and glutamate can activate the receptor like there is no tomorrow. In the long term, this damages the neurons, eventually leading to cell death. In the brain, that is not an easy situation to reverse or remedy."

What the author doesn't say is that the same mechanism is at play in the specialized cardiac cells that make up the electrical conduction pathways of the heart.

Many studies echo the *Psychology Today* summary of

magnesium's role in glutamate inhibition. Wikipedia shared the following: "Excessive synaptic receptor stimulation by glutamate is directly related to many conditions. Magnesium is one of many antagonists at the glutamate receptor, and magnesium deficiencies have demonstrated relationships with many glutamate receptor-related conditions."

I believe that the solution to food sensitivity is not to avoid more and more foods but to enhance the body's ability to handle these foods. Well-absorbed magnesium, multiple minerals, and unrefined sea salt, pink Himalayan salt, or Celtic sea salt in your drinking water help the underlying structure, function, and electrical activity of your body and allow your body to adapt to your environment and your diet. More is involved, of course, but begin with magnesium and then fill in the gaps with minerals, probiotics, methylated B vitamins, and taurine once you are saturated with magnesium.

Some individuals sensitive to MSG and glutamates find relief by taking taurine. The probable cause is that glutamate competes with the amino acid cysteine for uptake in the body. Cysteine converts into taurine; with too much glutamate, there won't be enough cysteine to make taurine. One result is heart irritability, since taurine helps regulate the heartbeat; it is an inhibitory neurotransmitter, has antioxidant activity, and helps make bile to digest fats. Taurine is found in my ReAline formula.

11. **Heart attack.** The heart is one big muscle. The highest amount of magnesium in the whole body is found in the heart. When magnesium is deficient, the heart muscle can go into spasm, causing angina or a heart attack. When a heart attack occurs, heart muscle cells die and are replaced with scar tissue. If that scar tissue is located in or around an area containing the heart's elec-

trical system, an arrhythmia can be triggered if the heart
is deficient in magnesium.

12. **Abnormal heart valves.** One type of heart valve ab-
    normality, mitral valve prolapse, is associated with mag-
    nesium deficiency. Without magnesium, the valve, which
    consists of two flaps coming together, becomes rigid and
    can't close properly, allowing leakage of blood through
    the partially open valve. If you have enough magnesium,
    the flaps of the valve are relaxed and close completely,
    preventing blood from escaping. Another type of abnor-
    mality is aortic valve calcification. Body parts do not cal-
    cify unless there is too little magnesium to keep calcium
    in solution.

13. **High blood pressure.** When the smooth muscles
    lining the blood vessels go into spasm from having too
    much calcium inside the cells and not enough magne-
    sium, the diameter of the blood vessels decreases and
    the blood pressure increases. Unfortunately, most pa-
    tients with high blood pressure are put on calcium chan-
    nel blocking drugs instead of the body's natural calcium
    channel blocker—magnesium. Calcium channel block-
    ers drain magnesium, as do most drugs, but diuretics
    drain magnesium even more. Most people end up on
    three or four drugs for blood pressure, which in many
    cases just worsen the problem because the drugs de-
    plete magnesium—thus making a person susceptible to
    AFib.

14. **Heart structural changes.** Changes in the heart's
    normal size or structure may affect its electrical system.
    Examples of such changes include an enlarged heart due
    to high blood pressure or advanced heart disease.

15. **The holidays.** You arrive at your destination tired and
    jet-lagged (travel is its own trigger, listed below), and if
    it's a gathering like Thanksgiving, you have all the stress-

ors of family interaction, overeating, too much alcohol, and not enough sleep.

16. **Hypoglycemia.** Low blood sugar can cause an attack of atrial fibrillation. When blood sugar drops below a certain level, mechanisms come into play that trigger the adrenal glands to release adrenaline in order to activate and release glycogen (sugar stores) in the liver. That same adrenaline surge can elevate the heart rate and trigger an AFib attack.

17. **Infections.** Viral infections cause fever, increase metabolism, and raise the heart rate. Infection with the bacterium *H. pylori,* which causes stomach ulcers, can contribute to AFib. Investigate mastic gum as a stomach ulcer treatment; it is highly effective and avoids the side effects of antibiotics. If you have stomach symptoms, you can rule out *H. pylori* infection by testing. What is the mechanism by which *H. pylori* triggers AFib? Some say this infection causes inflammation (indicated by an increase in C-reactive protein). We know that magnesium is a superb anti-inflammatory. The question arises—do these infections mostly occur in magnesium-deficient people? The answer is likely yes, because not everyone who has an infection suffers AFib.

18. **Inflammation.** High levels of CRP are a strong indicator of inflammation. CRP is twice as high in people with AFib compared to people without that condition. Magnesium is the body's most important anti-inflammatory nutrient.

19. **Lung disease.** People with asthma have a higher rate of AFib than those without. Asthma is a magnesium deficiency condition because the smooth muscles lining the bronchial tract go into spasm, cutting off the airways. A recent client told me her pulmonologist states that cough definitely can cause the arrhythmia but her cardiologist

says a cough absolutely cannot cause arrhythmia. She herself was unable to tell which came first, the cough or the arrhythmia. Neither of them mentioned that she could have vagus nerve irritation due to magnesium deficiency.

The vagus nerve and its branches innervate the trachea, lungs, heart, esophagus, and stomach. Thus a "trigger-happy" vagus nerve can cause you to cough as your heart beats erratically. I had those exact symptoms, which allows me to recognize them in others.

Another client told me that doctors thought she was crazy when she said a cold drink of water could leave her anxious and gasping for breath with an attack of arrhythmia. She was very grateful when I explained that her vagus nerve may be hyperirritable as a result of magnesium deficiency and could cause these symptoms when irritated by cold water or even cold food.

20. **Medications.** The list of medications that can cause AFib is very long, so I'm not going to include it here. You must look up the side effects of the medications you are on and see if atrial fibrillation is listed. The most bizarre one that I've found is flecainide, which is an antiarrhythmia drug—yet it causes fast, irregular, pounding, or racing heartbeat or pulse. I think it's because this drug contains six fluorine atoms, making it a fluoride compound. Fluorine binds irreversibly to magnesium, making it unavailable to the body. Paradoxically, digoxin, calcium channel blockers, beta-blockers, and anti-arrhythmia drugs can all worsen heart arrhythmia. Over-the-counter cough and cold medications are stimulants that can raise your blood pressure and increase your heart rate, which can trigger AFib. Recreational drugs such as marijuana can raise your heart rate for several hours. Cocaine can also trigger an abnormal heartbeat.

21. **Intense physical activity.** Doctors say that intense physical activity causes the release of adrenaline, which triggers AFib. The more likely cause is magnesium depletion, leading to heart spasms and AFib.

22. **Obesity.** Studies show that obesity can result in enlargement and stretching of the atria, which can trigger atrial fibrillation. There are reports that people who simply lose weight become free of their atrial fibrillation.

23. **Potassium deficiency.** Unlike magnesium deficiency, a deficiency in potassium may be found on a blood test. If you have low magnesium and low potassium, your potassium level won't improve when you take potassium supplements unless you also take magnesium. Because doctors don't use an accurate test for magnesium, they never find the underlying problem.

24. **Exposure to stimulants.** Artificial sweeteners such as aspartame (NutraSweet), sucralose (Splenda), and acesulfame potassium (Sunett) are stimulants, as are caffeine, cola, and tobacco. They can speed up your heart rate, and if you are also magnesium deficient, the two factors together can cause AFib.

25. **Sick sinus syndrome.** This condition is defined as improper functioning of the heart's natural pacemaker. This is another syndrome that is poorly understood. It is said to occur due to scarring, degeneration, or damage to the heart from aging, cardiovascular disease, heart attack, and high blood pressure. All these conditions are triggered or worsened by magnesium deficiency.

26. **Sleep apnea.** In my article "An Epidemic of Sleep Apnea," I associate the rise in sleep apnea with the increasing epidemic of magnesium deficiency and weight gain. Treating both can reduce the incidence of sleep apnea and that of AFib as well.[66]

27. **Stress that leads to anxiety and panic attacks.**
    Stress burns magnesium, which depletes the adrenal
    glands and leads to erratic firing of adrenaline, trigger-
    ing bouts of tachycardia and AFib. Stress in the form
    of a very active or scary dream can set off AFib. One
    client asked me why her AFib attacks usually hit her in
    the middle of the night. I told her that even dreams can
    trigger an adrenaline surge because the mind thinks you
    are "under attack." The adrenaline pumps your heart
    rate, which triggers an attack.

28. **Surgical procedures.** Heart surgery is a major trigger
    for atrial fibrillation. I think it's because the heart loses
    magnesium under that type of stress, and since IV mag-
    nesium is not a standard treatment during heart surgery,
    atrial fibrillation can be a direct result. However, even
    minor surgical or medical procedures can be a physical
    and emotional trigger. Just think of white-coat syndrome,
    where your blood pressure can soar and your pulse can
    increase when a doctor or nurse takes your blood pres-
    sure. Surgery can also expose you to medications that
    drain magnesium and leave you susceptible to AFib. In
    the presence of a magnesium deficiency, that racing and
    increased pressure can set off atrial fibrillation. Let your
    doctor know about your atrial fibrillation history before
    you have any medical procedure, even a minor one.

29. **High-sugar diet.** Sugar depletes magnesium, so high
    sugar intake will ultimately cause magnesium deficiency.
    Such a diet can cause episodes of low blood sugar. It can
    also contribute to obesity.

30. **An overactive thyroid gland.** Thyroid hormone
    regulates metabolism. If your thyroid gland produces
    too much hormone, or you are taking too much thyroid
    medication, your metabolism speeds up—and that in-

cludes heart rate. If you are also magnesium deficient, the two factors together can cause AFib.

31. **Travel.** The TSA, jet lag, dehydration, poor eating habits, problems sleeping, more alcohol than usual, late-night meals, and forgetting to take your magnesium can all combine to become one big trigger for AFib. Do your best to plan your trip to avoid stressors, and take more magnesium to counteract all the above.

32. **Vitamin D.** We've barely gotten the word out that calcium supplements carry a higher risk of heart disease and now doctors are pushing vitamin D as the next supplement fad. Yes, of course, vitamin D is necessary in the body, but they don't seem to realize that in high doses it pulls too much calcium into the body and requires more magnesium to convert it from the supplement form to the active form. I've had many people complain that when they begin taking high-dose vitamin D (above 2,000 IU per day) they experience magnesium deficiency symptoms. Some of these symptoms can be severe and very worrisome, especially when you don't know their origin.

33. **Yeast overgrowth.** This condition is the culmination of a high-sugar diet, too many antibiotics and steroid medications, and layers of stress that affect so many. Many practitioners and researchers also consider yeast the main cause of inflammation in our body. Inflammation can trigger AFib. Yeast produces 178 different metabolic by-products with far-ranging side effects. One of the by-products is alcohol. Dr. K. Iwata in Japan diagnosed "drunk" disease in people who had not consumed any alcohol but appeared to be intoxicated, and traced it to yeast overgrowth.

Another by-product of the digestion of sugar by yeast is acetaldehyde. It's also the main breakdown (oxidation) product of alcohol and is believed to be the actual cause of the many problems arising from excessive alcohol consumption. You may find that if you have yeast overgrowth and also drink alcohol, you are hit with a double dose of acetaldehyde hangover or brain fog.

I had no idea there were so many triggers for AFib until I began to do the research. This extensive list will have some people complaining that anything can cause AFib. But what I'm actually saying is that magnesium deficiency can cause everything and make it look like it's the fault of other conditions, for which you are given magnesium-draining drugs. It should come as a relief to you that your AFib is treatable.

NOTE: I never tell clients that they have to stop taking their AFib medications before starting to remineralize. People should feel better and have fewer and fewer symptoms before working with their doctor to wean off their medications.

CORONARY ARTERY CALCIUM IN AFIB

Allopathic medicine keeps finding more clues that magnesium deficiency is a cause of AFib. A recent study, "Coronary Artery Calcium Progression and Atrial Fibrillation," in the journal *Circulation: Cardiovascular Imaging*,[67] reported that "CAC [coronary artery calcium] progression during an average of 5–6 years of follow-up is associated with an increased risk for AF [atrial fibrillation]. The associated risk is greater in individuals with faster CAC progression." When they factored out all other possible causes, including cholesterol, the researchers found a 55 percent increased risk of AFib related to the buildup of calcium in the coronary arteries. This study truly confirms the role of calcium as a cause of AFib and, in my world, the treatment of AFib with magnesium. I've reported many times that magnesium dissolves calcium and directs it to the bones, where it is needed. If you

don't have enough magnesium to do that, calcium will precipitate into soft tissues, including blood vessels. Maybe this
study will also convince doctors that cholesterol is not the
bad guy in coronary artery disease—calcium is.

Of course, the researchers could not explain why elevated coronary artery calcium was associated with AFib.
Medscape reported on this study and commented that "inflammation could be the 'missing link' because chronic-low
grade inflammation causes atherosclerosis, which could lead
to atrial fibrosis."[68] More to the point, inflammation is a potent initiator of calcification,[69] which to me means that when
you are deficient in magnesium, calcium precipitates out into
arteries and other tissues. Researchers never mention that
the major cause of inflammation in the body is magnesium
deficiency in the face of calcium excess.

CORONARY ARTERY CALCIFICATION

What should clinicians do when a patient has an elevated
CAC score? Researchers even warn doctors not to screen for
CAC because they admit they have no effective therapies to
alter disease progression. A paper in the *Journal of the American College of Cardiology* concluded, "Despite promising early
data, such interventions (most notably with statin therapy)
have not been shown to slow the progression of CAC in any
randomized controlled trial to date. . . . Thus, routine quan-
tification of CAC progression cannot currently be recommended in clinical practice."[70]

In fact, another paper in the same journal found that
patients with coronary artery disease who take statins experience an increase in coronary calcification, an effect that is
independent of plaque progression or regression.[71] None of
this information stops doctors from using this ineffective and
harmful therapy to treat and prevent their favorite risk factor
for heart disease—elevated cholesterol. Doctors actually try

to defend statins by saying they are hard at work stabilizing plaque by converting softer, cholesterol-laden plaques that are prone to rupture into more stable calcified plaques that are relatively inert. Common sense should tell you that any buildup of calcium in the arteries is not a good thing. Unfortunately, because statins promote calcium buildup, the CAC score is now impossible to use as a means to follow the progression or improvement of coronary artery disease in people who take statin drugs.

Korean researchers found that low serum magnesium is associated with CAC in a Korean population at low risk for cardiovascular disease.[72] Of course they say that further studies are needed to confirm this finding and to verify the causal relationship between low serum magnesium and CAC. Nevertheless, it is a step in the right direction toward using magnesium as a first line of treatment to prevent CAC. Another study using a diet survey found that the less magnesium in the diet, the greater the coronary artery calcification.[73]

There is much more to the CAC story. Although they say they have no idea why, researchers report that CAC is associated with multiple age-related chronic diseases in the Multi-Ethnic Study of Atherosclerosis.[74] An elevated CAC score was associated with non-heart-related conditions such as cancer, chronic kidney disease, chronic obstructive pulmonary disease, and hip fractures. A CAC score of zero appears to protect a person from cardiovascular disease and other chronic diseases.

The story continues with a report that drinking at least one sugar-sweetened carbonated beverage per day may increase coronary artery calcium.[75] This study identified 22,000 adults in South Korea without prior coronary heart disease who consumed five or more regular soft drinks per week and had an elevated CAC score compared to those who did not consume soft drinks. The investigators concluded, "Our findings indicate that the cardiovascular hazards of carbonated-beverage consumption are evident even in the subclinical stages of atherosclerosis." This finding of coronary heart disease risk was added to the other risks ascribable to sugary beverages, including a higher risk of type 2 diabetes, obesity, and cardiovascular disease. One reason for the added risk is the extra magnesium that is required to metabolize sugar (as I mention in Chapter 8). Another is the high amount of phosphorus in soft drinks, a contributing factor in calcification.

While reading these studies and the Medscape article, I can be seen jumping up and down on the sidelines holding up a sign that says "Please Use Magnesium for the Therapeutic Treatment of CAC." A person with CAC needs therapeutic doses of magnesium to dissolve calcium in the arteries. However, I have found that magnesium supplements in high doses will cause a laxative effect before reaching therapeutic levels, except for ReMag.

DIET ADVICE FOR AFIB

Any mention of what to eat and what not to eat when you have a chronic health condition is fraught with inconsistencies and inaccuracies. My general diet recommendations are as follows:

- Eliminate alcohol, coffee, white sugar, white flour, gluten, fried foods, trans fatty acids (found in margarine and in baked, fried, and processed foods made with partially hydrogenated fats).
- If you eat animal protein, choose organically raised grass-fed beef, free-range chicken and eggs, and fish (especially wild-caught salmon).

- For vegetarian protein, choose fermented dairy, lactose-free cheese, and ReStructure Meal Replacement (it has no casein, very-low-lactose whey protein, and pea and rice proteins).
- Vegan protein choices include legumes, gluten-free grains, nuts, and seeds.
- Eat healthy carbs such as a variety of raw, cooked, and fermented vegetables, two or three pieces of fruit a day, and gluten-free grains.
- Include magnesium-rich foods listed in Appendix A and calcium-rich foods listed in Appendix B.
- For fats and oils, choose butter, olive oil, flaxseed oil, sesame oil, and coconut oil.

The above basic dietary advice can be followed by anyone with any chronic disease. However, in my AFib book, I created the following expanded diet guidelines and detailed explanation for AFib and other forms of heart disease, kidney disease, and most chronic disease in general:

1. **Salt.** The standard medical advice is to cut back on salt because it's supposed to cause high blood pressure. However, hypertension is still rampant in spite of decades of salt restriction. Also, doctors are talking about table salt (pure sodium chloride), which is nothing like the sea salt that our ancestors used.

   I do recommend limiting your intake of canned soups and processed meats because of the high sodium content, but also because they are so overly processed that there is barely any nutrition left. Instead of table salt, I recommend unrefined sea salt, pink Himalayan salt, or Celtic sea salt taken in drinking water. But many people are confused because they think salt is bad. Sea salt is very healthy because it includes seventy-two minerals; table salt is not healthy because it's refined and contains only sodium chloride.

Here are my water, sea salt, and mineral intake guidelines:

Water: Drink half your body weight (in pounds) in ounces of water. If you weigh 150 pounds, you will drink 75 ounces.

Unrefined sea salt, pink Himalayan salt, or Celtic sea salt: Add ¼ tsp to every quart of drinking water. To one of those bottles you will later add ReMag and ReMyte.

2. **Alcohol.** "Holiday heart syndrome," first described in 1978, is the name given to an attack of AFib coming after binge drinking. The risk for AFib is increased with moderate and heavy drinking. I think magnesium deficiency and yeast overgrowth make you doubly susceptible. If you have AFib, then the amount of alcohol you can safely drink is zero.

3. **Caffeine.** Caffeine has a stimulatory effect on the heart similar to alcohol. I agree with the medical recommendation that if you have AFib symptoms, it's wise to eliminate coffee and strong tea. Some large studies say that there is no association, but most of my clients say that caffeine speeds up their heart rate and they don't want to take the chance that it will trigger an AFib attack.

4. **Fruits and vegetables.** For a healthy heart and a healthy weight, fruits and vegetables provide the most nutrition, fiber, minerals, and vitamins for the least amount of calories. Eat organic as much as possible and aim for five servings of fruits and vegetables per day.

5. **Meat and dairy.** Doctors tell patients that in order to protect their heart they should avoid the saturated fats in butter, cheese, whole milk, ice cream, and fatty meats as well as processed and fried foods. I do agree with

avoiding ice cream, processed foods, and foods fried in vegetable oils. However, fermented dairy (yogurt, kefir) made from organic milk can be very healthy and provide you with natural probiotics. The latest high-protein diet, the Paleo diet, finds that a diet high in animal protein can be very healthy for weight loss and treating yeast overgrowth. But Paleo proponents definitely advise free-range sources to avoid the hormones and antibiotics fed to factory-farmed animals.

6. **Cholesterol.** Your doctor, bending to the prevailing attitude toward cholesterol, would have you limit your intake of eggs or just eat egg whites. Read Chapter 6 to find out why cholesterol is not the enemy. You can experiment with your diet and periodically do your own cholesterol testing through RequestATest.com. Order their Lipid Panel (cholesterol test, lipid test, FLP) for $29.

7. **Fish.** Fish oils from fresh fish have been shown to reduce the risk for heart disease. However, you also need to choose fish that are low in mercury. The Natural Resources Defense Council (NRDC) is a good resource. The NRDC's safe fish list includes anchovies, catfish, flounder, hake, haddock, herring, salmon, trout, whitefish, pollock, mackerel, sardines, and butterfish. NRDC says that farmed salmon should be avoided because it can contain high levels of PCBs.

8. **Whole grains.** Just when most of the natural health world is abandoning whole grains, the medical community is encouraging you to give up white bread for whole-wheat bread and pasta. My advice lies somewhere in between. I suggest that you avoid gluten-containing grains but hang on to millet, quinoa, brown rice, buckwheat, and amaranth. Oats do not contain gluten but they may be processed in facilities that also handle gluten, possibly becoming contaminated with molecules of

gluten and affecting people who have severe cases of gluten intolerance (celiac disease).

9. **Glutamate and MSG.** Remember what I said above about AFib triggers: glutamate and glutamic acid are considered GRAS substitutes for salt. It's important to avoid these additives, which are most often known as MSG. Because of the backlash against MSG, some companies are giving MSG different names. There is a very long list of MSG-contaminated foods at the MSGTruth website.[76] This is an active site that was created in 2002 by former food process engineer and food scientist Carol Hoernlein, who wants to tell the truth about food additives.

10. **Portion control.** The supersize servings that we get in restaurants and second helpings at home are the best way to gain weight. Smaller meals and waiting four to six hours between meals are both great weight-loss solutions. If your body wants some calories during that time, it will metabolize stores of glucose, called glycogen, from your liver. I call it liver-snacking!

11. **Cooking clean.** Steaming, roasting, broiling, and boiling keep you from frying with unhealthy vegetable oils. If you do want to sauté or fry an egg, use coconut oil.

12. **Diet and medications.** You may be told by your doctor that if you are taking warfarin (Coumadin), a blood thinner for your AFib, that you have to avoid green leafy vegetables because they are high in vitamin K, which can block the action of warfarin. Don't drink grapefruit juice or eat grapefruit when you are taking medications. Grapefruit juice contains a substance called naringenin, which can interfere with the effectiveness of antiarrhythmia drugs such as amiodarone (Cordarone) and dofetilide (Tikosyn). Grapefruit juice can also speed up certain

detoxification pathways in the liver and break down your medications more quickly, making them less effective.

13. **Magnesium.** It would be wonderful if we could obtain enough magnesium from our diet. However, that's just not possible because the soil is depleted of magnesium and no longer supplies our food with enough magnesium to cover our needs. Most people cannot eat 3.5 oz of kelp a day, and many consider 3.5 oz a day of nuts too fattening. That's why I advise taking magnesium in supplement form. See Chapter 18 for my recommendations.

14. **Potassium.** This electrolyte mineral is important, along with magnesium, for proper electrical transmission in the heart. Potassium deficiency is not common in people who eat vegetables daily. Deficiency can be created by the use of diuretics for high blood pressure, eating hospital food, taking medication, and prolonged periods of sweating, mostly in athletes. Chronic potassium deficiency can cause heart arrhythmia, low blood pressure, and constipation. For low blood levels of potassium, I recommend ReMyte and potassium broth (the broth recipe is in Appendix E).

MEDICAL TREATMENT OF PVCS

The Cardiac Arrhythmia Suppression Trial was a double-blind, randomized, controlled study designed to test the hypothesis that suppression of premature ventricular complexes with antiarrhythmic agents after a myocardial infarction would reduce mortality. The study ran from 1986 to 1998 and included more than 1,700 patients in twenty-seven centers.

The study used two treatment arms: encainide and flecainide or placebo, and moracizine or placebo. The investigators found that the drugs increased the death rate instead of lowering it, as was expected. Encainide was pulled from the marketplace in 1991 because it caused too many arrhythmias instead of preventing them. Moracizine was finally withdrawn from the market in 2007. Flecainide is still used, but I have personally red-flagged it because it's a fluoride compound with six fluorine atoms attached that can bind with magnesium, making it unavailable to the heart. Its side effects include tachycardia and arrhythmia.

Here is a detailed case history of a man in his late forties who began having symptoms when he was twelve. Just before our consult, he was making out his will and writing letters to his children because he was convinced he was dying.

While playing baseball around the age of twelve, after reaching to catch a ball my heart began beating very fast. I had to go to the emergency room and back then they couldn't do anything for me but wait out the attack. I was in tachycardia with my heartbeat in the 200s. It was scary. After twenty-four hours, with a priest's blessing, my heart went back to normal rhythm.

They sent me home to follow up with a cardiologist. He put me on Lanoxin 0.25 mg [which is not used in AFib anymore because it is linked with a higher risk of death] and a beta-blocker, Inderal 10 mg, at the ripe old age of twelve. I was also told to avoid all exercise.

Over the following years, I had periods of tachycardia that required medical attention in the ER. As the years went on they were able to stop the tachycardia with verapamil, a calcium channel blocker.

Eventually I changed cardiologists and was put on flecainide (Tambocor), which I now know is a fluoride compound and causes further magnesium depletion. I was advised to have an electrical heart study at Columbia Presbyterian in New York City. At this point it was

1995, I was thirty, and I had been on medication for eighteen years. Also, during this time I developed severe panic attacks, which are another symptom of magnesium deficiency probably caused by the flecainide robbing my body of magnesium. During that appointment at Columbia they identified an accessory nerve pathway that they said was causing the tachycardia and they did an ablation, which was successful. I was taken off all drugs and the doctors said I would not need them anymore.

In 2003, while working in the yard, my heart went into tachycardia again, and now they told me that sometimes ablation needs to be done again. This time I had it done at St. Michael's in Newark, New Jersey, and all went well. No more tachycardia and no more meds. However, I would still get PVCs [premature ventricular contractions] but no sustained tachycardia.

There were times over the years following the second ablation in 2003 that the PVCs would just start out of nowhere and stay for a few weeks, sometimes months. It was then I started looking at the Internet for some help and started taking magnesium in pill form. The magnesium seemed to improve my symptoms and I had very few PVCs.

Then, one day in 2014 I had an extreme urge to pee and after I did, the extreme urge did not go away. This went on for several weeks. I did go to a urologist, who checked my blood and prostate, and he said everything was normal. I also had an MRI that showed a very small stone in my ureter and he advised me to drink tons of water and eventually I think it passed. I realize now that kidney stones and perhaps slightly calcified bladder tissue led to these symptoms.

In retrospect, I realized that a short time before the

bladder symptoms and kidney stone episode, I had a doctor's appointment and he said I was low in vitamin D and recommended I take 4,000 IU. So I depleted my magnesium even more and my PVCs and spasms got much worse. I only took the vitamin D for a few months and without realizing why at the time, my PVCs were better after I stopped the vitamin D.

In the meantime, because my PVCs were worse, I went to the cardiologist and they admitted me to the hospital, where I had a stress test and a new echocardiogram. All was normal except for the PVCs, which occurred every third beat. It was so scary and frustrating. They prescribed metoprolol, a beta-blocker, and Cardizem, a calcium channel blocker, but they did not help.

It was at this time that I found Dr. Dean's website. I immediately ordered ReMag and began taking it. I felt some relief within the first day or two and after several days I was only getting the occasional spasm. At the same time, I went to see an arrhythmia specialist and he said that ablation would not be recommended for the PVCs. He prescribed flecainide but I would not take it because I learned that it's a fluoride drug that could further compromise my magnesium. I was already feeling better and feeling hopeful for the first time, and I know that magnesium is the missing link to my health.

I'm now twenty-six months into taking my ReMag, ReMyte, ReAline, and RnA Drops and I am no longer on any medication. Thank you!

MITRAL VALVE PROLAPSE

I mention mitral valve prolapse (MVP) in the list of atrial fibrillation triggers above, but certainly not everyone with

MVP develops AFib. Magnesium deficiency has been implicated in MVP, a disorder in which the mitral valve fails to
completely close off one of the heart chambers during heart
contraction. It is also called floppy valve syndrome. Blood
rushing through the open valve can be heard as a heart murmur with a stethoscope. When cardiac ultrasound became
more commonplace, the diagnosis of MVP escalated, especially in young women who went to their doctor because
they felt strange sensations in their heart.

There is no allopathic treatment for the condition, and
in mild and even moderate cases it rarely causes any symptoms. However, patients are given this diagnosis, which often
makes them feel they have a heart condition. Also, they are
warned that they should take antibiotics when having dental
work done, to prevent the possibility of bacteria from the
gums being picked up in the bloodstream and lodging on the
prolapsed valve, causing infection. This is a very rare occurrence and some doctors disapprove of this overuse of antibiotics, but it remains a potential liability threat to dentists
who don't warn and protect their patients. This overuse of
antibiotics has contributed to the overgrowth of yeast in the
population.

Dr. Melvyn Werbach, author of *Nutritional Influences on
Disease*, believes that MVP is overdiagnosed and also maintains it is a magnesium deficiency disease that is well treated
by magnesium. The valves of the heart are pulled tight by
muscles, which, like any other muscle in the body, depend on
magnesium for proper functioning. The mitral valve pro-
lapses because excess calcium relative to magnesium causes
it to go into spasm and not close properly, allowing back-
ward flow of blood, which is heard as a murmur.

Dr. Mildred Seelig reported that low magnesium levels
have been found in as many as 85 percent of MVP patients.[77]

Sixty percent of 141 individuals with strongly symptomatic MVP had low magnesium levels, compared to only 5 percent of the control group. Magnesium supplementation given for five weeks reduced the symptoms of chest pain, palpitation, anxiety, low energy, faintness, and difficulty breathing by about 50 percent in this group.[78] Many clients and customers have told me that their cardiologist could no longer detect an MVP murmur after they began taking supplemental magnesium.

AORTIC STENOSIS

From my medical training I always assumed aortic valve stenosis (AS) was a condition that had to be treated with surgery and was beyond the scope of nutritional medicine. However, AS is actually better defined as aortic valve calcification, where calcium deposits form on the heart's aortic valve. The narrowing that these deposits create is called stenosis, which reduces blood flow through the valve.

A 2013 study commented that AS is a common disease and valve replacement is the only established treatment.[79] However, the intent of this study was to investigate and characterize the mineral deposits in AS in order to understand the mechanism of aortic valve calcification and stenosis. Samples were taken from thirty aortic valves that had been surgically removed and replaced, and were analyzed using spectrometers. The removed aortic valves showed inflammation and deposits of calcium phosphate. When magnesium salts were introduced into the valve tissue in a test tube, the magnesium ions substituted for the calcium ions, removing calcium buildup. The investigators concluded, "Treatment of these patients with magnesium salts maybe could reduce the progress of aortic valve stenosis after valve replacement." And, I cry out in the wilderness, why not take magnesium supplements to prevent calcium from building up in the first place—why protect an artificial heart valve when you can protect the real thing?

All four heart valves—tricuspid, pulmonary, mitral, and aortic—can become calcified, but the aortic valve is affected the most.

CHELATION THERAPY

Alternative medicine could also make more use of magnesium in the treatment of atherosclerosis. Chelation therapy is an intravenous or oral treatment with a chemical, such as EDTA, DMPS, or DMSA, that pulls out heavy metals and (apparently) calcium from the plaque built up on the arterial walls. I think it's a very aggressive and expensive treatment that is more allopathic than alternative. I know a lot has been written about it and many people have benefited from chelation therapy, and I'm sorry to be so dismissive of it. It's because I feel it would make more sense and be much less expensive to take magnesium preventively, to keep calcium from building up in the first place. Balanced amounts of magnesium keep calcium dissolved in the blood and unable to deposit in arterial plaque or kidney stones and gallstones.

The downside of chelation therapy is that other minerals besides calcium will be removed and have to be replaced with IV minerals. My concern is that not all the minerals taken out are properly replaced, thus leading to long-term mineral deficiencies. With the availability of ReMag, which is even more effective than IV magnesium, and ReMyte, a completely absorbed multiple-mineral supplement, we have an alternative to chelation, and a safer addition to chelation therapy when that is needed.

DIET ADVICE FOR HEART DISEASE

Please follow the guidelines in the section "Diet Advice for AFib" earlier in this chapter.

SUPPLEMENTS FOR HEART DISEASE

- **ReMag:** With picometer, stabilized ionic magnesium you can reach therapeutic amounts without laxative effects. Start with ¼ tsp (75 mg) and work up to 2–3 tsp (600–900 mg) per day. Add ReMag to a liter of water and sip all day to achieve full absorption.
- **ReMyte:** Picometer twelve-mineral solution. Take ½ tsp three times a day, or add 1½ tsp to a liter of water with ReMag and sip throughout the day.
- **Vitamin E, as mixed tocopherols:** 400 IU twice a day, preferably Grown by Nature brand.
- **Crategus tincture:** 20 drops two or three times a day.

For high cholesterol and atherosclerosis add:

- **Niacin (vitamin B_3):** Begin with a dose of 250 mg a day and work up to a maximum of 4 grams daily under doctor's supervision. Do not use time-release niacin, which has been associated with liver damage.
- **ReAline:** B vitamin complex plus amino acids. Take 1 capsule twice per day. Contains food-based B_1 and four methylated B vitamins (B_2, B_6, methylfolate, and B_{12}), plus L-methionine (precursor to glutathione) and L-taurine (which supports the heart and weight loss).
- **Vitamin C complex:** 200 mg twice a day, from a food-based source, or make your own liposomal vitamin C (see Appendix D for a liposomal vitamin C recipe), and ascorbic acid, 1,000 mg twice a day.

- **Vitamin D$_3$:** 1,000 IU or 20 minutes in the sun daily or Blue Ice Royal (from fermented cod liver oil and butter oil) for vitamins A, D, and K$_2$, 1 capsule twice per day.
- **ReCalcia:** Picometer, stabilized ionic calcium, boron, vanadium. Take 1–2 tsp per day (1 tsp provides 300 mg calcium) if you don't obtain enough calcium from your diet. It can be taken with ReMag and ReMyte.

Obesity, Syndrome X, Diabetes

Obesity, syndrome X, and diabetes are part of a continuum of illness that may progress to heart disease if not headed off by good diet, supplements (especially magnesium), exercise, and stress reduction. They are not really separate diseases, as you may think, and underlying all this misery we find magnesium deficiency. In fact, there has been a recent addition to our medical vocabulary—*diabesity*. That word reflects the recognition that if someone is about thirty pounds overweight for more than a decade, diabetes will likely occur. People with syndrome X are obese, have insulin resistance that puts them on the road to diabetes, and also have hypertension, elevated cholesterol, and high levels of triglycerides.

Unfortunately, our current medical system has no interest in primary prevention. Doctors wait until your blood pressure is high, your cholesterol is elevated, and your blood sugar is above normal before they recommend drug therapy to suppress symptoms. Actually, they do talk more about prevention now, but that involves trying to talk patients into taking drugs to keep you from developing high blood pressure, high cholesterol, and high blood sugar.

I'm convinced that the billions spent on clinical trials for ineffective drugs could save millions of lives if spent on creating healthy, mineralized farmland, access to organic foods, popular exercise clubs, and a reduced workweek. But who am I kidding? That's not the way our capitalist, market economy runs. It's every person for him-/herself, which means you have to take very seriously what I'm telling you—magnesium deficiency is one of the, if not the, major causes of death and disability on the planet.

THREE THINGS YOU NEED TO KNOW ABOUT MAGNESIUM AND OBESITY

1. Magnesium helps the body digest, absorb, and utilize proteins, fats, and carbohydrates.
2. Magnesium is necessary for insulin to open cell membranes for glucose entry.
3. Magnesium helps prevent obesity genes from expressing themselves.

THE WEIGHT CONNECTION

Magnesium and the B-complex vitamins are energy nutrients: they activate enzymes that control digestion, absorption, and the utilization of proteins, fats, and carbohydrates. Lack of these necessary energy nutrients causes improper utilization of food, leading to such far-ranging symptoms as hypoglycemia, anxiety, and obesity.

Food cravings and overeating can be simply a desire to continue eating past the point of fullness because the body is, in fact, craving nutrients that are missing from processed food. You continue to eat empty calories that pack on the pounds but get you no further ahead in your nutrient requirements.

Magnesium is also necessary in the chemical reactions

that allow insulin to usher glucose into cells, where it is shunted into pathways that make energy for the body. If there is not enough magnesium to do this job, both insulin and glucose become elevated in the bloodstream outside the cells. That excess glucose gets stored as fat and contributes to obesity. Having excess insulin puts you on the road toward diabetes and tissue damage.

The connection between stress and obesity cannot be overlooked. The stress chemical cortisol signals a metabolic shutdown that makes losing weight almost impossible. It's as if the body feels it is under attack, such that it must hoard all its resources, including fat stores, and not let go of them under any circumstances. As you read in Chapter 3, magnesium can neutralize the effects of stress.

There is a flurry of research uncovering the inflammatory connection with obesity. The article "Recent Advances in the Relationship Between Obesity, Inflammation, and Insulin Resistance" provides an excellent overview.[1] I'll summarize the paper, which you can also read online. The authors say that current research shows that obesity is associated with chronic activation of the immune system, leading to low-grade inflammation of white adipose tissue, consequent insulin resistance, and impaired glucose tolerance, which can proceed to diabetes. Lab testing shows increased production of many different types of inflammatory molecules, which produce local and systemic effects throughout the body. These inflammatory markers decrease after weight loss—but not before they do damage to the body. One marker, interleukin-6 (IL-6), "may induce hepatic CRP [C-reactive protein] synthesis and may promote the onset of cardiovascular complications."

Numerous studies show that magnesium, with its antioxidant activity, lowers levels of the inflammatory markers CRP, tumor necrosis factor alpha (TNF-α), and IL-6.[2] It also supports adiponectin, a hormone made in fat cells that helps regulate inflammation within these cells and thus helps prevent weight gain, type 2 diabetes, and heart disease. As your weight increases, adiponectin levels go down; by contrast, weight loss helps boost adiponectin. A *Journal of Nutrition* study shows that magnesium is vital in maintaining adiponectin levels,[3] which is another reason magnesium is important for maintaining normal weight.

OBESITY, MORE THAN BAD GENES

The public has been told that obesity is inherited, which makes you think that you don't have a hand in creating this problem and can continue your bad habits and just blame your genes. However, you do have a role in creating this problem—and thus also in curing it.

Animal experiments show that if a mouse with an obesity gene is deprived of B vitamins, the gene will be expressed and the mouse will become obese. But if it is fed plenty of B vitamins, the gene will stay unexpressed and the mouse will remain thin. Every metabolic function in the body requires vitamins and minerals as metabolic cofactors; without them, symptoms develop. A 2014 study found that mice fed a fast-food diet—high in fat and sugar, low in fiber, B vitamins, and vitamin D—became obese and developed diabetes.[4] The investigators also found alterations in DNA methylation that can escalate into type 1 and type 2 diabetes.

The authors of a study published in the *American Journal of Clinical Nutrition* about magnesium's effect on genes reached several important conclusions.[5] One is that magnesium appeared to decrease fasting insulin concentrations. And here is their conclusion about the effects of magnesium on genes: "Gene expression profiling revealed up-regulation of 24 genes and down-regulation of 36 genes including genes related to metabolic and inflammatory pathways." Let me emphasize that the above study confirms that magnesium has an important effect on gene expression. This is a huge breakthrough in obesity research, but I imagine not many doctors have read this study or would begin using magnesium even if they had.

ABDOMINAL OBESITY

Gaining weight around the middle, aka belly fat, is related to magnesium deficiency and an inability to properly utilize insulin. It also sets the stage for syndrome X. You only need a tape measure to diagnose a predisposition to syndrome X—a waist size above 40 inches in men and above 35 inches in women puts you at risk.

In *The Magnesium Factor,* authors Seelig and Rosanoff present research showing that over half the insulin in the bloodstream is directed at abdominal tissue.[6] They theorize that as more and more insulin is produced to deal with a high-sugar diet, abdominal girth increases to process the extra insulin.

Most conditions associated with obesity are related to inflammation. A 2010 article "Magnesium, Inflammation and Obesity in Chronic Disease" brought in the magnesium connection.[7] The authors reported that people with moderate or even marginal magnesium deficiency exhibit chronic inflammatory stress, which may contribute "significantly to the occurrence of chronic diseases such as atherosclerosis, hypertension, osteoporosis, diabetes mellitus, and cancer."

SYNDROME X

Many believe that syndrome X is just another fancy name for the consequences of long-standing nutritional deficiency, especially magnesium deficiency. The set of conditions associated with syndrome X includes high cholesterol, hypertension, obesity, elevated triglycerides, and elevated uric acid.

High triglycerides are usually found when cholesterol is elevated and can be raised when someone is on a high-sugar diet, as with daily consumption of cakes, pastries, and sodas sweetened with high-fructose corn syrup. Even excessive amounts of fruit in the diet can elevate triglycerides.

High uric acid is due to incomplete breakdown of protein from lack of B vitamins and digestive enzymes. The complex of factors seen in syndrome X collectively appears to be caused by insulin resistance, which is a product of disturbed insulin metabolism (initiated by magnesium deficiency) and can eventually lead to diabetes, angina, and heart attack.

As previously noted, magnesium is required in the metabolic pathways, such as the Krebs cycle, that allow insulin to usher glucose into cells, where glucose participates in making ATP energy for the body. If magnesium is deficient, the doorway into the cells does not open to glucose, resulting in the following events:

1. Glucose levels become elevated.
2. Glucose is stored as fat and leads to obesity.
3. Elevated glucose leads to diabetes.
4. Obesity puts a strain on the heart.
5. Excess glucose becomes attached to certain proteins (the proteins become glycated), leading to kidney damage, neuropathy, blindness, and other diabetic complications.
6. Insulin-resistant cells don't allow magnesium into the cells.
7. Further magnesium deficiency leads to hypertension.
8. Magnesium deficiency leads to cholesterol buildup, and both these conditions are implicated in heart disease.

Syndrome X, according to Dr. Gerald Reaven, who coined the term, may be responsible for a large percentage of the heart and artery disease that occurs today. Unquestionably, magnesium deficiency is a major factor in the origins of each of the syndrome's signs and symptoms, from elevated triglycerides and obesity to disturbed insulin metabolism.[8, 9] As I've explained before, doctors do not learn about magnesium metabolism in medical school, so they remain oblivious to the effects of magnesium deficiency that can manifest as syndrome X.

INSULIN RESISTANCE

Insulin's job is to open up receptor sites on cell membranes to allow the influx of glucose, the cell's source of fuel. Cells that no longer respond to the advances of insulin and refuse the entry of glucose are called insulin-resistant. As a result, blood glucose levels rise and the body produces more and more insulin, to no avail. Glucose and insulin rampage throughout the body, causing tissue damage that results in overuse and wasting of magnesium, an increased risk of heart disease, and type 2 diabetes.

One of the major reasons the cells don't respond to insulin is lack of magnesium.[10] Studies do show that chronic insulin resistance in patients with type 2 diabetes is associated with a reduction of magnesium because magnesium is necessary to allow glucose to enter cells.[11] Studies also confirm that when insulin is released from the pancreas, magnesium in the cell normally responds and opens the cell to allow entry of glucose, but in the case of magnesium deficiency combined with insulin resistance, the normal mechanisms just don't work.[12] However, the higher the levels of magnesium in the body, the greater the sensitivity of the cells to insulin and the higher the possibility of reversing the problem.[13]

CARDIOVASCULAR METABOLIC SYNDROME (CVMS)

Dr. Larry Resnick of Cornell University, involved in heart and magnesium research for nearly thirty years, has another name for syndrome X: cardiovascular metabolic syndrome (CVMS), which was shortened to metabolic syndrome. Dr. Resnick is closer to the truth about this condition when he says it is characterized by a high calcium-to-magnesium ratio.[14] Remember, too much calcium automatically creates a magnesium deficiency.

Americans in general have a high calcium-to-magnesium ratio in their diet and consequently in their bodies. Finland, which has the highest incidence of heart attack in middle-aged men in the world, also has a high calcium-to-magnesium ratio in the diet: 4:1.8 (in part because Finland's cheese consumption is third-highest in the world—and cheese is very high in calcium).[15] The U.S. ratio in this study is said to be 3.5:1.

With a dietary emphasis on a high calcium intake without sufficient magnesium, according to magnesium expert Dr. Mildred Seelig, we will soon be faced with a 6:1 ratio in our population. The conventional recommended dietary ratio of calcium to magnesium, 2:1, has been debunked, as I have previously noted. To reverse syndrome X, it may be necessary to obtain 600 mg per day of calcium from dietary sources and 600 mg of magnesium in supplement form.

MAGNESIUM DEFICIENCY AND SYNDROME X

According to Dr. Resnick, syndrome X is caused not by chronically elevated insulin levels but by a low level of magnesium ions—because insufficient magnesium is the original cause of insulin resistance.[16] As previously explained, insulin opens the cells to glucose only if the cells have sufficient amounts of magnesium, and without magnesium, insulin resistance occurs. Studies clearly show that animals deprived of dietary magnesium develop insulin resistance, and the human population has the same risk.[17] Some researchers conclude that hypertension and insulin resistance may just be different expressions of deficient levels of cellular magnesium.[18] The various conditions that make up syndrome X, CVMS, or metabolic syndrome (its most recent designation) all have similar origins in magnesium deficiency. But most doctors separate all the risk factors and treat each separately with different drugs.

The magnesium deficiency in syndrome X comes from a combination of our magnesium-deficient diet and the well-documented loss of magnesium in the urine caused by elevated insulin. A vicious cycle creates further magnesium losses, causing more symptoms of syndrome X. In a fifteen-year study of 5,000 young adults, it was found that the more magnesium in the diet or taken as supplements, the lower the likelihood of developing metabolic syndrome.[19]

NOTE: To my mind, it's too confusing to have all these different names that mean the same thing: syndrome X, insulin resistance, cardiovascular metabolic syndrome, and metabolic syndrome. The reason none of them are household words or diagnostic criteria is because medicine doesn't have a drug to treat them. Allopathic medicine wants to label a disease and match it with a drug. Since these conditions are mostly related to lifestyle, diet, and mineral deficiency, with no one drug to treat them, they are, for the most part, ignored.

The cornerstone of both prevention and treatment of any of these syndromes is to restore magnesium to normal levels. Unfortunately, for many, the ravages of diabetes, hypertension, and high cholesterol have taken their toll. But even then, magnesium taken along with medications can play a beneficial role in controlling and reducing symptoms.[20, 21]

People often ask me, "How long will it take to get rid of my magnesium deficiency?" It's impossible to say because everyone's magnesium deficiency occurs for different reasons. However, a group of overweight individuals were given a daily 350 mg magnesium supplement for twenty-four weeks. Their serum magnesium levels increased and arterial stiffness was reduced.[22] Of note, testing at twelve weeks showed no change in serum magnesium; changes were only evident after six months. The authors conclude, "This gives some indication of the length of time it may take to increase a person's magnesium levels and their magnesium stores."

DIABETES

Diabetes has come up a lot in the above conversation about insulin resistance, syndrome X, CVMS, and metabolic syndrome, but let's focus on this condition specifically.

Diabetes is the seventh-leading cause of death in this country. There are 16 million diabetics in the United States, with the numbers increasing dramatically as the population gets older and as more young people succumb to a high-sugar diet.

There are two main types of diabetes. About 10 percent of diabetics are labeled type 1 and are dependent on insulin. Type 1 diabetes usually develops in children. They may have suffered a viral infection of the pancreas resulting in impaired or absent insulin production, and they require insulin injections to replace their loss.

Type 2 diabetics tend to be non-insulin-dependent, overweight, and between forty-five and sixty-five years old at onset. In type 2 diabetes, insulin is readily available—in fact, it is usually elevated—but the cells of the body appear to be resistant to it. Insulin is unable to do its job of opening up the cell membrane to allow the passage of glucose into the cell to create energy.

THREE THINGS YOU NEED TO KNOW ABOUT MAGNESIUM AND DIABETES

1. Magnesium deficiency is an independent predictor of diabetes.
2. Diabetics both need more magnesium and lose more than most people.
3. Magnesium is necessary for the production, function, and transport of insulin.

GESTATIONAL DIABETES

A third type of diabetes, gestational diabetes, is usually short-lived. This glucose intolerance may have been present subclinically before pregnancy but remained undetected. It usually develops due to the stresses of pregnancy and perhaps occurs more in women who are already magnesium deficient, because not every woman who gets pregnant develops gestational diabetes.

Ionized magnesium testing demonstrates the presence of magnesium depletion in pregnancy itself and to a greater extent in gestational diabetes. However, ionized magnesium testing remains available only as a research tool; the next best option is a magnesium RBC test, which is important in diagnosing magnesium deficiency in gestational diabetes. See Chapter 16 for more on magnesium testing.

Magnesium depletion, or relative calcium excess, may predispose women to vascular complications of pregnancy and needs to be addressed.[23] Intervention with magnesium supplements can greatly improve the outcome for both mother and baby. If the magnesium depletion continues throughout pregnancy, the woman can suffer preeclampsia or eclampsia (fluid retention, high blood pressure, seizures), which is effectively treated with IV magnesium.

DIABETES TYPE 1 AND TYPE 2

The signs and symptoms of diabetes are polydipsia (excessive thirst), polyuria (excessive urination), and polyphagia (excessive eating). In type 1 diabetes, weight loss may be the first sign, but type 2 diabetics are usually overweight. The excessive urination carries both sugar and magnesium out of the body. The excessive sugar, excreted through the urine and sweat, provides food for the yeast organism *Candida albicans,* resulting in rashes on the skin (especially under the breasts and in the groin area), yeast vaginitis in women, and yeast penile discharge in men.

Common complications of diabetes include nerve damage, called diabetic neuropathy, which mostly affects the feet, with symptoms of numbness, tingling, burning, and pain; atherosclerosis and heart attacks; damage to small blood vessels in the eyes and kidneys, causing vision loss (diabetes is the leading cause of blindness in the United States) and kidney disease; diabetic foot ulcers, with increased susceptibility to infection, gangrene, and amputation; and impotence in men. All these complications relate to magnesium deficiency and demonstrate the need for sensitive magnesium testing and magnesium supplementation for all diabetics.[24]

BEWARE THE POLYPILL

The American Heart Association (AHA) is very concerned about the increasing incidence of heart disease in diabetics. Their website reports the following statistics, confirming a strong correlation between cardiovascular disease and diabetes:

- At least 68 percent of people age sixty-five or older with diabetes die from some form of heart disease, and 16 percent die of stroke.
- Adults with diabetes are two to four times more likely to have heart disease or a stroke than adults without diabetes.
- The AHA considers diabetes to be one of the seven major controllable risk factors for cardiovascular disease.

The AHA lists the following risk factors:

- High blood pressure
- Abnormal cholesterol and high triglycerides
- Obesity
- Lack of physical activity
- Blood sugars too high, or out of normal range
- Smoking

What is the solution? Most doctors want to medicate diabetics to prevent heart disease and hypertension because that's what they are trained to do. The authors of a 2016 paper called "Usefulness of the Polypill for the Prevention of Cardiovascular Disease and Hypertension" want to create "a low-cost polypill containing four to five generic drugs with known effectiveness in the reduction of the CVRFs [cardiovascular risk factors]."[25] Taking drugs to prevent disease when those drugs have known side effects does not seem viable. The investigators even admit that they are getting only "fairly good results" with this approach.

"Fairly good results" does not give me any confidence that we should give four or five drugs to diabetics to prevent cardiovascular disease. I'm very concerned that the polypill will cause greater magnesium excretion and will be the actual cause of cardiovascular disease in diabetics. According to all the available scientific literature, including the over 600 references in this book, I think the polypill is the worst way to treat this condition, which should be addressed with diet, exercise, and magnesium.

MAGNESIUM PREVENTS AND TREATS DIABETES AND DIABETIC SYMPTOMS

A 2016 review paper gives an excellent summation of what we know about magnesium and diabetes.[26] The reviewers confirm that doctors have known for decades that magnesium deficiency has been strongly associated with type 2 diabetes. They know that if magnesium levels are low, the disease progresses rapidly, with a greater likelihood of complications. Research also shows that patients with low levels of magnesium have reduced pancreatic β-cell activity, therefore producing less insulin, and making the cells more insulin resistant.

They report that supplementation with magnesium improves glucose metabolism and insulin sensitivity. The many actions of magnesium are complex but include regulation of glucokinase, KATP channels, and L-type calcium channels in pancreatic β-cells, preceding insulin secretion. Also, the necessary addition of phosphorus to insulin receptors depends on magnesium, making it a direct factor in the development of insulin resistance.

This is not just a one-way relationship, because insulin is an important regulator of magnesium ion homeostasis. In the kidneys, insulin activates the renal magnesium channels that determine how much urinary magnesium is excreted. As a result, patients with type 2 diabetes and hypomagnesemia enter a vicious circle in which low magnesium causes insulin resistance and insulin resistance reduces serum magnesium.

The paper ends by providing "novel directions for future research and to identify previously neglected contributors to hypomagnesemia." After all that brilliant evidence showing the need for magnesium in diabetes, why can't the researchers just say, "Please take your magnesium"? In my opinion, there is no more need for costly research—that money would be better spent on handing out magnesium supplements to needy people.

There are so many papers that support the conclusions of this 2016 review that instead of discussing each study, I'll just list several references that you can read if you are interested.[27, 28, 29, 30, 31, 32, 33, 34, 35, 36, 37, 38, 39] I notice that many of these papers are written outside the United States, where people are falling into Western-style diets and lifestyle and developing chronic diseases such as diabetes, and doctors are trying to find out why.

NOTE: Please get in touch with me if any medical doctor ever tells you to take magnesium because of your diabetes. I'll regard that as a red-letter day, because I don't think doctors are paying any attention to magnesium research and applying it clinically.

The most important points regarding diabetes and magnesium are:

- Magnesium levels are low in diabetics.
- Diabetics are predisposed to heart disease, hypertension, obesity, insulin resistance, and high cholesterol.
- Magnesium prevents and treats heart disease, hypertension, obesity, insulin resistance, and high cholesterol.

There aren't many clinical trials studying the effects of magnesium supplementation on blood glucose levels. One 2015 clinical trial gave evidence that magnesium can lower glucose levels. It was a randomized double-blind placebo-controlled trial of 116 men and non-pregnant women, ages thirty to sixty-five, with low magnesium levels and newly diagnosed with prediabetes.[40] Subjects received either 30 mL of $MgCl_2$ 5 percent oral solution (equivalent to 382 mg of magnesium) or an inert placebo oral solution once daily for four months. Results showed that magnesium supplementation reduced plasma glucose levels and improved the glycemic status of adults with prediabetes and hypomagnesaemia. Hopefully these results will encourage doctors to advise magnesium supplementation for all their prediabetic and diabetic patients.

TYPE 2 DIABETES AND CHILDREN

Type 2 diabetes is increasingly diagnosed in younger people. One study said that young people accounted for 20 percent to 50 percent of new-onset diabetes patients.[41] Researchers suggest that this rise is a result of an increase in the frequency of obesity in pediatric populations. They write that obesity in youth has been increasing since the 1960s. The investigators offer no advice, just that more studies are required to determine the causes of these increases. Common sense tells us that kids sitting around all day on their cell phones, playing computer games, and ingesting junk food and sugary drinks gain weight, which puts a strain on their pancreas and leads to insulin resistance.

Dr. Milagros Gloria Huerta, an endocrinologist in Florida, has determined that magnesium deficiency is one reason for the increased incidence of diabetes. She and her team found that magnesium deficiency is associated with insulin

resistance in obese children. When checking the dietary intake of magnesium and serum magnesium levels, Dr. Huerta
and her colleagues tested obese and non-obese children and
found that obese children had lower dietary magnesium intake and lower serum magnesium compared to non-obese
children.[42] She concludes, "Magnesium supplementation or
increased intake of magnesium-rich foods may be an important tool in the prevention of type 2 diabetes in obese children."

DIABETIC COMPLICATIONS AND MAGNESIUM

Lack of magnesium increases the risk of cardiovascular disease, eye symptoms, and nerve damage in diabetics, whereas
supplementation can prevent them.[43, 44, 45] Most important
for diabetics is that insulin's main job requires magnesium,
and without magnesium, insulin is not properly secreted
from the pancreas, and what does get into the bloodstream
doesn't work correctly. Magnesium is also a necessary cofactor in the production of energy from sugar stores in the muscles and liver. That can explain why diabetics often complain
of low energy.

At the cellular level, magnesium is required to open pathways into the cell for the entrance of blood sugar. If magnesium is in short supply, sugar stays in the bloodstream, and
as it becomes elevated, symptoms of diabetes appear. One of
the symptoms of diabetes is copious urination; magnesium
levels are elevated in diabetic urine, which means greater
losses and more symptoms in a vicious cycle of depletion.

Studies show that even moderate improvement of blood
sugar control in patients with type 1 diabetes reduces the loss
of magnesium, increases serum HDL cholesterol (the "good"
cholesterol), and decreases serum triglycerides. These reductions in magnesium loss and serum triglycerides and the el-

evation of good cholesterol may reduce the risk of developing cardiovascular disease in patients with type 1 diabetes.[46]

HOW DID WE BECOME
A NATION OF DIABETICS?

In non-Western cultures, where most traditional diets are composed largely of unprocessed foods and are low in sugar, it takes only one generation of people eating a more typical Western diet high in sugar and refined flour to develop diabetes. This is true of people around the world, from the Inuit to secluded African peoples and people in India and China. The immediate advice given to a newly diagnosed diabetic is to stop eating sugar and other refined carbohydrates. It is only common sense that avoiding these unhealthy nonfoods as a preventive measure could greatly reduce the incidence of diabetes, yet the medical community has been slow to promote this advice.

Partly as a result of a poor diet, both obesity and type 2 diabetes are on the rise in children. In the last decade, soft drink consumption has almost doubled among kids, adding an average of 15 to 20 extra teaspoons of sugar a day just from soda and other sugared drinks. These all-too-popular beverages account for more than a quarter of all drinks consumed in the United States. More than 15 billion gallons were sold in 2000.[47] In 2011, the Beverage Marketing Commission reported that the average American drank 44 gallons of soft drinks, which is a decline from 1998, when we drank an average of 58 gallons.

A 2001 report by Dr. D. Ludwig in the prestigious medical journal the *Lancet* revealed that each additional soft drink a day gives a child a 60 percent greater chance of becoming obese.[48] In a commentary in the same edition of the *Lancet*, Dr. France Bellisle, of France's Institute of Health and Medical Research, said Ludwig's study provided convincing new evidence about the relationship between sugar and weight gain in children.[49] She said that before Ludwig's report, "many epidemiological studies [had] concluded that intake of carbohydrate (CHO) or even sucrose bears no relation with body adiposity. . . . [and that c]hildren and adults who ingest large amounts of CHO, sucrose, or both are leaner than their peers." Past research, most of it funded by the sugar industry, continually put the blame of childhood obesity on lack of exercise. The worst that sugar could do, they said, was cause dental cavities.

I consider it quite unfortunate that it took so long for the first study on sugar and weight gain to be funded and published. Too many children and adults are already addicted to sugar, and there is no turning back.

After Ludwig's research, a flurry of studies and a 2016 meta-analysis came to the same conclusion: "Our systematic review and meta-analysis of prospective cohort studies and [randomized controlled trials] provides evidence that [sugar-sweetened beverage] consumption promotes weight gain in children and adults."[50] However, the researchers offered no solutions.

LABORATORY FINDINGS IN DIABETES

- Blood glucose greater than or equal to 200 mg/dL (11.1 mmol/L) two hours after an oral dose of 75 g of glucose dissolved in water
- Incidental blood glucose greater than or equal to 200 mg/dL (11.1 mmol/L) in someone with signs and symptoms of diabetes
- High cholesterol and low HDL levels
- Low magnesium levels in the blood

We know from other important research that obese children develop insulin resistance, a precursor to diabetes, fifty-three times more frequently than normal kids. The CDC's webpage on childhood obesity quoted 2012 statistics saying that:

- Childhood obesity had more than doubled in children and quadrupled in adolescents over the previous thirty years.
- The percentage of U.S. children ages six to eleven who were obese increased from 7 percent in 1980 to nearly 18 percent in 2012.
- The percentage of adolescents ages twelve to nineteen who were obese increased from 5 percent to nearly 21 percent over the same period.
- In 2012, more than one-third of children and adolescents were overweight or obese.

We are eating more and more sugar per person each year, so it is no wonder that more and more people are developing symptoms of diabetes and insulin resistance and suffering from magnesium deficiency. Dr. Mehmet Oz, in his book *You on a Diet*, says, "The average person consumes 150 pounds of sugar per year—compared to just 7½ pounds consumed on average in the year 1700. That's 20 times as much! When typical slightly overweight people eat sugar, they on average store 5 percent as ready energy to use later, metabolize 60 percent and store a whopping 35 percent as fat that can be converted to energy later." Even more shocking are studies in both animals and healthy adults that demonstrate a greatly depressed immune response to infection that lasts for more than five hours after the ingestion of 20 teaspoons of sugar.[51, 52, 53]

Part of the danger with sugar is that you may not even realize how much you are ingesting. On ingredient labels, the measurements are given in grams. However, most Americans think in teaspoons, so our eyes may not even register the amounts. People are stunned when told that there are 8 to 10 teaspoons of sugar in an ordinary soda (1 tsp of sugar is equivalent to 4.2 g). Even more shocking is the amount of sugar found in most single servings of sweetened yogurt, which most people think of as a health food.

Sugar overload can cause magnesium deficiency in several ways. Processed sugar is devoid of vitamins and minerals, leaving empty calories that provide no valuable nutrients. Nutritional research reported by Dr. Abram Hoffer (the originator, with Linus Pauling, of orthomolecular medicine) shows that the refining of sugar removes 93 percent of chromium, 89 percent of manganese, 98 percent of cobalt, 83 percent of copper, 98 percent of zinc, and 98 percent of magnesium. All these minerals are essential to life. In addition, the body has to tap into its own reserves of minerals and vitamins to ensure sugar's digestion.

According to Natasha Campbell-McBride in her book *Gut and Psychology Syndrome,* twenty-eight atoms of magnesium are required to process one molecule of glucose.[54] If you are trying to break down a molecule of fructose, you need fifty-six atoms of magnesium. That's an extremely unbalanced and unsustainable equation. Inability to utilize sugar results in the formation of an excess of products such as pyruvic acid and other sugars that accumulate in the brain, nervous system, and red blood cells where they interfere with cell respiration and hasten degenerative disease.

Adding sugar to the diet also produces an excessively acid condition in the body. To neutralize acidity, the body has to draw upon its stores of the alkaline minerals magnesium, calcium, and potassium. If the acidic condition is severe, magnesium and calcium may even be taken from the bones and teeth, which can lead to tooth decay and softening, and ultimately osteoporosis.

In summary, magnesium plays a pivotal role in the secretion and function of insulin; without it, diabetes is inevitable. Measurable magnesium deficiency is common in diabetes and in many of its complications, including heart disease, eye damage, high blood pressure, and obesity. When the treatment of diabetes includes magnesium, these problems are prevented or minimized.[55] We also know that magnesium-rich water in certain communities confers a protective effect against diabetes.[56, 57]

Magnesium supplementation improves insulin response, improves glucose tolerance, and reduces the stickiness of red blood cell membranes. Magnesium is also essential in the treatment of peripheral vascular disease associated with diabetes.[58] With long-term damage, however, many symptoms may be irreversible, even with adequate magnesium and associated nutrients.

DIET ADVICE FOR DIABETES

Any mention of what to eat and what not to eat when you have a chronic health condition is fraught with inconsistencies and inaccuracies. My general diet recommendations are as follows:

- Eliminate alcohol, coffee, white sugar, white flour, gluten, fried foods, trans fatty acids (found in margarine and in baked, fried, and processed foods made with partially hydrogenated fats).
- If you eat animal protein, choose organically raised grass-fed beef, free-range chicken and eggs, and fish (especially wild-caught salmon).

- For vegetarian protein, choose fermented dairy, lactose-free cheese, and ReStructure Meal Replacement (it has no casein, very-low-lactose whey protein, and pea and rice proteins).
- Vegan protein choices include legumes, gluten-free grains, nuts, and seeds.
- Eat healthy carbs such as a variety of raw, cooked, and fermented vegetables, two or three pieces of fruit a day, and gluten-free grains.
- Include magnesium-rich foods listed in Appendix A and calcium-rich foods listed in Appendix B.
- For fats and oils, choose butter, olive oil, flaxseed oil, sesame oil, and coconut oil.
- Use the safe sugar substitute stevia. It's made from the leaves of a plant that grows in South America. You can find it in health food stores or online.
- Don't use the sugar substitute aspartame, which can worsen blood sugar control and cause weight gain, headaches, nerve damage, and eye damage because it is made partly from wood alcohol, which breaks down into formaldehyde.
- Fiber, from sources such as oat bran, flaxseed, and apples, has a positive effect on keeping blood sugar balanced.
- Alternative medicine practitioners recommend that you identify any existing food allergies by eliminating likely suspects (dairy, gluten, corn) from the diet for a week and then eating several meals of one of the suspected foods in one day to test your reaction and your blood sugar, which will be elevated if you are allergic.

Warning: Do not test meals consisting of foods to which you have reacted strongly in the past. Simply keep avoiding them.

SUPPLEMENTS FOR DIABETES

- **ReStructure Protein Powder:** A low-glycemic, whey, pea, and rice protein powder, complex carb, and fat-balanced meal replacement. Use 1–2 servings per day.
- **ReMag:** With picometer, stabilized ionic magnesium you can reach therapeutic amounts without laxative effects. Start with ¼ tsp (75 mg) and work up to 2–3 tsp (600–900 mg) per day. Add ReMag to a liter of water and sip all day to achieve full absorption.
- **ReMyte:** Picometer twelve-mineral solution. Take ½ tsp three times a day, or add 1½ tsp to a liter of water with ReMag and sip throughout the day.
- **ReCalcia:** Picometer, stabilized ionic calcium, boron, vanadium. Take 1–2 tsp per day (1 tsp provides 300 mg calcium) if you don't obtain enough calcium from your diet. It can be taken with ReMag and ReMyte.
- **ReAline:** B vitamin complex plus amino acids. Take 1 capsule twice per day. Contains food-based B_1 and four methylated B vitamins (B_2, B_6, methylfolate, and B_{12}), plus L-methionine (precursor to glutathione) and L-taurine (which supports the heart and weight loss).
- **Vitamin E, as mixed tocopherols:** 400 IU twice a day.
- **Vitamin C complex:** 200 mg twice a day, from a food-based source, or make your own liposomal vitamin C (see Appendix D for a liposomal vitamin C recipe), and ascorbic acid, 1,000 mg twice a day.
- **Vitamin D_3:** 1,000 IU or 20 minutes in the sun daily; Blue Ice Royal (from fermented cod liver oil and butter oil) for vitamins A, D, and K_2, 1 capsule twice per day.
- **Omega-3 fatty acids:** 3 g daily.
- **Garlic:** 1 or 2 cloves daily.

9

PMS, Dysmenorrhea, Menopause, PCOS

Maureen didn't know what came over her every month, but she would get anxious and irritable and go on a chocolate binge. She tried to keep it to herself, but lately the other women at work had begun to make not-so-subtle comments and tease her about her "evil twin." Then Anna sat with her over lunch one day and told her about a support group she was leading for women with premenstrual syndrome. One of their self-help methods was to keep a journal of symptoms.

Maureen's journal for the next couple of months clearly showed that her symptoms of anxiety, fluid retention, sugar and chocolate cravings, mood swings, irritability, bloating, edema, headache, and sore breasts escalated before her pe-riod and lifted the minute her period began.

Taking magnesium supplements may be the solution for PMS, advises Melvyn Werbach, M.D. One study showed that of 192 women taking 400 mg of magnesium daily for PMS, 95 percent experienced less breast pain and had less weight gain, 89 percent suffered less nervous tension, and 43 percent had fewer headaches.[1] Dr. Werbach and several other researchers also advise that women should take 50 mg of vitamin B_6 daily with the magnesium to assist in magne-sium absorption. However, I'm not in favor of high-dose B vitamins because they are all synthetic. I would rather see people take methylated B vitamins, like the ones found in my ReAline product, or food-based B vitamins or nutritional yeast flakes, which are high in B vitamins.

Magnesium RBC tests show low levels of magnesium in women with PMS.[2] Even serum magnesium levels, which are low only when there is a severe magnesium deficiency, diminished significantly in the premenstrual week in a group of forty women.[3] In a small trial of thirty-two women, oral magnesium was found to be an effective treatment for pre-menstrual symptoms related to mood changes.[4] Treatment with magnesium eases headaches, sugar cravings, low blood sugar, and dizziness related to PMS.[5, 6]

In another innovative research study, magnesium ion levels were tested at several times during normal menstrual cycles to determine magnesium and calcium levels in rela-tion to menstrual phases.[7] There was a comparatively high magnesium ion level in the first week after the onset of the period, a statistically significant decrease in magnesium ions midcycle, around the time of ovulation, and a large decrease in ionized magnesium and serum magnesium when the serum progesterone concentration peaked in the third week.

There was also a significant increase in the serum calcium-to-magnesium ratio both at the time of ovulation and in the fourth week after the onset of the period. That calcium-to-magnesium imbalance can cause premenstrual symptoms during the last week of the menstrual cycle. The good news is that you can take care of PMS easily with the right amounts of calcium and magnesium. For most women this translates into 500–700 mg calcium (from dietary sources) and 600–900 mg of magnesium a day in divided doses. Calcium food sources include dairy, greens, whole grains, nuts, seeds, and bone broth (see Appendix C). If you don't eat dairy and can't get enough calcium from food, you can get 300–600 mg of calcium from ReCalcia.

An elegant study demonstrates that estrogen and progesterone, the female sex hormones, influence magnesium ion levels in the body, which may help explain why magnesium relieves symptoms of PMS, including migraine, bloating, and edema.[8]

Exposure of cultured smooth muscle cells from brain blood vessels to a low concentration of estrogen did not interfere with the level of magnesium ions. However, exposure to increased concentrations of estrogen induced significant loss of magnesium ions. At the highest concentration, the level of magnesium ions decreased approximately 30 percent in comparison with controls. Exposure of the cultured cells to a low concentration of progesterone resulted in an increased level of magnesium ions. However, when these cells were exposed to higher concentrations of progesterone, cellular levels of magnesium ions decreased significantly. The higher the estrogen or progesterone concentration, the lower the levels of magnesium ions.

The data in this experiment indicate that the normally low concentrations of the female sex hormones estrogen and progesterone help cerebral vascular smooth muscle cells sustain normal concentrations of magnesium ions, which are beneficial to vascular function, whereas high levels of estrogen and progesterone significantly deplete magnesium ions, possibly resulting in cerebral vessel spasms and reduced cerebral blood flow—thus leading to premenstrual syndrome, migraine, and possible risk of stroke. These findings help to explain why more women than men suffer migraines and why migraines occur more frequently in the second half of the menstrual cycle, when estrogen and progesterone are both elevated. It stands to reason that elevated levels of progesterone and estrogen in the birth control pill can cause magnesium depletion and a similar list of symptoms.

The late Guy Abraham, M.D., an obstetrician and gynecologist, was a widely published author who pursued major research on premenstrual syndrome. Dr. Abraham identified four types of PMS, each of which has distinct characteristics related to hormonal fluctuations. Unfortunately, his criteria are not widely recognized.

1. PMS-A (anxiety): Symptoms of mood swings, nervous tension, irritability, and anxiety. Related to high estrogen, low progesterone.
2. PMS-C (craving): Symptoms of increased appetite, headache, fatigue, dizziness, fainting, and palpitations. Related to increased carbohydrate intake and decreased prostaglandin E1–type foods (from fish, nuts, seeds).
3. PMS-D (depression): Symptoms of depression, crying, forgetfulness, confusion, insomnia, and excess hair growth. Related to low estrogen, high progesterone, elevated testosterone.
4. PMS-H (hyperhydration): Symptoms of fluid retention,

weight gain, swollen extremities, breast tenderness, abdominal bloating. Related to excess aldosterone (a kidney hormone that causes fluid retention).

Maureen had symptoms from three of the four groups. Her successful treatment involved balancing hormones and replacing deficient nutrients. She began to take a daily tablespoon of flaxseed oil, which contains omega-3 essential fatty acids, along with magnesium, vitamin B$_6$, and increased her dietary calcium. Essential fatty acids are necessary building blocks for hormone production as long as they have magnesium and B vitamins as cofactors.

PMS AND DEPRESSION

Women can get depressed before their period, but it's a biochemical depression caused by fluctuating hormones and magnesium deficiency. Yet PMS is usually considered by medical doctors and pharmaceutical companies to be a psychiatric condition suitable for treatment with selective serotonin reuptake inhibitors such as fluoxetine (Prozac, Sarafem).

Remember, a lack of fluoxetine does not cause PMS symptoms; a lack of magnesium does. The replacement of magnesium in the body will treat PMS and cause no side effects. In fact, it has also been found that magnesium relieves the depression of premenstrual syndrome by positively influencing serotonin activity naturally. Sarafem can make no such claim. There is more to the Sarafem story, however. It is a fluoride drug with three fluorine ions in every molecule of Sarafem. When Sarafem breaks down in the body, it can release fluorine ions that can bind with magnesium and make the symptoms of PMS worse. What some people say about the effects of these drugs is that they don't take away your symptoms; they just make you not care about them anymore!

DIET ADVICE FOR PMS

Any mention of what to eat and what not to eat when you have a chronic health condition is fraught with inconsistencies and inaccuracies. My general diet recommendations are as follows:

- Eliminate alcohol, coffee, white sugar, white flour, gluten, fried foods, and trans fatty acids (found in margarine and in baked, fried, and processed foods made with partially hydrogenated fats).
- Limit animal protein, especially the week before your period. Red meat contains arachidonic acid, which suppresses progesterone production and causes symptoms of inflammation that worsen PMS and can lead to painful periods. When you do eat animal protein, choose organically raised grass-fed beef, free-range chicken and eggs, and fish (especially wild-caught salmon). Estrogen dominance can occur when you eat, drink, or breathe in synthetic hormones, pesticides, or other chemical residues that mimic estrogen.
- For vegetarian protein, choose fermented dairy, lactose-free cheese, and ReStructure Meal Replacement (it has no casein, very-low-lactose whey protein, and pea and rice proteins).
- Vegan protein choices include legumes, gluten-free grains, nuts, and seeds.
- Healthy carbs include raw, cooked, and fermented vegetables, and two or three pieces of fruit a day.
- Essential fatty acids—from food sources: fish, nuts, and seeds, including flaxseed—are much healthier than from

processed supplements. They help prevent PMS, unless you have a magnesium deficiency. Without magnesium, essential fatty acids are not metabolized properly and are not able to calm the irritability and inflammation of PMS and painful periods.

- For fats and oils, choose butter, olive oil, flaxseed oil, sesame oil, and coconut oil.

A diet survey comparing PMS sufferers with women without PMS showed that the PMS group had an extremely high intake of sugar, more carbs, more dairy, more sodium, and less magnesium, zinc, and iron with the following percentages:[9]

- 275 percent higher in refined sugar
- 79 percent higher in dairy products
- 78 percent higher in sodium
- 77 percent lower in magnesium
- 63 percent higher in refined carbohydrates
- 53 percent lower in iron
- 52 percent lower in zinc

Ounce for ounce, chocolate has more magnesium than any other food, and the irresistible urge to consume chocolate is a sure sign of magnesium deficiency. Premenstrual chocolate craving is widespread because magnesium is at its lowest around the time of a woman's menses. The answer is not to eat more chocolate laced with sugar and fat, however, but to increase magnesium intake by eating raw cacao, more nuts, whole grains, seafood, and green vegetables, and by taking magnesium supplements. The chocolate cravings will vanish when there is enough magnesium in the diet. Then you can just be a chocolate lover and enjoy my recipe for Chocolate Frozana.

CHOCOLATE FROZANA

1 tbsp cacao powder
2 tbsp coconut oil
¼ tsp Just Like Sugar, stevia, or maple syrup powder
Six 2-inch pieces of frozen banana

Mix the first three ingredients in a small shallow dish and drop in a 2-inch piece of frozen banana and coat. You can coat the banana once or several times. The oily cacao will harden immediately around the frozen banana. Repeat with the remaining banana pieces. You can either eat immediately or return to the freezer for another time—if you can wait that long! It's crunchy, creamy and so tasty. You could also add grated coconut or crushed nuts to the chocolate sauce for even more enjoyment.

SUPPLEMENTS FOR PMS

- **ReMag:** With picometer, stabilized ionic magnesium you can reach therapeutic amounts without laxative effects. Start with ¼ tsp (75 mg) and work up to 2–3 tsp (600–900 mg) per day. Add ReMag to a liter of water and sip all day to achieve full absorption.
- **ReMyte:** Picometer twelve-mineral solution. Take ½ tsp three times a day, or add 1½ tsp to a liter of water with ReMag and sip throughout the day.
- **ReCalcia:** Picometer, stabilized ionic calcium, boron, vanadium. Take 1–2 tsp per day (1 tsp provides 300 mg calcium) if you don't obtain enough calcium from your diet. It can be taken with ReMag and ReMyte.
- **ReAline:** B vitamin complex plus amino acids. Take 1 capsule twice per day. Contains food-based B_1 and four methylated B vitamins (B_2, B_6, methylfolate, and B_{12}), plus L-methionine (precursor to glutathione) and L-taurine (which supports the heart and weight loss).

- **Vitamin E, as mixed tocopherols:** 400 IU daily, preferably Grown by Nature brand.
- **Essential fatty acids (EFA):** I recommend a combination: (1) Blue Ice Royal (from fermented cod liver oil and butter oil), for vitamins A, D, and K_2, 1 capsule twice per day; (2) flaxseed oil, 1 tbsp twice per day (store the bottle in the freezer); (3) wild-caught fish.
- **Milk thistle:** 250 mg three times a day, to detox the liver.
- **Progesterone cream:** Before using progesterone cream, have a naturopathic or holistic doctor evaluate your hormones by testing saliva levels. Retest every three to six months to avoid overdosing, which can deplete magnesium.

DYSMENORRHEA (PAINFUL PERIODS)

Calcium can act like a painkiller and muscle relaxant, but it might be that it accomplishes this by driving magnesium out of the cells and into the bloodstream to balance out the extra calcium. While in the bloodstream, it is then directed toward ailing tissues to treat pain. So taking calcium can alleviate menstrual cramps—until eventually you become even more magnesium-depleted. However, taking magnesium without calcium before your period may forestall the pain altogether. A series of European studies with small groups of women who suffered painful periods consistently showed relief of symptoms when they took high doses of magnesium.[10, 11, 12]

Take 600 mg of dietary calcium along with 600 mg of supplemental magnesium, preferably therapeutic, non-laxative ReMag. I favor food sources of calcium or my Re-Calcia because, in general, calcium supplements are poorly absorbed, at the cellular level. Therefore, they often end up precipitating out into soft tissue, organs, and arteries causing calcification in such conditions as atherosclerosis, gallstones, kidney stones, breast tissue calcification, and fibromyalgia.

Extra magnesium can also be taken when the pain is at its worst (300 mg several times a day for a total of 900–1,200 mg). Or put 3 tsp (900 mg) of ReMag in a liter bottle of sea-salted water and sip throughout the day. See more about magnesium therapy in Chapter 18.

Some women find that decreasing their intake of red meat before their period helps prevent cramps. What may not be obvious is that when you cut back on meat you have a better chance of eating more magnesium-rich foods that will ease symptoms of painful periods.

MAGNESIUM AND MENOPAUSE

At a time when all menopausal women are only told to take lots of calcium supplements, the following report offers great hope. A reader of my blog wrote to me about her experience with magnesium and menopause. She said that in her research she found that most of the thirty-four symptoms of menopause are actually identical to the symptoms of magnesium deficiency. So she put herself on a magnesium supplementation regime.

Within three days she began to feel more normal. Her daytime hot flashes had dropped from twenty or so a day to fewer than ten, and they were milder. Her episodes of night sweats fell from more than ten per night to three or less. Her insomnia disappeared and her terrible anxiety, rapid heartbeat, and depression all started to fade away, as did skin-crawling sensations and aches and pains. Having suffered progressively with worsening symptoms since entering menopause three years prior, she said that ten days after starting supplementation she was basically symptom free. She ended by saying, "Magnesium is a miracle, and everyone, particularly menopausal women, should be made aware of it." Unfortunately, when women of menopausal age are prescribed calcium and no magnesium, their menopausal symptoms can become worse.

POLYCYSTIC OVARIAN SYNDROME

Polycystic ovarian syndrome (PCOS) patients have a high incidence of insulin resistance and glucose intolerance—two clear symptoms of magnesium deficiency. In a recent telephone consultation, a young woman told me she had been advised to go on a drug for diabetes, not because she has diabetes but because she has PCOS and the drugs were supposed to lower her insulin resistance. PCOS patients also tend to be at risk for hypertension, diabetes, and heart disease.

Since a low magnesium ion level and a high calcium-to-magnesium ratio are associated with insulin resistance, cardiovascular problems, diabetes mellitus, and hypertension, a study was done with a group of PCOS patients to determine the effects of magnesium intervention. Significantly lower levels of ionized magnesium and serum magnesium and a significantly higher calcium-ion-to-magnesium-ion ratio were found in the PCOS patients compared with the controls, which gave me enough evidence to recommend she speak to her doctor about taking a magnesium supplement of at least 300 mg twice per day to treat her insulin resistance and possibly her PCOS as well.[13]

Infertility, Pregnancy, Preeclampsia, Cerebral Palsy

Advice passed down through generations of midwives includes giving Epsom salts (magnesium sulfate) throughout pregnancy. Therefore, it comes as no surprise that magnesium is an important part of the whole miracle of ushering new life into the world. Conception, pregnancy, and delivery are times when nature, nutrients, and nurturing are the prescription, not drug intervention. I learned this important lesson from the astonishing results in the delivery suite when IV magnesium was used to stop eclamptic fluid retention, high blood pressure, and seizures. This powerful yet safe natural medicine can do much more than we currently allow.

INFERTILITY

The Pottenger Cat Study is very instructive on the absolute requirement for good nutrition in pregnancy. Francis M. Pottenger, M.D., beginning in 1932, ran a ten-year nutritional experiment on several groups of cats. He fed one group heat-processed food and another group raw meat and raw milk. The cats fed cooked food became infertile by the third generation, in contrast to those eating the raw food diet. This simple study underscores the importance not just of magnesium but of all nutrients necessary in producing a viable pregnancy. I don't know if these results can be translated into human experience, but we do know that heating food past the boiling point destroys vitamins and burns off magnesium and enzymes. Some minerals may be left, but the vital balance with other nutrients is ultimately lost.

Dr. Sherry Rogers, a diplomate in family practice, allergy-asthma-immunology, and environmental medicine and a fellow of the American College of Nutrition, says that just as migraines are caused by spasms in the brain arteries, smooth muscle spasms in the fallopian tubes cause infertility. This may explain why so many infertile women get pregnant when they go on a whole-foods diet and take supplements including magnesium.[1] Magnesium is required in higher amounts during pregnancy.[2, 3] So taking it to enhance conception also creates a healthier pregnancy.

It also appears that male infertility is associated with magnesium deficiency. Both magnesium and zinc are found in very significant amounts in seminal fluid. However, infertile men have much lower levels of magnesium, especially when they also have chronic prostatitis or prostate infection.[4]

PREECLAMPSIA, ECLAMPSIA, AND MAGNESIUM

Marie was not having an easy pregnancy. She had gained too much weight, she had headaches, and her ankles and hands were swollen. She also felt a tightness in her head and shortness of breath. At her eight-month visit to the doctor, her blood pressure was elevated, she had hyperactive reflexes, and her urine showed protein—all symptoms of preeclampsia (also called pregnancy-induced hypertension or toxemia). Preeclampsia occurs in 7 percent of all pregnancies and, according to the Preeclampsia Foundation, is responsible for at least 76,000 maternal deaths worldwide each year. A rapidly progressive condition characterized by high blood pressure, hyperactive reflexes, edema, headaches, changes in vision, and protein in the urine, preeclampsia can escalate and cause seizures, at which point it is called eclampsia.

Eclampsia is a serious condition that can cause premature labor, premature birth, and cerebral palsy in the newborn. Marie's doctor said that bed rest was the only solution to lower her blood pressure but that if she continued to have high blood pressure around the time of delivery, he would give her intravenous magnesium. Even knowing that magnesium would be the treatment, he didn't think to order magnesium blood levels or to offer magnesium therapy before her symptoms worsened.

According to the Preeclampsia Foundation, 1,400 women die each day—that's more than 500,000 each year—worldwide from pregnancy-related causes. On their website, they say that for most women, symptoms of preeclampsia are erroneously attributed to the shifts and changes of simply being pregnant. However, headaches, blurred vision, upper abdominal pain, and unexplained anxiety can be the prelude to more serious symptoms of eclampsia. All of these symptoms may be due to magnesium deficiency.

Where preeclampsia ends and eclampsia begins is a matter of degree and requires astute clinical observation. High blood pressure, seizures, dramatic fluid retention, decreased urine output, blurry vision, nausea, and abdominal pain must be assessed by your doctor. According to the Preeclampsia Foundation, the only cure for eclampsia is delivering the baby. Otherwise, they just recommend bed rest and monitoring.

Almost as an afterthought, the foundation mentions a 2002 study by the Magpie Trial Collaborative Group. In this study, investigators found that "magnesium sulfate ($MgSO_4$) can ease the symptoms of preeclampsia and has reduced seizures stemming from eclampsia by 56 percent when given intravenously in a controlled environment by trained staff." Their next statement should have been the first thing mentioned in the treatment section: "Magnesium sulfate has been a standard treatment option in the U.S. since the 1950s; however, it is not widely used internationally."

The Magpie Trial was in 2002; it took another decade to produce a study assessing magnesium levels in preeclampsia.[5] The study was conducted by researchers in Bangladesh who were concerned that, in spite of numerous studies, they were no closer to finding the cause of or the cure for preeclampsia. A total of 108 subjects were assessed and 66 were diagnosed with preeclampsia. The mean serum magnesium of women with mild preeclampsia to severe preeclampsia was significantly decreased compared with controls. A greater decrease in serum magnesium was also found in subjects with severe preeclampsia compared to those with mild preeclampsia. The investigators concluded that reduction in serum levels of magnesium during pregnancy might be a possible contributor in the etiology of preeclampsia and supplementation may be of value to prevent preeclampsia. Note that serum magnesium was the test of choice. If more accurate testing was used (magnesium RBC or ionized magnesium), I'm sure that more women would have been diagnosed with preeclampsia and properly treated.

Although IV magnesium is the treatment of choice for pregnancy-induced hypertension, magnesium should be used throughout pregnancy as an oral supplement to prevent symptoms of preeclampsia and eclampsia. Many researchers and clinicians recommend that pregnant women be followed with magnesium RBC testing and take 300–600 mg of supplemental magnesium.[6, 7, 8]

NOTE: Always check with your obstetrician or health care provider before adding any supplement, but know that magnesium has a long history of safety for both mother and child.

If pregnant mothers routinely take oral magnesium throughout pregnancy, studies suggest that it can prevent complications during delivery and postpartum and help prevent premature births.[9] Clinical trials have demonstrated that mothers supplementing with magnesium oxide have larger, healthier babies and lower rates of preeclampsia, premature labor, sudden infant death, cerebral palsy, and birth defects.[10] What has become apparent in recent studies, however, is that only 4 percent of magnesium oxide is absorbed and utilized in the body. Forms of magnesium that are better absorbed would likely have even more beneficial effects.

Fortunately, Marie consulted a midwife specializing in preeclampsia, who was familiar with the use of magnesium in pregnancy. They checked the label of Marie's prenatal supplement and found that it contained only 150 mg of magnesium; she really needed at least 360 mg just to meet the RDA for pregnant women. The midwife recommended that Marie take a magnesium supplement to give her a total of 400 mg of elemental magnesium per day and that she increase her intake of magnesium-rich foods.

MEDICATING ECLAMPSIA

Magnesium sulfate given intravenously for eclampsia has been used successfully since the early 1900s.[11] In the 1960s, the advent of new diuretics and anticonvulsant drugs threatened to displace magnesium sulfate. Drug companies continue to run expensive clinical trials to compare their newest antihypertensives and anticonvulsants to magnesium sulfate. Most studies show that magnesium is, in fact, more effective than synthetic medications, as it decreases both infant and maternal mortality, and is extremely safe. As one researcher remarked, "The significant improvement in fetal outcome with dietary magnesium supports the concept of magnesium supplementation during pregnancy."[12]

On her new regimen, Marie noticed many positive changes. She had less back and neck tension, was no longer constipated (a common side effect of pregnancy), had more energy, and lost her edema and puffiness. Finally, the tightness in her head lessened and her blood pressure began to go down. When she told all this to her obstetrician, he actually apologized for not being more aware of her magnesium status and said it was a good reminder for him to be more diligent about the amount of magnesium his patients were taking.

SIDS

Magnesium deficiency has been implicated in sudden infant death syndrome (SIDS), which has features in common with the sudden cardiac death of adults[13] and may be prevented by giving adequate magnesium to the mother and child.[14] An episode of muscular tension, spasm, or weakness induced by magnesium deficiency could physically prevent a distressed infant from turning its head when lying facedown and thus result in suffocation.[15]

The triple-risk model for SIDS describes the intersection of three potential risks: (1) a vulnerable newborn who is magnesium deficient, (2) a critical adjustment and development period in a newborn displaying hyperirritability and unsettled cardiovascular and respiratory control (magnesium deficiency symptoms), and (3) inability to cope with an outside stressor such as high-pitched noise, excessive motion or handling, chill, fever, or vaccination (magnesium deficiency symptoms). Together, these three risks may trigger a shock-like episode of apnea, unconsciousness, and slow heart rate. Researchers feel that it is likely that a high proportion of SIDS deaths could be prevented by simple oral magnesium supplementation to infants during the first critical weeks and months of life.[16] Magnesium could easily be given in the form of liquid ReMag in a baby bottle of water.

Dr. Jean Durlach, a professor at St. Vincent de Paul Hospital in Paris and president of the International Society for the Development of Research on Magnesium (SDRM), states, "This simple and cheap supplementation with doses of 300 milligrams per day to the mother is ethically justifiable. Furthermore, the beneficial effects of magnesium supplementation are well established for the mother, for fetal development, and for the baby at birth." He calls for a large clinical trial of magnesium supplementation in pregnant and breast-feeding women.[17] My recommendation is for pregnant and breast-feeding women to not wait for another clinical trial but to simply take magnesium, which is a safe and important nutrient that is necessary for a healthy pregnancy.

CEREBRAL PALSY

Cerebral palsy (CP) can occur in an infant who suffers a brain hemorrhage during the last stages of pregnancy, either because of the mother's high blood pressure or through another mechanism that prevents oxygen from getting to the developing baby's brain. It can also be caused by low birth weight and prematurity. In cerebral palsy, the brain is damaged in such a way that it is unable to properly direct muscle function. The brain gives the muscles contradictory signals, and as a result, the muscles lock and become spastic or go limp, creating a disabling and incurable condition.

Close to half the infants born with CP also have mental handicaps. Very-low-birth-weight babies (less than 1,500 g, or 3.3 lbs) are a hundred times more likely to have disabling CP than infants of average birth weight (3,000–3,500 g); more than 25 percent of all CP occurs in very-low-birth-weight babies. More than half a million Americans suffer from CP, with estimated medical costs of $5 billion a year.

Since there is no treatment for CP, preventing cerebral palsy would be "very desirable indeed," asserts neurologist Karin B. Nelson of the National Institutes of Health (NIH) in Bethesda, Maryland. Dr. Nelson and her colleagues concluded a groundbreaking study in 1995 showing that very-low-birth-weight babies in four centers in California had a lower incidence of cerebral palsy when their mothers were treated with magnesium sulfate shortly before giving birth.[18]

"This intriguing finding means that use of a simple medication could significantly decrease the incidence of cerebral palsy and prevent life-long disability and suffering for thousands of Americans," said Zach W. Hall, Ph.D., who at the time was director of the National Institute of Neurological Disorders and Stroke. The researchers calculated that magnesium sulfate reduced the prevalence of cerebral palsy by an astounding 90 percent and reduced the prevalence of mental retardation by about 70 percent. They speculated that magnesium may play a key role in brain development and possibly prevent cerebral hemorrhage in preterm infants.

Dr. Diane Schendel found very similar results the following year while studying a population in Atlanta.[19] Those mothers receiving magnesium sulfate delivered infants with a 90 percent lower prevalence of cerebral palsy and a 70 percent lower prevalence of mental retardation. The researchers reported that at one year of age, only 1 out of 113 babies whose mothers received magnesium sulfate had developed cerebral palsy. Only two of the babies had mental handicaps. In contrast, 30 of the 405 children whose mothers did not receive magnesium sulfate had cerebral palsy and 22 had handicaps. The investigators theorized that magnesium may prevent fetal brain hemorrhage or block the harmful effects of a diminished oxygen supply to the brain. As for those babies exposed to too much oxygen in an attempt to overcome intrauterine deficits, magnesium protects the lungs.[20] A 2000 literature review suggests that magnesium chloride may be even more protective for the developing brain than magnesium sulfate.[21, 22]

Beyond magnesium supplementation, which should be given to all expectant and breastfeeding mothers, there are certain interventions that can prevent some of the subsequent brain damage to low-birth-weight infants. One therapy is specialized craniosacral massage provided within hours or days of birth by licensed practitioners. Naturopaths can help identify food or airborne allergies that can worsen symptoms, and can recommend a wholesome diet and supplement program to the breastfeeding mother. Be warned that many over-the-counter supplements for children contain the synthetic sweetener aspartame, a potent neurotoxin. You should never expose your child to this chemical.

SUPPLEMENTS FOR CHILDREN
WITH CEREBRAL PALSY

- **ReMag:** With picometer, stabilized ionic magnesium you can reach therapeutic amounts without laxative effects. Start with ¼ tsp (75 mg) and work up to 1 tsp (300 mg) per day. Add ReMag to a bottle or cup of water or juice and have the infant or child sip all day to achieve full absorption.
- **ReMyte:** Picometer twelve-mineral solution. Take ¼ tsp twice per day, or add ½ tsp to a bottle or cup of water or juice with ReMag and sip throughout the day.
- **ReAline:** B vitamin complex plus amino acids. Take 1 capsule per day, mixed in applesauce or some other food. Contains food-based B_1 and four methylated B vitamins (B_2, B_6, methylfolate, and B_{12}), plus L-methionine (precursor to glutathione) and L-taurine (which supports the heart and weight loss).
- **Vitamin C complex:** 200 mg twice a day, from a food-based source, or make your own liposomal vitamin C (see Appendix D for a liposomal vitamin C recipe), and ascorbic acid, 1,000 mg twice a day.
- **Essential fatty acids (EFA):** Blue Ice Royal (from fermented cod liver oil and butter oil), for vitamins A, D, and K_2. Open 1 capsule and put contents in food once per day.

Osteoporosis, Arthritis, Kidney Stones, Kidney Disease

THREE THINGS YOU NEED TO KNOW ABOUT MAGNESIUM, OSTEOPOROSIS, AND KIDNEY STONES

1. Magnesium is just as important as calcium to prevent and treat osteoporosis.
2. Magnesium keeps calcium dissolved in the blood so it will not form kidney stones or precipitate in soft tissues of the body.
3. Taking calcium for osteoporosis (without magnesium) can promote kidney stones.

Muriel wondered how she managed to have soft bones and kidney stones all at the same time. Her recent bone density test showed obvious osteoporosis, yet she was now in the hospital with her third kidney stone attack. A young intern explained that she was losing calcium from her bones, which was being deposited in her kidneys and flushed out as hard, jagged crystals that were excruciatingly painful to pass. The high doses of calcium that she was taking for her osteoporosis were only making matters worse.

Muriel's urologist did an analysis on her kidney stones and told her to stop eating all dairy products and to avoid calcium supplements, but Muriel was very concerned that her osteoporosis would worsen.

When she consulted with me, I was able to explain that there are approximately seventeen nutrients essential for healthy bones, including magnesium, the most important mineral along with calcium. Susan Brown, Ph.D., director of the Osteoporosis Education Project in Syracuse, New York, warns that "the use of calcium supplementation in the face of magnesium deficiency can lead to a deposition of calcium in the soft tissue such as the joints, promoting arthritis, or in the kidney, contributing to kidney stones."[1] Dr. Brown recommends a daily dose of 450 mg of magnesium for the prevention and treatment of osteoporosis.

Women with osteoporosis have lower-than-average levels of magnesium in their diets, according to survey reports. Magnesium deficiency can compromise calcium metabolism and also hinder the body's production of vitamin D, further weakening bones.

The following is an expansion of the list that I've already mentioned in Chapter 2. It shows magnesium's multifactorial role and bears repeating:

- Adequate levels of magnesium are essential for the absorption and metabolism of calcium.
- Magnesium stimulates a particular hormone, calcitonin, that helps to preserve bone structure and draws calcium out of the blood and soft tissues back into the bones, preventing some forms of arthritis and kidney stones.
- Magnesium suppresses another bone hormone called parathyroid hormone, preventing it from breaking down bone.
- Magnesium converts vitamin D into its active form so that it can help calcium absorption.

- Magnesium is required to activate an enzyme that is necessary to form new bone.
- Magnesium regulates active calcium transport.
- It is also important to mention that vitamin K_2, along with magnesium, plays an important role in helping direct calcium to the bones, where it belongs.

With all these roles for magnesium to play, it is no wonder that even a mild deficiency can be a risk factor for osteoporosis. Furthermore, if there is too much calcium in the body, especially from calcium supplementation, as in Muriel's case, magnesium absorption can be greatly impaired, resulting in worsening osteoporosis and the likelihood of kidney stones, arthritis, and heart disease as well as gall stones, heel spurs, and breast tissue calcification.

Most people, including M.D.'s, do not understand the importance of balancing calcium and magnesium at the cellular level. Calcium cannot build bones or prevent osteoporosis without adequate levels of magnesium. It's as simple as that. If our bones were made entirely from calcium, they would become brittle and could shatter just like a stick of chalk falling on the sidewalk. However, with the right percentage of magnesium, bone has the proper density and matrix that actually makes it flexible and more resistant to shattering. I'm afraid many elderly people are suffering bone fractures because they have too much calcium and not enough magnesium.

Other factors that are important in the development of osteoporosis include diet, drugs, endocrine imbalance, allergies, vitamin D deficiency, and lack of exercise. A detailed review of the osteoporosis literature shows that chronically low intake of magnesium, boron, folic acid, and vitamins D, K_2, B_{12}, and B_6 leads to osteoporosis. Similarly, chronically

high intake of protein, table salt, alcohol, and caffeine adversely affects bone health.[2, 3] The typical Western diet (high
in protein, table salt, and refined and processed foods) combined with an increasingly sedentary lifestyle contributes to
the epidemic incidence of osteoporosis.

Minerals make up 60 percent of bone, mostly calcium
and phosphate. Magnesium provides the resilience factor.
Bone also includes water and a matrix of proteins such as
collagen, which form the scaffold for minerals to deposit.
Collagen is the most abundant protein in the body and
makes up about 90 percent of this bone matrix. Collagen has
its own list of requirements for proper structure and function, and you can obtain those in a good diet that includes
animal protein along with well-absorbed minerals and vitamins from organic food sources.

The animal-based collagen requirement for bone was
not even addressed in a 2014 review called "Can Vegans
Have Healthy Bones?"[4] The authors found that vegan diets
can be deficient in protein, calcium, and vitamin D. They
caution, as so many others have in the past, that vegans must
take great care in planning their diet so that they meet all
their nutrient requirements. They concluded, "More research is needed in order to understand more fully the impact of veganism on bone health."

Looking at her lifestyle, Muriel saw how much she had
contributed to her own condition. She averaged five cups of
coffee, three glasses of wine, and twenty cigarettes a day.
This was causing calcium and magnesium, and the other
nutrients that have to deal with toxins, to be overworked or
flushed out of her body. Her diet was mostly nutrient-deficient
fast food because she was constantly on the run. Muriel also
drank lots of soda, which is high in sugar and phosphorus,
both of which cause calcium and magnesium to be elimi-

nated. She also avoided the sun and therefore got little vitamin D.

Instead of becoming discouraged, Muriel was able to look on the bright side. At least now she knew what lifestyle habits she had to change and what supplements to take. Her kidney stones soon became a thing of the past, her overall health dramatically improved, and after two years she had not just stopped losing bone but there was actually a measurable increase in her bone density.

OSTEOPOROSIS MISUNDERSTOOD AND MISTREATED

Osteoporosis is neither a normal nor inevitable consequence of aging. Our bones were designed to last a lifetime. Popular wisdom, however, is that osteoporosis in women is due to a lack of calcium and declining estrogen levels with age. To treat osteoporosis, therefore, doctors rely on estrogen, calcium, and drugs that keep bone cells from breaking down. The NIH "Osteoporosis Prevention, Diagnosis, and Therapy Consensus Statement of 2000" was developed from a conference including eighty experts, but no mention of magnesium deficiency as a causative factor in osteoporosis was made in the final report.[5]

However, a 2014 meta-analysis confirmed the association between serum magnesium levels and postmenopausal osteoporosis.[6] Seven studies involving 1,349 postmenopausal women were identified. Overall, postmenopausal osteoporotic women had lower serum levels of magnesium than the healthy controls. The investigators concluded that low serum magnesium seems to be a risk factor for osteoporosis among the postmenopausal group.

With drug companies funding most of the osteoporosis

research, there are no large clinical trials investigating the magnesium connection in bone production, and there probably never will be. As long as people are given false hope that there is some magic bullet in the pharmaceutical pipeline that will "cure" osteoporosis, or any other chronic disease, they will ignore the underlying diet- and nutrient-related reasons for their health problems.

Reports that Fosamax causes jawbone deterioration is evidence that this osteoporosis drug, and likely all bisphosphonates, cause brittle bones. This side effect of jawbone deterioration has dentists refusing to place dental implants in women who are on Fosamax. Fosamax works by destroying osteoclasts, the cells that break down bone as it ages. These cells also sculpt the bone as new bone forms, shaping it into a strong and stable matrix. Fosamax prevents bone from breaking down—but the drug companies did not reckon with the necessary bone-remodeling function of the osteoclast. Without osteoclasts, bones have no blueprint to follow and calcium is deposited helter-skelter. X-rays of bones under the influence of Fosamax may appear dense at a glance, but when you look closely, you see that without the remodeling capacity of osteoclasts, the bones' internal structure is in complete disarray. These bones are brittle and they break more easily.

Instead of cozying up to Fosamax, doctors should read a 2013 study in the *Journal of Nutritional Biochemistry* showing that magnesium has a direct influence on increasing the formation of osteoclasts.[7] In the previous edition of *The Magnesium Miracle*, I reported that animal research proves that magnesium depletion alters bone and mineral metabolism, which results in bone loss and osteoporosis.[8, 9] In this 2013 study, investigators acknowledged that magnesium deficiency occurs frequently and leads to loss of bone mass, abnormal bone growth, and skeletal weakness. But they wanted to determine how this occurs. Using an animal model, they found that magnesium deficiency inhibited the activity of osteoclasts—which is the mechanism of action of Fosamax. They concluded that altered osteoclast numbers and activity may contribute to the bone changes that are seen in magnesium-deficient patients.

Magnesium deficiency is very common in women with osteoporosis compared to controls.[10] But what happens when women take enough magnesium?

- In one study, postmenopausal women with osteoporosis were able to stop the progression of the disease with 250–750 mg of magnesium daily for two years. Without any other added measures, 8 percent of these women experienced a net increase in bone density.[11]
- A group of menopausal women given a magnesium hydroxide supplement for two years had fewer fractures and a significant increase in bone density.[12]
- Another study showed that by taking magnesium lactate to provide 180–300 mg of elemental magnesium daily for two years, 65 percent of the women were completely free of pain and had no further degeneration of spinal vertebrae.[13]
- Magnesium in conjunction with hormonal replacement improved bone density in several groups of women compared to controls.[14, 15]
- Another study showed that if you take estrogen and have a low magnesium intake, calcium supplementation may increase your risk of thrombosis (blood clotting that can lead to a heart attack).[16]

It is unfortunate that decades ago the treatment for osteoporosis was simplified into the single battle cry "take calcium." Calcium still dominates every discussion about osteoporosis, is used to fortify dozens of foods (including orange juice and cereal), and is a top-selling supplement, but its day in the sun seems to be over. One author in the late 1990s cited scientific studies that did not support large doses of calcium after menopause, as soft tissue calcification could be a serious side effect.[17] All that extra calcium was being deposited in soft tissue, causing atherosclerosis, gallstones, kidney stones, heel spurs, and breast tissue calcification, instead of being directed to the bones.

This warning has been bolstered by the work of Dr. Mark Bolland, who I reported on in Chapter 2 in the section "The Failure of Calcium." Bolland found that women who take calcium supplements are at greater risk for heart disease as calcium builds up in arteries causing atherosclerosis. The point to make here is that all the calcium supplementation in the past two decades has not prevented the epidemic of osteoporosis that we are suffering today.

I want to mention again that bones are not just about magnesium—although you might get that impression because of my focus. Sixty percent of bone is made up of minerals, mostly calcium and phosphate, along with magnesium (which provides the resilience factor), water, and an organic matrix of proteins, especially collagen. Our bones are a dynamic interweaving of minerals and protein that we can't hope to manipulate by introducing only one or two variables. Instead, we should do our best to eat a good diet, exercise, and take a range of absorbable nutrients, and let the body and our bones take care of themselves.

OSTEOPOROSIS DRUGS

I was curious to see what the National Osteoporosis Guideline Group in the United Kingdom would suggest for osteoporosis therapy in light of the connection between calcium and heart disease that I discussed above and in Chapter 2.[18] I was very disappointed, however, because in their 2013 report there is no mention of magnesium. Although calcium was downplayed, that just meant there will be much more drug intervention in women's bone health. The significance of magnesium in bone health cannot be underestimated, yet it is overlooked every day in most doctors' offices.

The British guidelines began with a list of the main drugs that drug companies claim lower the risk for vertebral fracture (and for hip fracture in some cases). These include bisphosphonates, denosumab, parathyroid hormone peptides, raloxifene, and strontium ranelate. The authors of the guidelines acknowledged the dangers inherent in these drugs, as they:

1. Cautioned against mixing two or more of these drugs together because of unknown side effects
2. Mentioned the high cost of some of the drugs
3. Warned that withdrawing bisphosphonates (e.g., Fosamax) is associated with rebound decrease in bone mineral density and bone turnover. This implies that once you are on Fosamax you should stay on it forever or else experience even more bone loss and deterioration.

At the end of the report were the guidelines about calcium and vitamin D, which read, "Calcium and vitamin D supplementation is widely recommended for older persons who are housebound or live in residential or nursing homes and is often recommended as an adjunct to other treatments for osteoporosis." And then came the caveat: "Potential adverse cardiovascular effects of calcium supplementation are controversial, but it may be prudent to increase dietary calcium intake and use vitamin D alone rather than using both calcium and vitamin D supplementation."

There was no mention of magnesium anywhere in the guidelines. Neither did they mention testosterone, which is a known bone builder in men and also in women. However, you don't have to rush into the unknown world of testosterone hormone replacement just yet.

MAGNESIUM AND TESTOSTERONE

A 2011 study found that in a group of 399 older men, magnesium levels are strongly and independently associated with testosterone and another anabolic hormone, insulin growth factor-1 (IGF-1).[19] Any increase in testosterone will automatically increase estrogen since it comes after testosterone in the natural steroid pathway of the adrenals and sex glands.

In another study, three groups of men were studied. Two groups took the same amount of magnesium, 10 mg/kg/day.[20] One group was composed of sedentary men. The second group were tae kwon do athletes, who worked out 1.5–2 hours per day. The third group were also tae kwon do athletes but took no magnesium supplements. The group that took magnesium and practiced tae kwon do had the greatest increase in free and total testosterone. The sedentary group who took supplements also saw significant increases in testosterone.

A 2015 study investigated the "relationship between serum magnesium concentration and metabolic and hormonal disorders in middle-aged and older men."[21] The researchers found that magnesium was higher in men who had normal total testosterone levels. Subjects with metabolic syndrome had lower serum magnesium compared to patients without metabolic syndrome. Serum magnesium concentration in men with type 2 diabetes was lower compared to men without diabetes. The same was found in patients with arterial hypertension—serum mag-

> nesium concentration was lower than in patients without hypertension. The higher the magnesium concentration, the lower the body mass index, waist-to-hip ratio, abdominal circumference, and arterial blood pressure. Higher concentration of magnesium was associated with higher total testosterone, lower LDL, and lower total cholesterol. The investigators concluded that "lower serum magnesium levels may be conducive to the development of total testosterone deficiency, arterial hypertension, diabetes, and therefore metabolic syndrome."

Natural estrogen produced by the body is also important for bone formation. I emphasize natural estrogen because the synthetic forms do not have the same bone-building effects and there is the added risk of cancer when using synthetic estrogen replacement therapy.

Why am I so concerned about the inappropriate treatment of osteoporosis? Statistics on osteoporosis incidence show that in spite of the increased use of calcium supplementation for this condition, the incidence continues to climb. How is that even possible when we have led a war on osteoporosis for so long? The answer is that we chose the wrong weapons, and now those weapons have turned against us.

In a report on the national trends in osteoporosis for the years 1988–2003 researchers tracked osteoporosis treatment and doctors' visits.[22] They reported that physician visits increased fourfold between 1994 (1.3 million visits) and 2003 (6.3 million visits). This increase coincided with the widespread use of calcium supplements and the availability of oral daily bisphosphonates (Fosamax) and the selective estrogen receptor modulator raloxifene. Prior to 1994, the main therapeutic choices were calcium and estrogens. Between 1994 and 2003, bisphosphonate prescriptions for osteoporosis increased from 14 to 73 percent and raloxifene prescriptions for osteoporosis increased from 0 to 12 percent.

MAGNESIUM FOR CHILDREN'S BONES

When a child is taken off dairy for allergies, constipation, bowel upsets, or frequent infections, parents will exclaim, "How can my kids get calcium for their bones if I don't give them dairy?" But not once do they ask about magnesium. Finally, a 2013 study shows that the amount of magnesium consumed and absorbed is the key predictor of a child's bone health.[23] The researchers found that intake of dietary calcium was not significantly associated with total bone mineral content or density. This study, presented at the annual meeting of the Pediatric Academic Societies in Washington, D.C., validates magnesium's vital importance. It confirms that magnesium works synergistically with calcium. Magnesium regulates the proper amount of calcium in a child's body and marches it straight into the bones. Calcium, if it's not balanced with magnesium, ends up depositing in a child's kidneys, coronary arteries, and cartilage, not in the bones and teeth, where it is needed the most.

Lead researcher Steven A. Abrams, M.D., F.A.A.P., professor of pediatrics at Baylor College of Medicine in Houston, said, "Calcium is important, but, except for those children and adolescents with very low intakes, may not be more important than magnesium." For researchers to boldly state that calcium "may not be more important than magnesium" represents a huge breakthrough in helping people grasp the importance of magnesium in bone health. Until now, it's been all about calcium for both children and adults.

TREATMENT OF OSTEOPOROSIS

Osteoporosis is generally a progressive disease, and some say it is incurable, but if you avoid the risk factors that are under your control, take a good range of bone-building nutrients, and exercise, you can halt the condition even if you have symptoms. Of course, prevention is the best defense, the key elements of which are:

- Eat a balanced, high-protein, nutrient-rich diet.
- Obtain your calcium from your diet and ReCalcia, take ReMag for magnesium, and bone support factors from ReMyte and ReAline.
- Practice some form of exercise every day.
- Avoid caffeine, alcohol, and tobacco.

DIET ADVICE FOR OSTEOPOROSIS

Any mention of what to eat and what not to eat when you have a chronic health condition is fraught with inconsistencies and inaccuracies. My general diet recommendations are as follows and include a high-protein diet, lots of vegetables, and gluten-free grains containing large amounts of magnesium, calcium, and potassium, which contribute to maintaining bone mineral density.[24]

- Eliminate alcohol, coffee, white sugar, white flour, gluten, fried foods, and trans fatty acids (found in margarine and in baked, fried, and processed foods made with partially hydrogenated fats).
- If you eat animal protein, choose organically raised grass-fed beef, free-range chicken and eggs, and fish (especially wild-caught salmon).

- For vegetarian protein, choose fermented dairy, lactose-free cheese, and ReStructure Meal Replacement (it has no casein, very-low-lactose whey protein, and pea and rice proteins).
- Vegan protein choices include legumes, gluten-free grains, nuts, and seeds.
- Eat healthy carbs such as a variety of raw, cooked, and fermented vegetables, two or three pieces of fruit a day, and gluten-free grains.
- Include magnesium-rich foods listed in Appendix A and calcium-rich foods listed in Appendix B.
- For fats and oils, choose butter, olive oil, flaxseed oil, sesame oil, and coconut oil.

SUPPLEMENTS FOR OSTEOPOROSIS

- **ReMag:** With picometer, stabilized ionic magnesium you can reach therapeutic amounts without laxative effects. Start with ¼ tsp (75 mg) and work up to 2–3 tsp (600–900 mg) per day. Add ReMag to a liter of water and sip all day to achieve full absorption.
- **ReMyte:** Picometer twelve-mineral solution. Take ½ tsp three times a day, or add 1½ tsp to a liter of water with ReMag and sip throughout the day.
- **ReCalcia:** Picometer, stabilized ionic calcium, boron, vanadium. Take 1–2 tsp per day (1 tsp provides 300 mg calcium) if you don't obtain enough calcium from your diet. It can be taken with ReMag and ReMyte.
- **ReAline:** B vitamin complex plus amino acids. Take 1 capsule twice per day. Contains food-based B_1 and four methylated B vitamins (B_2, B_6, methylfolate, and B_{12}), plus L-methionine (precursor to glutathione) and L-taurine (which supports the heart and weight loss).
- **Vitamin C complex:** 200 mg twice a day, from a food-

based source, or make your own liposomal vitamin C (see Appendix D for a liposomal vitamin C recipe), and ascorbic acid, 1,000 mg twice a day.

- **Essential fatty acids:** I recommend a combination: (1) Blue Ice Royal, from fermented cod liver oil and butter oil, for vitamins A, D, and K_2, 1 capsule twice per day; (2) flaxseed oil, 1 tbsp twice per day (store the bottle in the freezer); (3) flaxseed oil and omega-3 fatty acids from Re-Structure Protein Powder; (4) wild-caught fish.
- **Vitamin D_3:** 1,000 IU or 20 minutes in the sun daily. Blue Ice Royal.

HORMONE THERAPY

Some doctors recommend progesterone for postmenopausal women. Only consider hormone therapy after testing to determine deficiency. Please find a doctor who does hormone testing—preferably saliva testing—and who can prescribe bioidentical progesterone.

ARTHRITIS

In the first edition of *The Magnesium Miracle* I did not even have a section on arthritis. Since then, research has caught up with some of the wonderful testimonials I receive from people who are treating their arthritis with magnesium.

One particularly amazing testimonial is from Joe, who came on my radio show during Thanksgiving week, 2016, to give thanks for his new body. Joe suffered with ankylosing spondylitis since age fifteen. At age fifty-two, Joe said his arthritis was terrible, his sedimentation was through the roof, he could barely get out of bed in the morning, and had to crawl to the bathroom. He said he could no longer work but he was on tons of medication that he could no longer afford and he was just getting worse. By some miracle, he ran into a friend who told him that all he needed was ReMag and RnA Drops from Dr. Dean. He took the advice and got on my Total Body ReSet program with five of my Completement Formulas and within six months, he shocked everyone by riding around the neighborhood on a bicycle. Joe thought he would never be able to work out at the gym, but he said with the Completement Formulas, and especially ReStructure protein powder, he's working out with more energy and stamina than guys half his age.

Many people think that having arthritis comes with the territory as you get older. But that's just not true. Arthritis only means inflammation of the joints: *arthr-* is Latin for joint and *-itis* means inflammation. Arthritis is just a word, not a disease. But often if we get an ache or a pain we start labeling it arthritis and let it take hold in our body because we think it's par for the course.

One very unfortunate result of being diagnosed with arthritis is that you are often prescribed steroid shots or nonsteroidal anti-inflammatory drugs (NSAIDs) for pain relief. Be aware that these drugs are now associated with atrial fibrillation, atrial flutter, heart attack, and stroke. In fact, back in 2005, the FDA put out a warning that NSAIDs such as ibuprofen and naproxen increased the risk of having a heart attack or stroke, but I don't think anyone paid attention.

In 2015 the FDA escalated the warning to cover even short term use of NSAIDs in what Dr. Gregory Curfman of the *Harvard Health Blog* called an unusual step because NSAIDs are so widely used.[25] Dr. Curfman wrote that for over fifteen years, experts have known that NSAIDs increase the risk of heart attack and stroke. He said that research shows these drugs may also elevate blood pressure and cause heart failure. A single drug, Vioxx, was responsible for at least 140,000 heart attacks in one five-year period. Vioxx was finally removed from the market in 2004 and the heart disease risk was eventually studied thoroughly and seen in all NSAIDs.

The 2015 FDA warning extends to the short-term use of NSAIDs, as the risk of heart attack and stroke may begin within a few weeks. The higher the dose and the longer the prescription, the greater the risk. The risk is even worse in people who already have heart disease. A 2011 study in the *British Medical Journal* concluded that NSAIDs are associated with increased risk of atrial fibrillation and atrial flutter.[26] The association was strongest for new users of the drugs, who experienced a 40–70 percent increased risk.

I think NSAIDs target the heart because they deplete magnesium, and they probably exhibit this side effect to a greater extent in people who are already magnesium deficient. When magnesium is very deficient, atrial fibrillation and atrial flutter can occur. Joint inflammation can be caused by magnesium deficiency. If you have arthritis and your joints are inflamed because of magnesium deficiency, the very drugs you are prescribed can often make you worse and harm your heart. It becomes a vicious, unstoppable cycle.

Here's a case history sent to me by a seventy-eight-year-old woman suffering from arthritis:

As I reached my seventy-eighth birthday last winter, it was no surprise that my hands suffered an attack of arthritis. The pain was mostly at the base of my thumbs, and the left hurt a lot more than the right because I am left-handed and use it more in my massage practice.

It got so bad I could hardly use the hand at all. So, in February, although I hated the idea, I agreed to a steroid shot. That solved the immediate problem and the left thumb is fine now, but in the last two months my right thumb has been getting more painful.

I didn't want to take the steroid path again. So last week, I decided to spray my right thumb every morning and night with two bursts of ReMag. Guess what? Not only is the pain pretty much gone but the thumb, which seemed to be shortening as the tendons tightened, now has a longer stretch. Maybe not a miracle, but pretty close to it! I still get twinges, but feel much more freedom in the hands, which is indispensable, as I use them to access the tensions of others all the time.

For this edition of *The Magnesium Miracle* I found the latest research showing that science has caught up with people's experience regarding magnesium in the prevention and treatment of arthritis.

A 2016 paper in *Life Science* called "Unraveling the Role of Mg^{++} in Osteoarthritis"[27] reveals the importance of magnesium in the treatment of osteoarthritis. The researchers said that magnesium deficiency is considered to be a major risk factor for the development and progression of osteoarthritis. They found that magnesium deficiency is "active in several pathways that have been implicated in OA, including increased inflammatory mediators, cartilage damage, defective chondrocyte biosynthesis, aberrant calcification and a weakened effect of analgesics." They referenced laboratory and clinical evidence in animal studies that suggested nutritional supplementation of magnesium could provide effective therapies for osteoarthritis.

The *Journal of Rheumatology* published a 2015 study called "Relationship Between Serum Magnesium Concentration and Radiographic Knee Osteoarthritis."[28] There were 2,855 subjects in this cross-sectional study. The investigators measured magnesium using the inferior serum magnesium test and arthritis was determined by specific X-ray criteria. They found a significant association between serum magnesium concentration and osteoarthritis, concluding that as serum magnesium levels fell, the incidence of osteoarthritis of the knee increased. The same study found that the lower the dietary intake of magnesium, the higher the incidence of knee osteoarthritis.

KIDNEY STONES

Kidney stones are more common than we think. About 10 percent of the population will have a kidney stone in their lifetime. The Norman Parathyroid Center is the world's leading authority on parathyroid glands, parathyroid disease, and parathyroid surgery; they also know a lot about high blood calcium, which is a sign of hyperparathyroidism and a sign of kidney stones.

Their webpage on kidney stones states, "Hyperparathyroidism is the number one cause of kidney stones and thus every person with a kidney stone MUST be tested for a problem with their parathyroid glands. Nearly half of all people with kidney stones have a benign parathyroid tumor in their neck that must be removed or the kidney stones will return." See Chapter 2 for more information on hyperparathyroidism.

Kidney stones occur when the microscopic debris excreted in the urine becomes too concentrated to pass freely through the kidneys into the bladder. Kidney stones are quite common in the general population but most of them pass as tiny bits of "gravel" without you even knowing. Risk factors for kidney stones include a history of hypertension, rapid weight loss, chronic dehydration, and a low dietary intake of magnesium.[29]

One percent of autopsies reveal stones in the urinary tract, confirming that they are very common and also confirming that most are small enough to pass unnoticed. Up to

15 percent of white males and 6 percent of all women will develop one stone, with recurrence in about half of these people. Approximately one person in a thousand in the United States is hospitalized annually with excruciatingly painful stones trapped in their urinary passages. The pain begins in the lower back and can radiate across the abdomen or into the genitals or down the inside of the thigh.

Most kidney stones are made up of calcium phosphate, calcium oxalate, or uric acid. The kind of stones you have can only be determined by collecting the stones (the doctor will have you urinate into a fine sieve) and having the material analyzed. Calcium stones are seen chiefly in men, often with a family history. Calcium phosphate and calcium oxalate alone are responsible for almost 85 percent of all stones; uric acid stones make up 5–10 percent. Uric acid stones are also seen mostly in men, half of whom have gout. The remaining 5 percent are rare stones that can be formed during kidney infections.

Diagnosis is made by urinalysis and X-ray. If there are only a few calcium crystals or small stones, often no treatment may be needed, but pain caused by their passing may be relieved with painkillers and muscle relaxants. Larger stones are treated with surgery or with lithotripsy (the breakdown of the stones into little pieces using special ultrasound machines).

Several factors can be involved in stone formation:

1. Elevated calcium in the urine is caused by a diet high in sugar, fructose, alcohol, coffee, and meat. These acidic foods presumably pull calcium from the bone, to neutralize acidity, and excrete it through the kidneys. Calcium supplementation without magnesium also causes elevated calcium in the urine.

2. Higher-than-normal levels of oxalate found in the urine may relate to a high dietary intake of oxalic-acid-containing foods: rhubarb, spinach, chard, raw parsley, chocolate, tea, and coffee, among others. The oxalic acid in them promotes stone formation by binding to calcium, creating insoluble calcium oxalate. But don't forsake all greens and lose out on their beneficial nutrients. There are plenty of low-oxalate greens to make up for the ones you have to avoid.[30] However, when you are saturated with enough magnesium, it can bind with oxalate in a much more soluble magnesium oxalate and be excreted without incident.

3. Dehydration concentrates calcium and other minerals in the urine. Drinking half your body weight (in pounds) in ounces of water each day (to which you add ¼ tsp of sea salt per quart) is essential to flush the kidneys properly. Increased sweating and not drinking enough water create concentrated urine.

4. Soft drinks containing phosphoric acid encourage kidney stones in some people by pulling calcium out of the bones and depositing it in the kidneys.

5. A diet high in purines (substances found in alcohol, meat, and fish) can cause uric acid kidney stones.

Kidney stones and magnesium deficiency share the same list of causes, including a diet high in sugar, alcohol, oxalates, and coffee. An important animal study shows that a high dietary intake of fructose (from high-fructose corn syrup sweeteners) significantly increases kidney calcification, especially when dietary magnesium is low.[31]

The U.S. Department of Agriculture warns that young people, especially, derive too many of their daily calories from high-fructose corn syrup in sodas and eat few greens that are rich in magnesium. The phosphoric acid in soft drinks is also punishing to the magnesium in the body and depletes magnesium stores while wearing away bone.[32, 33]

One of magnesium's many jobs is to keep calcium in solution to prevent it from solidifying into crystals. Even in times of dehydration, if there is sufficient magnesium, calcium will stay in solution.

Magnesium is the pivotal treatment for kidney stones. If you don't have enough magnesium to help dissolve calcium, you will end up with various forms of calcification. This translates into stones, muscle spasms, fibrositis, fibromyalgia, atherosclerosis (calcification of the arteries), and breast tissue calcification, which in some cases may be mistaken for DCIS (ductal carcinoma in situ) and vice versa. My concern is that breast tissue calcification from overuse of oral calcium supplements can be mistaken for DCIS and involve rounds of X-rays, mammograms, and breast tissue biopsies to rule out cancer.

Many decades ago, Dr. George Bunce clinically proved the relationship between kidney stones and magnesium deficiency.[34] As early as 1964, Bunce reported the benefits of administering a daily 420 mg dose of magnesium oxide to patients who had a history of frequent stone formation.

When there is more calcium than magnesium in the blood, kidney stones can form. Let's look at that simple experiment from Chapter 2 again to prove the point. Open a capsule of calcium powder and see how much dissolves in 1 ounce of water; a goodly amount settles in the bottom of the glass. Then open a capsule of magnesium powder and slowly stir it into the calcium water. When you introduce the magnesium, the remaining calcium dissolves; it becomes more water-soluble. If there is enough magnesium to properly dissolve calcium in the blood, then it won't form crystals in the kidney.

Several older studies show the benefits of magnesium hydroxide in preventing stone formation.

- Fifty-five patients with a combined 480 stones in the previous ten years were placed on 500 mg of magnesium hydroxide daily. Patients were followed for two to four years. The mean stone episode rate decreased from 0.8 to 0.08 stones per year on treatment and 85 percent of the patients remained free of recurrence during follow-up, whereas 59 percent of the patients in the control group continued to form stones.[35]

- A study using magnesium oxide and vitamin B_6 (a natural diuretic) showed a decrease in stone formation for 149 patients, who went from an average of 1.3 stones per year to 0.1 stones. Patients were followed for between four and a half and six years.[36]

- In another study, fifty-six patients were given 200 mg of magnesium hydroxide twice per day. At the two-year mark, forty-five were free of kidney stone recurrence; of thirty-four patients not taking magnesium, fifteen had recurrences after two years.[37]

- Other studies show that urinary magnesium concentration is abnormally low and urinary calcium concentration is abnormally high in more than 25 percent of patients with kidney stones. Supplemental magnesium intake corrects this abnormality and prevents the recurrence of stones. The investigators acknowledge that magnesium oxide or magnesium hydroxide therapy cause a considerable lessening of kidney stone recurrence in men and feel that soft tissue calcifications can be stopped and even prevented by magnesium therapy.[38]

- Magnesium seems to be as effective against stone formation as diuretics, the major drug treatment for kidney stones.[39] I think magnesium therapy would be more effective, since diuretics will deplete magnesium, increasing the chances of calcium kidney stones. Avoidance of calcium, taking diuretics, and mechanical intervention constitute the current allopathic medical approach to kidney stones with no attention paid to magnesium.

- A 2005 review paper notes that while magnesium oxide and magnesium hydroxide had been looked upon favorably for the treatment of kidney stones, magnesium citrate proved to be far superior in double-blind, randomized, placebo-controlled trials, reducing the occurrence of kidney stones by 90 percent.[40]

- Epidemiological findings round out the picture of kidney stone occurrence and its association with low magnesium intake. For example, the disease pattern in Greenland includes a low incidence of heart disease and kidney and urinary tract stones, few cases of diabetes mellitus, and little osteoporosis, all of which may be related to low calcium and high magnesium in the diet in Greenland.[41]

DIET ADVICE FOR KIDNEY STONES

Hydration is very important in the prevention of kidney stones.

- Hydrate your body by increasing your water intake. Drink half your body weight (in pounds) in ounces of water. If you weigh 150 pounds, you will drink 75 ounces.

- Add unrefined sea salt, pink Himalayan salt, or Celtic sea salt to your drinking water, ¼ tsp to every quart of drinking water.

I recommend a very strict diet in the beginning of your treatment protocol to see how effective diet alone can be. Then you can experiment with adding in some "forbidden foods" and see how your body reacts. My strictest diet recommendations are as follows:

- Eliminate alcohol, coffee, white sugar, white flour, gluten, fried foods, and trans fatty acids (found in margarine and in baked, fried, and processed foods made with partially hydrogenated fats).
- If you eat animal protein, choose organically raised grass-fed beef, free-range chicken and eggs, and fish (especially wild-caught salmon).
- For vegetarian protein, choose fermented dairy, lactose-free cheese, and ReStructure Meal Replacement (it has no casein, very-low-lactose whey protein, and pea and rice proteins).
- Vegan protein choices include legumes, gluten-free grains, nuts, and seeds.
- Healthy carbs include raw, cooked, and fermented vegetables, and two or three pieces of fruit a day. Include magnesium-rich foods listed in Appendix A. The foods that are high in calcium are usually abundant in magnesium as well; see the list of foods containing high amounts of calcium in Appendix B.
- For fats and oils, choose butter, olive oil, flaxseed oil, sesame oil, and coconut oil.
- If you have uric acid kidney stones, eliminate foods high in purines, such as alcohol, anchovies, herring, lentils, meat, mushrooms, organ meats, sardines, and shellfish.
- If you have oxalate stones, decrease consumption of foods high in oxalic acid: red beet tops, black tea, cocoa, cranberries, nuts, parsley, tomatoes, rhubarb, chard, and spinach.
- The citric acid in lemons, limes, oranges, pineapples, and gooseberries dissolves calcium oxalate and calcium phosphate, preventing stone formation.

SUPPLEMENTS FOR KIDNEY STONES

- **ReMag:** With picometer, stabilized ionic magnesium you can reach therapeutic amounts without laxative effects. Start with ¼ tsp (75 mg) and work up to 2–3 tsp (600–900 mg) per day. Add ReMag to a liter of water and sip all day to achieve full absorption.
- **ReMyte:** Picometer twelve-mineral solution. Take ½ tsp three times a day, or add 1½ tsp to a liter of water with ReMag and sip throughout the day.
- **ReAline:** B vitamin complex plus amino acids. For kidney stones, B_6 is important and it's contained in ReAline. Take 1 capsule twice per day. Contains food-based B_1 and four methylated B vitamins (B_2, B_6, methylfolate, and B_{12}), plus L-methionine (precursor to glutathione) and L-taurine (which supports the heart and weight loss).
- Use ReStructure, a low purine protein powder.

KIDNEY DISEASE

In the original edition of *The Magnesium Miracle* I did not have a specific section on kidney disease. That was mostly because for many decades the only nutritional advice for patients with kidney disease was to avoid magnesium! Over the years, however, I've learned that the kidneys need magnesium just like any other organ and the attack on magnesium has little scientific merit. Magnesium is a biological necessity, and the blanket avoidance of it in kidney disease has led to untold suffering.

The NIH acknowledges a "growing burden of kidney disease." Statistics show a sharp increase in kidney disease affecting one in ten American adults. But how are doctors diagnosing kidney disease these days? Perhaps they are setting the diagnostic criteria for kidney disease (in this case, filtration rates) at a lower level, much as they are doing with blood pressure and cholesterol. By having broader criteria, more people find themselves being diagnosed with pre-diabetes, pre-hypertension, and now pre–kidney disease and are terrified because they are being told they are developing chronic diseases for which there is no cure.

Catching more people in the net of pre–kidney disease means these patients will be offered medications for associated conditions, like heart disease, high blood pressure, and diabetes, that seem to go hand in hand with kidney disease.

I think part of the increase in kidney disease is due to the rampant use of prescription medications. But doctors do not want to admit that their treatments are causing harm. One paper published in 2009 thoroughly reviewed the problem of drug-induced kidney disease, finding that the kidneys can be damaged by a large number of therapeutic agents.[42] Linda Fugate, Ph.D., lists the top ten classes of drugs that cause kidney damage and references the 2009 review article.[43] Since that time, many more drugs have been implicated and the evidence is mounting that chronic use of medications instead of judicious short-term use is causing cumulative harm.

Top Ten Drug Families That Cause Kidney Damage

1. Antibiotics, including ciprofloxacin, methicillin, vanco-mycin, and sulfonamides.
2. Analgesics, including acetaminophen and nonsteroidal anti-inflammatory drugs (NSAIDs): aspirin, ibuprofen, naproxen, and others available only by prescription.
3. COX-2 inhibitors, including celecoxib (Celebrex). Two drugs in this class have been withdrawn from the market because of cardiovascular toxicity: rofecoxib (Vioxx) and valdecoxib (Bextra). COX-2 inhibitors were developed to be safer for the stomach, but have the same risk as other NSAIDs for kidney damage.

4. Heartburn drugs of the proton pump inhibitor class, including omeprazole (Prilosec), lansoprazole (Prevacid), pantoprazole (Protonix), rabeprazol (Rabecid, Aciphex), and esomeprazole (Nexium, Esotrex).

5. Antiviral drugs, including acyclovir (Zovirax), used to treat herpes infection, and indinavir and tenofovir, both used to treat HIV.

6. High blood pressure drugs, including captopril (Capoten).

7. Rheumatoid arthritis drugs, including infliximab (Remicade), chloroquine, and hydroxychloroquine (the latter two are used to treat malaria and systemic lupus erythematosus, as well as rheumatoid arthritis).

8. Lithium, used to treat bipolar disorder.

9. Anticonvulsants, including phenytoin (brand name Dilantin) and trimethadione (brand name Tridione), used to treat seizures and other conditions.

10. Chemotherapy drugs (including interferons, pamidronate, cisplatin, carboplatin, cyclosporine, tacrolimus, quinine, mitomycin C, bevacizumab) and antithyroid drugs (including propylthiouracil, used to treat overactive thyroid).

PROTON PUMP INHIBITORS
DEPLETE MAGNESIUM

A 2016 study gives evidence that proton pump inhibitors (PPIs), used to treat heartburn, may cause kidney injury.[44] The authors echo my sentiments that any drug should only be used when necessary, not as a preventive measure. They say, "The results emphasize the importance of limiting PPI use to only when it is medically necessary, and also limiting the duration of use to the shortest period possible. A lot of patients start taking PPIs for a medical condition and they continue much longer than necessary." Often doctors tell patients to keep taking drugs "just in case" their symptoms come back instead of instituting more natural measures to prevent recurrence of symptoms.

END-STAGE RENAL DISEASE

The number of patients enrolled in a Medicare-funded program to manage end-stage renal disease (ESRD) has increased from 10,000 in 1973 to a frightening 615,899 as of 2012.[45] Medicine says they are at a loss to explain why so many people are affected. And despite the magnitude of the resources committed to the treatment of ESRD and assuming there have been improvements in the quality of dialysis therapy, these patients continue to experience significant mortality and morbidity and a reduced quality of life. If dialysis is taking over the function of the kidneys, then people should be feeling much better than they are. One reason for the escalation of symptoms could be magnesium deficiency that only gets worse with time because magnesium supplementation is avoided in dialysis patients and the amount of magnesium in their dialysate fluids is too low.

Signs of kidney disease include high blood pressure, protein on urinalysis, and an elevated glomerular filtration rate. High blood pressure is a very common cause of kidney disease. But in my opinion, the most common causes of high blood pressure are magnesium deficiency and calcium excess. Why else would doctors prescribe calcium channel blockers for high blood pressure if calcium was not a problem? Kidney patients are told to keep their blood pressure under control, but how are you going to do that if you are warned to stay away from magnesium? Instead you are told to take blood pressure medications that drain more magnesium.

Protein in the urine is one of the earliest signs of kidney disease, especially if you also have diabetes. One of the known medical signs of diabetes is a low magnesium level. So if you have kidney disease and you can't take magnesium, your blood sugar levels are going to keep getting higher as your magnesium gets lower. And then you will be put on drugs for diabetes, which will cause more magnesium deficiency.

Doctors recommend kidney blood tests be done annually to help diagnose kidney disease early, so it can be treated. And what is the medical treatment? Using medications to prevent high blood pressure and diabetes. On all the medical websites I researched, there was no mention of using magnesium to prevent and treat high blood pressure or diabetes. These sites make it clear, however, that kidney disease is usually progressive, ending in kidney failure (end-stage renal disease) and heart failure. All the websites warn patients to avoid magnesium.

KIDNEYS NEED MAGNESIUM

I mentioned three kidney review papers in the Introduction that are opening the dialogue about magnesium and kidney disease. The first two reviews are from the *Clinical Kidney Journal*, February 2012 issue—"Magnesium in Disease" and "Magnesium Basics."[46, 47] In fact, there is a whole supplement section called "Magnesium—A Versatile and Often Overlooked Element: New Perspectives with a Focus on Chronic Kidney Disease," devoted to magnesium in kidney disease.[48] I'll list the titles of the articles in that supplement to show the scope of the dialogue. Most articles are freely available on the Internet, so you can share them with your doctor. You may be surprised to learn that giving a few articles from a peer-reviewed journal to your doctor could make all the difference in his or her acceptance of magnesium therapy.

Articles in "Magnesium—A Versatile and Often Overlooked Element"

1. Editorial: Whither Magnesium?
2. Magnesium Basics
3. Regulation of Magnesium Balance: Lessons Learned from Human Genetic Disease
4. Magnesium in Disease
5. Magnesium in Chronic Kidney Disease Stages 3 and 4 and in Dialysis Patients
6. Magnesium and Outcomes in Patients with Chronic Kidney Disease: Focus on Vascular Calcification, Atherosclerosis and Survival
7. Use of Magnesium as a Drug in Chronic Kidney Disease

"Magnesium and Dialysis: The Neglected Cation" is a 2015 review where the authors found that magnesium requirements need to be reevaluated in the treatment of kidney disease and the use of magnesium in dialysis patients.[49]

There was a much earlier attempt to evaluate the need for magnesium in kidney disease, in 1993. Here is the story that opened my eyes to the importance of magnesium in kidney disease, a story told to me by well-known magnesium researcher Dr. Burton Altura.

Many years ago Dr. Altura asked a colleague, a kidney disease specialist, Dr. Markell, to test his kidney patients for magnesium levels. It was agreed that both ionized magnesium and serum magnesium would be tested and compared in dialysis patients.[50] The results were that people with chronic kidney disease (of all varieties) had simultaneously the highest levels of serum magnesium and the lowest levels of ionized magnesium. It appeared that their magnesium was stuck in the bloodstream and not getting into their cells. It's not reported in the study, but when these patients took a liquid magnesium, their ionized magnesium levels improved, their serum magnesium levels became normal, their symptoms were alleviated, and their kidney function tests improved.

This anecdote explains for me why doctors fear magnesium. They just measure serum magnesium, see that the levels are elevated, and assume the worst. However, they don't test for and therefore don't notice that ionic magnesium is low, showing that the cells remain starved for magnesium. There is not enough magnesium in ionic form to get inside the cells to do its work. Unfortunately, the definitive test for magnesium, which measures ionized magnesium, is a research tool and not available to the public. You can read more about magnesium testing in Chapter 16. Also read in Chapter 18 about the stabilized ionic form of magnesium, ReMag, that is the only form that I recommend for people with kidney disease.

MAGNESIUM DEFICIENCY IN END-STAGE RENAL DISEASE

The following is a case history that emphasizes what end-stage renal disease patients are up against in their battle to stay well. This insightful correspondence is from a Ph.D. in health sciences who suffers from ESRD. She describes the magnesium deficiency caused by her dialysis and her self-treatment with ReMag.

I am a sixty-year-old ESRD patient on home hemodialysis for four years. I am a type 1 diabetic as well. When I began dialysis I gave the nurse my list of supplements, which included magnesium, and I was told in no uncertain terms that dialysis patients should not and cannot take magnesium, our kidneys could be harmed by it. So I complied with their fearful stance as I entered into the unknown realms of kidney failure care, assuming they knew what they were talking about.

Before I began home hemodialysis I started off with peritoneal dialysis, since they presented it as the more "natural" mode. (Fluid is introduced through a permanent tube in the abdomen and flushed out the same tube during the night.) I soon developed incredible itching all over my body that they said was from being underdialyzed. But now I also believe that as my magnesium bottomed out, my calcium and phosphorus soared and combined to form calcium phosphate crystals, which deposited in my skin. Dialysis people have lots of skin issues. Yes, they are due to toxins, but perhaps more importantly due to low magnesium.

I remember seeing things that looked like little white crystals in my skin, which I scratched until I bled. My own dialysis doctors were not even convinced this was due to dialysis! A nephrologist at Vanderbilt gave me a second opinion and had seen it. He said they call it the "crazy itch" and treat it by putting people under UV lights. Knowing what I do now, I presume the UV would be helpful by raising active vitamin D, which helps lower the calcium phosphate complex levels in the skin by sending the calcium and phosphorus into the bones.

I also began having horrendous nighttime calf and

foot cramping on peritoneal dialysis, having to jump out of bed at night to try to soothe the unbearable pain. I was still afraid to take magnesium, so I downed vitamin E, B complex, etc., and whatever else I could find as suggestions online.

Then I was switched to home hemodialysis and there must be more magnesium in the dialysis solution they use compared to peritoneal dialysis because my skin improved. However, over a year ago I began to have heart palpitations that would at first come and go but then worsened and became more constant. After reading many recent studies online, I believe that the dialysis liquid they are putting in me is actually pulling magnesium out of my blood and depleting me. I feel my heart begin to palpitate in my chest towards the end of every treatment. Many patients have leg cramping during treatment. Many dialysis patients have heart issues; it's the number one killer of dialysis patients, and most likely caused by magnesium deficiency.

During the four years since I have been on dialysis, I have broken bones in my feet three times; increased the level of calcification in my arteries (showed up on X-ray); had worsening palpitations, brain fog, and changes in my teeth; and who knows what else!

Thank goodness I found Dr. Dean's ReMag and have been supplementing with it. I find it hard to believe but it totally resolves my palpitations. Of course I bump heads with the powers that be who say magnesium is dangerous for kidney patients, but my kidney specialist is finally behind my decision to use it.

Besides eliminating my palpitations, since I have been taking ReMag, my phosphorus levels have dropped to nearer normal levels so they are reducing the phosphate binders that I take with every meal. My hope is to reach a point where I need no binders at all. I have the hope that supplementing with ReMag will reverse many of my symptoms.

Magnesium is rarely measured in the dialysis setting. I went through all kinds of red tape to get pre- and posttreatment magnesium RBC blood testing. This should be routine! To me this is unbelievable because I'm sure most patients are having their magnesium sucked away through their dialysis treatment. And sure enough, my magnesium levels were lower after dialysis than before it. So each treatment depletes my magnesium further and further.

The more I look into magnesium deficiency, the more I attribute the majority of my health problems, since beginning dialysis, to the depletion of my magnesium levels. When I bring this up, the dialysis staff gets quite defensive. I seem to know more than they do, which intimidates them, not to mention that it really is the fault of their dialysis liquid that I have suffered these symptoms. They know so little about magnesium and how it interacts with phosphorus, calcium, PTH, and vitamin D_3.

I just thank God I have found the studies online saying that I really do need magnesium and then I found ReMag, which really made such a difference, almost immediately. I sometimes wake up in the middle of the night with palpitations, and no way can I sleep with my heart bouncing around in my chest, so I pour a capful of ReMag in a few swallows of water, and I swear, within minutes my heartbeat returns to normal.

The 2015 review paper, "Magnesium and Dialysis: The Neglected Cation," that I mentioned above and in the Introduction should provide kidney specialists with enough updated information to accept magnesium as a necessary mineral for kidney health.[51] At the very least, it's an article that you can print out and give to your doctor to explain why you want to take magnesium even if you have kidney disease.

NOTE: I recommend only ReMag for people with kidney disease because it is so well absorbed into the cells that it's not going to build up to high levels in the blood.

VASCULAR CALCIFICATION IN KIDNEY DISEASE

Just as doctors are finding a buildup of calcium in the coronary arteries that they follow with coronary calcium scans to assess the risk of heart disease, kidney artery calcification is a sign of progressive kidney disease. A paper by Demer and Tintut in the journal *Circulation* discusses a complication of chronic kidney disease called vascular calcification that is causing widespread problems.[52]

The authors acknowledge the sad fact that most people over sixty years of age have "progressively enlarging deposits of calcium mineral in their major arteries." The calcium buildup causes stiffness of the arteries, which results in hypertension, aortic stenosis, cardiac enlargement, angina, intermittent claudication of the lower legs, and congestive heart failure. They conclude, "The severity and extent of mineralization reflect atherosclerotic plaque burden and strongly and independently predict cardiovascular morbidity and mortality."

I was shocked by the assertion in this paper that "progressively enlarging deposits of calcium mineral in their major arteries" is a fact of life in the over-sixty age group. Such a declaration goes hand in hand with the knowledge that most individuals over sixty have magnesium deficiency and the inability to keep calcium in solution!

Vascular calcification is gaining more recognition, but investigators are trying to distinguish it from atherosclerosis (hardening of the arteries), which is calcified fatty plaque that clogs up arteries. Personally, I think it's just another theory that keeps researchers funded while ignoring the fact that calcium buildup in the arteries in any form is a serious health problem and magnesium is the solution.

A 2014 study did find that magnesium minimizes the buildup of vascular calcification by directly antagonizing phosphate and also by suppressing absorption of dietary phosphate.[53] The investigators suggest that this action of magnesium allows it to act as a phosphate binder, which would be very helpful in dialysis patients who suffer excess phosphate levels. They do not mention the direct effects of magnesium on calcium—to keep it dissolved in solution in the body.

SUPPLEMENTS FOR KIDNEY DISEASE

- **ReMag:** With picometer, stabilized ionic magnesium you can reach therapeutic amounts without laxative effects. Start with ¼ tsp (75 mg) and work up to 2 tsp (600 mg) per day. Add ReMag to a liter of water and sip all day to achieve full absorption.
- **ReMyte:** Picometer twelve-mineral solution. Take ½ tsp three times a day, or add 1½ tsp to a liter of water with ReMag and sip throughout the day.
- **ReAline:** B vitamin complex plus amino acids. Take 1 capsule twice per day. Contains food-based B_1 and four methylated B vitamins (B_2, B_6, methylfolate, and B_{12}), plus L-methionine (precursor to glutathione) and L-taurine (which supports the heart and weight loss).

- **Vitamin C complex:** 200 mg twice a day, from a food-based source, or make your own liposomal vitamin C (see Appendix D for a liposomal vitamin C recipe), and ascorbic acid, 1,000 mg twice a day.
- **Vitamin D$_3$:** 1,000 IU or 20 minutes in the sun daily. Blue Ice Royal, from fermented cod liver oil and butter oil, for vitamins A, D, and K$_2$, 1 capsule twice per day.

The Research Continues

WHEN DRS. BURTON AND BELLA ALTURA WROTE THE FORE-word to the first edition of *The Magnesium Miracle,* they called it a "remarkable, almost encyclopedic, but very readable book." They offered more very complimentary comments and then, true and honest scientists to the end, they said, "As to the other interesting parts of the book, our qualifications allow us to comment only on the material pertaining to the scientific basis for the need of magnesium." At that time, in 1999, they had written more than 1,000 papers, mostly on magnesium, but they had not done research on the topics that I put in Part Three under the title "The Research Continues."

However, by 2016, the Alturas had completed even more research, especially on aging. I will comment in depth on their paper on telomeres and aging in Chapter 15. I have also updated the chapters on chronic fatigue syndrome, fibromyalgia, environmental illness, asthma, cystic fibrosis, Alzheimer's, and Parkinson's disease with more current research. The research does continue, and the evidence is now conclusive that magnesium deficiency contributes to all the above conditions and magnesium therapy can help prevent and help treat them.

MAGNESIUM RESEARCH ON THE RISE

The studies supporting magnesium's role as a necessary mineral for health have exploded in the past few years. I briefly mentioned almost a dozen recent magnesium review papers in the Introduction, but that's not even close to the complete works on magnesium. New reports on magnesium for memory, brain plasticity, life extension, chronic fatigue syndrome, diabetes, cancer, connective tissue, stroke, pancreatic enzyme function, neuroprotection in premature infants, prostate cancer, macular degeneration, and glaucoma all caught my eye.

MAGNESIUM AND CANCER

With one in two men and one in three women developing cancer in their lifetime, it's important to mention the relationship of this serious condition to magnesium deficiency. Many years ago, in 1993, Dr. Mildred Seelig wrote an extensive paper on cancer and its interaction with minerals and vitamins with a focus on magnesium. The paper, called "Magnesium in Oncogenesis and in Anti-Cancer Treatment," is available online.[1] Back then Seelig noted a relationship between magnesium deficiency and cancer, which should have alerted the cancer establishment to do further research.

J. I. Rodale wrote a chapter on cancer and magnesium in his 1963 publication, with evidence from doctors in France of the importance of magnesium for this set of diseases.[2] He extensively quoted French physician Dr. Delbet, who felt that magnesium acts as a "brake" on cancer cell replication.

He also observed that as the body grows older it grows more deficient in magnesium, and with this loss in magnesium there is a decrease in vitality, resistance, and cell regeneration.

The latest reports on the association of cancer and magnesium are particularly interesting. I don't believe it's a "cure" for cancer, but as Dr. Delbet says, it can be protective. Here is an overview of the current research.

- A 2015 study in the *British Journal of Cancer* called "Magnesium Intake and Incidence of Pancreatic Cancer: The Vitamins and Lifestyle Study" found that magnesium intake may be beneficial in preventing pancreatic cancer.[3] The study analyzed data on more than 66,000 men and women between the ages of fifty and seventy-six, looking at the direct association between magnesium and pancreatic cancer. Every 100 mg-per-day decrease in magnesium intake was associated with a 24 percent increase in the occurrence of pancreatic cancer. The researchers commented in a *Science Daily* article: "For those at a higher risk of pancreatic cancer, adding a magnesium supplement to their diet may prove beneficial in preventing this disease."

- Japan's National Cancer Center in Tokyo found that magnesium reduces a man's risk of colon cancer, but, surprisingly, this benefit did not extend to women. This was quite an extensive study of 40,830 men and 46,287 women (average age fifty-seven) who were followed for eight years. For men, a magnesium dietary intake of at least 327 mg per day was associated with a 52 percent lower risk of colon cancer, compared with men taking lower amounts.[4] Dietary intake was assessed using a food frequency questionnaire. The only way I can explain the lack of correlation in women is that they have a much higher need for magnesium to produce and process their hormones and would need more than 327 mg to achieve cancer protection.

- Meta-analyses have shown that a higher intake of dietary magnesium is associated with a lower risk of colorectal tumors. The research of Kuno and colleagues uncovered the mechanism: magnesium inhibits inflammation-related colon cancer in mice by modulating the proliferative activities and chromosomal instability of colorectal cancer cells.[5] The study authors recommend that clinical trials be funded to give magnesium to people with colon inflammation, who are at risk for colorectal cancer, with the expectation that it will show that magnesium prevents cancer from forming.

- A group of 1,170 women with confirmed breast cancer was followed for 87.4 months after diagnosis. It was found that higher dietary intake of magnesium was inversely associated with risk of all-cause mortality. That means the higher intake of magnesium, the lower the risk of death. The investigators concluded that "magnesium intake alone may improve overall survival following breast cancer, and the association may be stronger among those with high Ca:Mg intake ratio." That means the more calcium compared to magnesium, the worse your chance of survival.[6]

While research identifies magnesium deficiency as an associated causative factor (and increased magnesium as a curative factor) in aging, anxiety, arthritis, cerebral palsy, depression, diabetes, dysmenorrhea, head injury, heart disease, high cholesterol, hypertension, insomnia, kidney disease, menopause, obesity, PCOS, infertility, osteoporosis, pain, preeclampsia, pregnancy, stroke, and syndrome X, many investigators believe, as I do, that magnesium also plays an important role in chronic fatigue syndrome, fibromyalgia, and environmental illness. Other researchers say that more investigation needs to be done to prove definitively that magnesium deficiency is a contributing factor. I think the funding for these conditions is largely absent because these conditions have been called psychosomatic for decades. I also say that magnesium supplementation is safe and that people can do their own clinical study on their own body and not wait for science to catch up with reality.

THE MAGNESOME

After the human genome was decoded, human proteome research, to identify all human proteins, became the next frontier. In 2012 this research led to the discovery of the "human magnesome," the name given to a set of proteins containing multiple binding sites for magnesium ions. Using innovative technology, researchers found that magnesium binding sites are very common in proteins and help direct their structure and function.[7]

Early on in their research, Piovesan and his team concluded that "presently we can annotate some 5% of the human genome as inheriting the capability of binding magnesium ions." By 2012, researchers found that 27 percent of the human sequences studied (3,751 out of 13,689) carried magnesium binding sites. This was a much larger percentage than they expected.

I don't know how medicine will utilize this magnesome research. In fact, ever since I reported this study in the 2014 printing of *The Magnesium Miracle*, I've heard nothing more about the human magnesome and have not received a reply from the author to my queries. However, the research shows that magnesium is in a unique position to alter the structure and function of human proteins. Hopefully the discovery of the magnesome will herald a new wave of magnesium research and will highlight the biological supremacy of this regulatory mineral and its role in epigenetics—factors that turn genes on and off. Magnesome research helps us understand exactly why our genes are not in total control of our bodies—they depend on minerals and vitamins to alter their expression. I fervently hope that their research has not been scuttled dismissing magnesium as a vital nutrient simply because it won't lead to the development of new drugs.

The Human Genome Project was launched to identify all the genes in the human body and fulfill the dream that geneticists would be able to match individual genes to individual diseases and then modify those genes. Researchers assumed that if a person had a disease, it would be caused by a faulty gene, and all they would have to do is just snip that gene or a portion of that gene out of existence. Researchers were shocked to find only 23,000 genes in the human body, after many predictions that they would find three times that amount. The more important aspect of genetic research is the epigenetic control of genes by the environment, including nutrients in the environment like magnesium that can switch genes on and off.

MAGNESIUM IN THE PAST

Part Three offers an overview of what many clinicians and researchers already know about these conditions and the magnesium connection. Many of us are not waiting for the conclusions of this research to be "proven" over and over again because we see the beneficial results of magnesium therapy manifesting every day.

But first let's look at magnesium through the eyes of John I. Rodale, the founder of *Prevention* magazine, who in 1968 wrote *Magnesium: The Nutrient That Could Change Your Life*, available free online.[8] Rodale unearthed scientific and clinical research on the use of magnesium in treating infection, polio, epilepsy, alcoholism, prostate inflammation, cancer, and arthritis. Unfortunately, much of this research has been lost or ignored, but it deserves mention in order to reinforce what we already know, stimulate further discussion, and open doors to more investigation of the safety and effectiveness of magnesium.

The scientific research on magnesium that Rodale reported in his book highlighted the work of the brilliant French surgeon Pierre Delbet. His interest in magnesium spread to many other doctors in France, who expanded his work. Rodale gives a long list of French physicians who over the years verified Dr. Delbet's findings and produced new ones of their own. Delbet's magnesium research began while he was searching for a suitable antiseptic solution to apply to the wounds of soldiers injured in World War I. He discovered that magnesium chloride had wonderful healing properties when applied externally. We would do well to pick up Dr. Delbet's research where he left off. Instead it is completely ignored.

IMMUNE SYSTEM

After judging magnesium chloride to be a very effective antiseptic solution, Dr. Delbet began testing oral forms of it on dogs and then on his patients, finding it to be a powerful immune system booster. In a paper presented to the French Academy of Medicine in September 1915, Delbet describes the effect on white blood cells of a solution of magnesium chloride injected into the veins of dogs. White blood cells from blood samples taken before and after the injection were tested for their microbe-killing ability. Rodale reports that "five hundred white cells in the first sample destroyed 245 microbes. Five hundred white cells from the second destroyed 681 microbes. This increase in microbe-killing under the influence of magnesium chloride was 180 percent greater than the other solutions. More experiments were performed; in one there was an increase of 129 percent, in another, 333 percent."

POLIO

Chapter 5 in Rodale's book *Magnesium: The Nutrient That Could Change Your Life* describes the treatment of polio with magnesium.

Fortunately, polio is not the scourge it once was. However, back in the 1920s it was a terrible disease. A follower of Dr. Delbet, Dr. A. Neveu, published a booklet titled *Therapeutic Treatment of Infectious Diseases by Magnesium Chloride: Poliomyelitis.* The book described fifteen cases of polio effectively treated with magnesium chloride. Neveu was so convinced of the effectiveness of magnesium chloride that he insisted that every home should have a solution of magnesium chloride on hand to treat the first signs of sore throat, especially when stiffness of the neck was involved. His formula was 20 grams of magnesium chloride powder to 1 liter of water.

PROSTATE

There appears to be no medical cure for enlargement of the prostate (benign prostatic hypertrophy, or BPH), which leads to frequent nighttime urination. However, in 1930 Dr. Delbet and another doctor made two separate presentations to the Medical Academy of France showing that magnesium chloride could adequately treat this condition.

SENILITY AND AGING

It appears that the early French researchers were very aware of the problem caused by calcium precipitating into the tissues of the body. Dr. Delbet observed that with age, the body's tissues have three times more calcium than magnesium, and he concluded that magnesium deficiency plays a role in senility.

ALCOHOLISM

In his research more than a century ago, Dr. Delbet came to the conclusion that a major cause of alcoholism is magnesium deficiency. Presently there is little research being done on this association and even less on the clinical application of magnesium in the treatment of alcoholism. This is in spite of the fact that medical researchers are aware of the association of alcoholism with magnesium deficiency.

MAGNESIUM AND BODY ODOR

There are no scientific studies about the effects of magnesium on body odor, but Rodale reported in his book that Delbet considered body odor to be due to an imbalance in the normal intestinal bacteria and that magnesium somehow restored that balance. Rodale later collected many anecdotal reports about the reduction of underarm odor, stool odor, and general body odor in people taking magnesium.

Chronic Fatigue Syndrome, Fibromyalgia

THREE THINGS YOU NEED TO KNOW ABOUT MAGNESIUM, CHRONIC FATIGUE SYNDROME, AND FIBROMYALGIA

1. Magnesium deficiency is common in chronic fatigue syndrome and fibromyalgia sufferers.
2. Magnesium forms an important part of treatment for chronic fatigue syndrome and fibromyalgia.
3. Magnesium ameliorates the fatigue, muscle pain, and chemical sensitivity of chronic fatigue syndrome and fibromyalgia.

Over the past one hundred years, we have had a tremendous love affair with chemicals and electronics and a strange marriage with scientific methodology. It is safe to say that important advances in chemicals, pharmaceuticals, and science in general came out of the World War II effort and space research. The unseen potential risks to the public were presumably outweighed by the crisis of the time.

However, our sedentary lifestyle, consumption of synthetic foods, environmental chemicals, and polluted atmosphere have coincided with a greater frequency of chronic fatigue syndrome and fibromyalgia. On a parallel track, magnesium and other nutrients have become woefully depleted and, as we will see in Chapter 13, leave us unable to protect our bodies and brains from chemicals.

CHRONIC FATIGUE SYNDROME

Chronic fatigue syndrome (CFS) was formally recognized and defined as an illness by the Centers for Disease Control (CDC) in 1988. I began recognizing the condition in my practice around that time and worked with an immunologist gathering blood test data to try to find a cause.

In the early years of CFS, many doctors considered the condition psychological; some still do because there are no definite blood or biopsy markers to identify it. CFS goes by various names: Epstein-Barr, yuppie flu, and, in Britain, myalgic encephalomyelitis (which identifies the muscles and brain as sites of inflammation). Unfortunately, chronic fatigue syndrome is the name that has stuck in the United States, which makes it seem related to the generalized fatigue that anyone can suffer at one time or another. The name minimizes the global impact that this devastating disease can have on a person's life.

The symptoms of CFS are chronic headaches, swollen glands, periodic fevers and chills, muscle and joint aches and pains, muscle weakness, sore throat, and numbness and tingling of the extremities. The general feeling is one of incredible fatigue and inability to do even the simplest of tasks or to exercise without becoming exhausted, inability to cope with any stress, and insomnia.

There are many theories about the cause of CFS, but one triggering factor could be a reactivation of an already present mononucleosis-like virus called Epstein-Barr virus. Upward of 90 percent of the population already have antibodies to Epstein-Barr virus, meaning the virus infected them at some point in their lives. In most people the infection came and went like a normal cold or flu. But for some, the first infection or the reactivation of the virus can be quite severe and leave them feeling fatigued, run-down, and never truly healthy again.

If CFS is some type of infection presenting itself in a new way, then the people it affects most severely seem to be more run-down and stressed than average. It appears that this infection becomes chronic because the immune system is not strong enough to fight it off or because sufferers come in contact with a chemical or pollutant or allergen that undermines their resistance and allows them to succumb to the illness. One of the ways the immune system is stressed is by the generalized depletion of minerals and vitamins that it needs to function properly.

CHRONIC FATIGUE SYNDROME DIAGNOSTIC CRITERIA

Major Criteria
- New onset of fatigue, causing a 50 percent reduction in activity for at least six months
- Exclusion of other illnesses that can cause fatigue

Minor Criteria
- Presence of eight of eleven symptoms, or six of eleven symptoms and two of the three signs

Symptoms
- Mild fever
- Recurrent sore throat
- Painful lymph nodes
- Muscle weakness

- Muscle pain
- Prolonged fatigue after exercise
- Recurrent headache
- Migratory joint pain
- Neurological or psychological complaints: sensitivity to bright light, forgetfulness, confusion, inability to concentrate, excessive irritability, depression
- Sleep disturbance
- Sudden onset of symptom complex

Signs
- Low-grade fever
- Sore throat without signs of pus
- Palpable or tender lymph nodes

Sheila fit the profile of chronic fatigue syndrome. After suffering mononucleosis during college, she has never felt quite the same. The mono seemed to weaken her immune system and her adrenal glands. Sheila worked as a teacher and was constantly exposed to germs, coming down with every cold and flu that passed through the school. Because she traveled a lot, she received numerous inoculations, which further weakened her. In her spare time, she enjoyed furniture refinishing, which exposed her to tung oil, found in varnishes, paint strippers, and paint. Tung oil is made from euphorbia, a plant that produces phorbol esters, and has been proposed as a causative agent for chronic fatigue syndrome.[1]

After a trip to the Far East, Sheila became more and more fatigued and came down with a terrible month-long flu with a horribly achy head, muscles, and joints. Her doctor put her on one antibiotic after another, even though she had no bacterial infection. Her cough and chest pain finally cleared up, but she continued to have periodic fevers, a sore throat, and sore muscles. She couldn't exercise at all because she would end up in bed for days, and no matter how tired she was, she couldn't sleep. Sheila was depressed by this constant sickness. Sometimes she felt as if she were losing her mind: she couldn't concentrate, remember, or perform simple arithmetic. She couldn't teach and was so exhausted that she could do only the bare minimum to take care of herself.

Fortunately, Sheila's doctor was involved with a study at a local university looking into possible drug treatments for CFS. Sheila entered the blind study and did not know which treatment she was receiving. The three medications were an anti-inflammatory drug (ibuprofen), an antidepressant (amitriptyline), and magnesium. She had weekly visits with a nurse to assess her symptoms, twenty-four-hour urine collections, blood tests, and questionnaires. After two weeks her fatigue improved, as did her muscle weakness, twitching, poor concentration, and irritability.

At the end of the study, Sheila was told that her treatment had been 300 mg of elemental magnesium twice a day, that her magnesium had been very low at the beginning of the study, and that she could safely continue with the treatment if she wished. Sheila now had the energy to do more things to take care of herself: exercise, shop for the right foods, and prepare more meals from fresh foods. She knew she was on the road to recovery, thanks to magnesium. Several other studies confirm the efficacy of using magnesium for the treatment of chronic fatigue syndrome symptoms.[2, 3, 4, 5]

FIBROMYALGIA

It wasn't until 1990 that the American College of Rheumatology established diagnostic criteria for fibromyalgia, thereby giving it official status as an illness. *Fibro-* means "connective tissue" and refers to the thin tissue that wraps around muscles, and *myalgia* means "muscle pain." Sometimes called fibrositis, fibromyalgia is a close cousin of CFS and shares many of its symptoms: incapacitating fatigue, muscle and joint pain, neuralgia, sleep disorders, anxiety, depression, cognitive confusion, and digestive problems. (CFS sufferers, in addition, have mild fever, swollen glands, and a sore throat, which distinguishes them from fibromyalgia patients.)

Having a name, however, does not define the causes of the illness, and the American College of Rheumatology does not offer a curative treatment. I believe fibromyalgia is the latest label for an accumulation of toxins and infections from both environment and lifestyle. Twenty-six doctors who present their cases in a book on chronic fatigue and fibromyalgia agree.[6]

Our exposure to toxins, chemicals, and prescription drugs begins at birth. Substances we think are safe can break down our immune systems and deplete our nutrient reserves. I and many other doctors believe they lead to CFS, fibromyalgia, and environmental illness for a growing list of sufferers.[7] I'll continue the discussion about environmental illness in Chapter 13, but focus on CFS and fibromyalgia in this chapter.

FIBROMYALGIA DIAGNOSTIC CRITERIA

Major Criteria

- Generalized aches or stiffness of at least three anatomical sites for at least three months
- Six or more typical, reproducible tender points, called trigger points, in the muscles
- Exclusion of other disorders that can cause similar symptoms

Minor Criteria
- Generalized fatigue
- Chronic headaches
- Sleep disturbances
- Neurological and psychological complaints
- Joint swelling
- Numbness or tingling sensation
- Irritable bowel syndrome
- Variation of symptoms in relation to activity, stress, and weather changes

Below is a chronology of ailments and the kinds of medical treatments any one of us may receive over the course of a lifetime. Each treatment can trigger the next event and further drug intervention.

However, in my experience, a person with fibromyalgia can diminish his or her symptoms by at least 50 percent by taking the right amount and the right kind of magnesium. See Chapter 18 for more information on my magnesium recommendations. I've found that the other 50 percent of symptoms are related to yeast overgrowth and require a yeast detox protocol.

Health Chronology for CFS and Fibromyalgia Sufferers

- Diaper rash, caused by *Candida albicans* (yeast), is mistakenly treated with cortisone creams, which encourage further growth of the yeast.
- Childhood ear infections can begin at birth as yeast infections picked up from the mother during delivery. Most ear infections are treated with antibiotics.
- Ear infections may become chronic and require multiple courses of antibiotics, leading to diarrhea and intestinal yeast infections.

- Anesthetics used in surgery to place tubes in the ears add another toxin.
- Colic can develop due to antibiotics.
- Inability to digest milk due to an irritated bowel leads to frequent changes of formula and further irritation.
- Gas and bloating can result from hard-to-digest soy formula.
- Eczema, aggravated by food sensitivity, is suppressed with cortisone creams.
- Allergies to foods, especially yeast, wheat, and dairy, can arise from poor digestion.
- Asthma, which may be environmental, is treated with medications including corticosteroid inhalers.
- Multiple colds and flus are mistreated with many courses of antibiotics.
- Annual flu vaccines contain mercury preservative.
- Cravings for sweets can be caused by yeast overgrowth and may cause or aggravate hyperactive behavior in children.
- Dental cavities lead to multiple mercury amalgam fillings. Toxic mercury vapor may be inhaled or absorbed, disrupting enzymes in the brain, kidneys, and liver.
- Allergic reactions are treated with allergy shots, antihistamines, and cortisone sprays.
- Many adolescents take long-term oral antibiotics for acne.
- Many teens and young adults develop mononucleosis, and up to 20 percent never feel quite as healthy again.
- Bladder infections are treated with antibiotics, which cause yeast infections.
- Birth control pills cause chronic vaginal yeast infections, which are mistreated with antibiotic creams.
- Pregnancy hormones encourage vaginal yeast infections.
- Chronic sleep deprivation is common in all parents of small children and is a major stress on the immune system.

- Irritable bowel syndrome can develop after a bout of diarrhea (attributed to traveler's diarrhea or food poisoning) and is usually treated with antibiotics.
- Chronic sinus infections (97 percent are fungal, according to the Mayo Clinic) occur due to lowered immune system and are mistakenly treated with antibiotics.
- Hypothyroidism often occurs but remains undiagnosed and untreated.
- Adrenal exhaustion is common due to constant stress from all the above factors.
- Hospitalization for infections or surgery usually warrants intravenous antibiotics and a host of other drugs.
- Major colds and flus can lead to bronchitis and pneumonia, which are treated with strong antibiotics. A growing number of fibromyalgia sufferers lay the blame for their symptoms on Cipro.
- Chronic fatigue syndrome and fibromyalgia are treated with anti-inflammatories, sleeping pills, and antidepressants.
- Environmental allergies with extreme sensitivities to inhalants, especially perfumes, colognes, household products, pesticides, and molds, are treated with corticosteroid inhalers.
- Dysmenorrhea, irregular periods, infertility, and worsening premenstrual symptoms occur due to a buildup of toxins and lack of nutrients.
- Infertility is treated with an array of synthetic hormonal drugs.
- Depression, anxiety, panic attacks, and palpitations are treated with antidepressants and psychotherapy.
- Menopause is medicated with synthetic hormones.

Magnesium is depleted with every step of this scenario and results in a total body burden of drugs, toxins, and various stressors. The end result looks very much like chronic fatigue syndrome.

THE LAYERS OF FIBROMYALGIA

Let's look at the journey through life from the ground up to understand why we have become so nutrient-deficient and how this affects the immune system.

Plants grown on devitalized, overworked soil that has been poisoned by acid rain are poor in nutrients, including magnesium. The topic of magnesium-deficient soil is covered in Chapter 2. Synthetic foods, created by modern processing and refining, are devoid of natural vitamins, minerals, and fiber. They are "fortified" with useless synthetic vitamins and often no minerals except calcium or iron. Magnesium is the nutrient hardest hit by food processing.

A poorly nourished body is not able to adequately process junk food, with its dozens of chemical additives. It treats these chemical additives like foreign invaders and has to detoxify them in the liver. The intermediary metabolites are sometimes more toxic than the original substance, leaving the body hypersensitive and hyperimmune, sometimes turning on the body and creating autoimmune disease (such as multiple sclerosis or rheumatoid arthritis). Magnesium is depleted in the attempt to detoxify the body of these foreign chemicals.

There are thousands of medicinal drugs currently in use. Magnesium expert Dr. Mildred Seelig noted that the side effects of many drugs may be associated with magnesium deficiency because magnesium becomes depleted with the effort the body makes to try to detoxify these drugs.

DEVELOPING YEAST OVERGROWTH

With the discovery of antibiotics and the hope that they could cure all our infectious diseases, there has been an escalating overuse of these powerful drugs. When antibiotics kill bacteria, they cannot discriminate; they kill both good and bad bacteria. The good bacteria killed in the gastrointestinal tract are then replaced with yeast *(Candida albicans)*. A total of 178 different toxins produced by yeast over the course of its life cycle become foreign chemicals to an already beleaguered immune system.

The birth control pill, with its daily hormone surge, feeds yeast in the gut, as do sugar products. Yeast overgrowth results in episodes of alternating diarrhea and constipation. Magnesium is lost due to diarrhea and is drained by the constant demand to balance the pH of the body due to the acidity of soda pop and junk food.

The symptoms from yeast and its breakdown products are body-wide. Often these symptoms lead one to think that there are infections in the sinuses, throat, bladder, or vagina. A doctor will consequently prescribe more antibiotics for these symptoms, which merely perpetuates the problem. Overgrowth of yeast in the intestines can cause micropunctures in their lining, called leaky gut, thus allowing the absorption of incompletely digested food into the bloodstream. These undigested food particles add to the list of foreign bodies, and the immune system reacts by forming antibodies to try to get rid of them. The result is food sensitivities that may be misdiagnosed as food allergies.

Environmental allergies are created when inhaled chemicals and toxins irritate the mucous membranes of the nasal passages. They can trigger symptoms of asthma, which is made worse by magnesium deficiency.

Depression can be a direct result of accumulating chemicals in the body from drugs, synthetic food, and infections. When the brain is deficient in magnesium it is no longer protected from the onslaught of chemicals such as aspartame and MSG.

Because there are no medical tests to confirm that chemicals, drugs, and synthetic food are causing our symptoms, people who feel sick are often told that all their tests are normal, the implication being that their symptoms are all in their head. Having no proof of their illness is frustrating and depressing, making sufferers feel even more unwell. The majority of chronically ill patients who used to come to my office or now talk to me on my radio show have seen between six and thirty doctors for their complaints. Patients with fatigue or depression have usually been referred to a psychiatrist. Some patients have been prescribed thousands of dollars' worth of drugs and supplements annually to treat their multiple complaints, which usually have done no good and merely added to their toxin load.

THERE IS NO CFS OR FIBROMYALGIA DRUG

The complex nature of CFS and fibromyalgia is formidable. Even though more doctors understand and accept the existence of CFS, the focus of CFS research seems to be on finding one cause. And the treatments offered are only symptomatic: rheumatologists and psychiatrists treat sleeplessness with sleeping pills; pain with anti-inflammatory drugs, painkillers, and muscle relaxants; and anxiety and depression with antianxiety drugs and antidepressants. None of these medications seem to work, and they certainly don't cure the problem; in fact, people with CFS seem to be very sensitive to drugs and can develop many side effects, including magnesium deficiency.

No attention is paid to diet or nutrient deficiencies. Doctors ignore the possibility that there could be a nutrient imbalance, such as a magnesium deficiency, or coexisting conditions, such as a yeast infection, low thyroid, adrenal exhaustion, or allergies, that cause a complex of symptoms. They also tend to overlook possible toxicities, which allow common infections to appear more virulent as they take advantage of a weakened host. Yet magnesium deficiency is known to exacerbate all the symptoms of CFS and fibromyalgia, and increased magnesium intake has been effective in helping to restore health to many sufferers. Magnesium is also one of the best ways to strengthen the immune system and boost resistance against germs.

WORSE WITH EXERCISE

Exercise is often suggested for people suffering from fatigue, but even the mildest aerobic exercise is exhausting to people with CFS or fibromyalgia, who have no energy because their magnesium-driven energy system is bankrupt. Without magnesium to power the Krebs cycle, ATP is depleted. Exercise creates lactic acid buildup, which leads to more pain when it is not cleared by a particular enzyme that requires magnesium. Even the work of metabolizing pain medications depletes magnesium. This explains why chronic fatigue patients do not do well on most medications.

A buildup of lactic acid in the muscles causes pain and can be treated with 300 mg of elemental magnesium twice a day. If the joints accumulate toxicity, arthritis can occur; if the nerves are irritated by neurotoxins, they begin to lose their myelin sheath, and symptoms of multiple sclerosis can result. In fact, autoimmune disease may be the end stage of a buildup of toxicity exacerbated by a deficiency of nutrients, such as magnesium, that are designed to clear toxins from the body. According to some doctors, the definition of auto-immune disease as "disease against self" is not accurate; the disease process is, in fact, attacking a self that is altered by toxins and nutrient deficiencies.

Patients with fibromyalgia also have chronically low levels of serotonin, which greatly exaggerates their pain. Yeast overgrowth in the intestines can diminish the production of serotonin in the gut. As mentioned previously, magnesium is a necessary building block for both the production and uptake of serotonin by brain cells.

CFS AND FIBROMYALGIA WORSENED BY STRESS

Stress does worsen these conditions, which has led many doctors to call them psychosomatic diseases. But stress is just part of the whole picture. Acute episodes of CFS and fibromyalgia can be brought on by exposure to stress, whether emotional or physical. The consequent increase in adrenaline and stress chemicals hastens magnesium loss and can be a factor in both conditions. Low levels of magnesium intensify the secretion of the stress chemicals but in an erratic fashion, thus increasing the risk of adverse effects of stress and creating another vicious cycle.[8]

The overproduction of adrenaline due to stress leads to magnesium deficiency and therefore puts a strain on the magnesium-dependent energy system of the body, causing energy depletion that leads to fatigue. Fatigue is often reduced with magnesium supplementation. In fact, a major breakthrough occurred in CFS research when low magnesium levels were discovered in most sufferers. Of the many enzyme systems that require magnesium, the most important ones are responsible for energy production and energy storage.

MALIC ACID AND FIBROMYALGIA

Another nutrient, malic acid, which is found in apples, is important for the body's energy production, and some say it may be useful in the treatment of CFS and fibromyalgia. Malic acid is active in the seventh step of the Krebs cycle chain reaction that produces the energy molecule ATP. The last several steps of the Krebs cycle have succinate transitioning into fumarate, then into malate, and finally into pyruvate. All of these chemicals are substrates, not cofactors like magnesium. So some researchers have the idea that giving the body more malic acid substrate might produce more energy. Nobody really knows exactly if it does.

I do know that when I took a magnesium malate supplement years ago, it gave me the laxative effect and I didn't notice any positive effect. I think that giving extra substrate for a biochemical reaction can increase the need for the cofactors in that reaction, so I'm wary of that. Also, every chance I get I remind people that magnesium is required as a cofactor in six of the eight steps of the Krebs cycle, including the step between succinate and malate. So I think that well-absorbed magnesium is more important than just taking malic acid.

However, a study by Guy D. Abraham, M.D., done in 1995 did show positive results in the treatment of fibromyalgia with magnesium and malic acid supplementation in a very small group.[9] Fifteen patients with fibromyalgia who took magnesium (300–600 mg) and malic acid (1,200–2,400 mg) experienced improvement in their symptoms within the first forty-eight hours. Over an eight-week period of supplementation their degree of muscle tenderness and pain dropped from 19.6 points to 6.5 points, according to standardized medical scores. Unfortunately, there wasn't a control group who just took magnesium or another group that just took malic acid, so we have no way of knowing what really caused the improvement.

There are magnesium malate supplements available, but I do not think there is enough magnesium in the formulation to have lasting effects. I fall back on the evidence that therapeutic amounts of magnesium are required to improve the symptoms of fibromyalgia, and the best form of non-laxative magnesium is ReMag.

TREATMENT FOR CHRONIC FATIGUE AND FIBROMYALGIA

Diet and supplements should focus on building the immune system and the digestive system. In my experience, addressing yeast overgrowth and magnesium deficiency can result in an overall improvement of about 70–80 percent in CFS and fibromyalgia. Further improvement comes from treating low thyroid, weakened adrenals, estrogen dominance, and heavy metal toxicity. For these conditions I recommend my ReMag, ReMyte, and ReAline formulas.

Any mention of what to eat and what not to eat when you have a chronic health condition is fraught with inconsistencies and inaccuracies. My general diet recommendations for CFS and fibromyalgia are as follows:

- Eliminate alcohol, coffee, white sugar, white flour, gluten, fried foods, and trans fatty acids (found in margarine and in baked, fried, and processed foods made with partially hydrogenated fats).
- Limit red meat and dairy, which contain chemicals that increase inflammation in the body.
- If you eat animal protein, choose organically raised grass-fed beef, free-range chicken and eggs, and fish (especially wild-caught salmon).

- For vegetarian protein, choose fermented dairy, lactose-free cheese, and ReStructure Meal Replacement (it has no casein, very-low-lactose whey protein, and pea and rice proteins).
- Vegan protein choices include legumes, gluten-free grains, nuts, and seeds.
- Healthy carbs include raw, cooked, and fermented vegetables; increase yellow vegetables and green leafy vegetables, which contain substances that inhibit inflammation. Eat only one or two pieces of fruit a day, as fruit sugar feeds yeast. The skins of grapes (choose organic grapes) contain quercetin, which prevents histamine release and inhibits inflammatory products.
- Include magnesium-rich foods listed in Appendix A and calcium-rich foods listed in Appendix B.
- For fats and oils, choose butter, olive oil, sesame oil, and coconut oil.
- Increase intake of fish oils, seed and nut oils, cold-water fish (herring, sardines, salmon), flaxseed oil, and walnuts to reduce inflammation.
- Try a modified fast to decrease inflammation: use a whey, rice, or pea protein powder like ReStructure, a green drink, and/or fresh organic juices plus fiber for three days, followed by a vegetarian diet for four days.
- Get out of the rut of eating the same foods every day. To eliminate possible food allergies, avoid your top three favorite foods (people often crave foods they are sensitive to). Eggs, shellfish, and peanuts usually cause immediate sensitivity reactions; milk, chocolate, wheat, citrus, and food colorings cause delayed food reactions.
- Carefully check labels in the grocery store and speak up in restaurants to avoid even small amounts of potential allergic triggers such as MSG, aspartame, and sulfites.

SUPPLEMENTS FOR CHRONIC FATIGUE AND FIBROMYALGIA

- **ReMag:** With picometer, stabilized ionic magnesium you can reach therapeutic amounts without laxative effects. Start with ¼ tsp (75 mg) and work up to 2–3 tsp (600–900 mg) per day. Add ReMag to a liter of water and sip all day to achieve full absorption.
- **ReMag spray:** Transfer the ReMag to a spray bottle. Each drop of ReMag contains 2.5 mg of stabilized ionic magnesium, so 8 sprays = 20 mg = 1 ml.
- **ReMag Lotion:** Apply several times per day to affected areas. Each teaspoon contains 200 mg of ReMag.
- **ReMyte:** Picometer twelve-mineral solution. Take ½ tsp three times a day, or add 1½ tsp to a liter of water with ReMag and sip throughout the day.
- **ReCalcia:** Picometer, stabilized ionic calcium, boron, vanadium. Take 1–2 tsp per day (1 tsp provides 300 mg calcium) if you don't obtain enough calcium from your diet. It can be taken with ReMag and ReMyte.
- **ReAline:** B vitamin complex plus amino acids. Take 1 capsule twice per day. Contains food-based B_1 and four methylated B vitamins (B_2, B_6, methylfolate, and B_{12}), plus L-methionine (precursor to glutathione) and L-taurine (which supports the heart and weight loss).
- **Vitamin C complex:** 200 mg twice a day, from a food-based source, or make your own liposomal vitamin C (see Appendix D for a liposomal vitamin C recipe), and ascorbic acid, 1,000 mg twice a day.
- **Vitamin D_3:** 1,000 IU or 20 minutes in the sun daily. Blue Ice Royal from fermented cod liver oil and butter oil, for vitamins A, D, and K_2, 1 capsule twice per day.

Environmental Illness

**THREE THINGS YOU NEED TO KNOW ABOUT
MAGNESIUM AND ENVIRONMENTAL ILLNESS**

1. Symptoms of chemical sensitivity can be completely or partially produced by magnesium deficiency.
2. Magnesium helps detoxify toxic chemicals.
3. Magnesium binds with and helps eliminate heavy metals from the body.

Dr. Sherry Rogers is a diplomate in family practice, allergy-asthma-immunology, and environmental medicine and a fellow of the American College of Nutrition. In private practice for close to forty years, she treats very ill people from all over the world who have environmental toxicity and chemical sensitivity. The condition is called multiple chemical sensitivity (MCS) because a susceptible person usually has sensitivities to more than one chemical.

One of Dr. Rogers's basic maxims is that symptoms of chemical sensitivity can be wholly or partly due to magnesium deficiency. She has tested enough people over the decades to know this to be a fact. Part of her success derives from implementing magnesium therapy for all her patients. Dr. Rogers notes that Dr. Frederica P. Perera, professor of environmental health sciences and director of the Columbia Center for Children's Environmental Health, has indicated that there is as much as a 500-fold difference in the ability of individuals to detoxify the same chemical.[1] One of the key markers of this difference is each individual's magnesium level.

CFS and fibromyalgia are actually aspects of environmental illness. In Chapter 12, we saw how these conditions develop over time in a toxic environment. Now we will take a closer look at some environmentally sensitive people and the chemicals they encountered.

Natalie, sometimes in jest but more often in anger, would call what she experienced a "chemical warfare attack." It happened when she stepped out onto her driveway and was enveloped by a cloud of chemical spray from a lawn care truck treating her neighbor's yard. She could neither breathe nor speak. Her lungs were on fire, and her head felt as though it were exploding. She felt dizzy and shaky. She managed to stagger into the house, where she collapsed on the floor. Her husband found her a few minutes later and took her to the hospital, where they could do very little except give her oxygen and tell her to rest.

Natalie had been the picture of health—athletic, active, and happy. Now she was chronically fatigued. She became hypersensitive to every chemical she came in contact with. She couldn't even read; magazines and newspapers reeked of ink. Perfume samples that came in magazines were a nightmare. She had to find natural substitutes for cleaning products and cosmetics. Plants with moldy-smelling dirt had to go. She became allergic to wool. Her husband had to do all the cooking because she was sensitive to the gas fumes from their stove. Her diet became increasingly limited, as she reacted to many foods. When she couldn't even use the telephone because holding the plastic receiver gave her hives, she became a prisoner in her own home with no contact with the outside world.

Elizabeth, Ted, and their children developed an array of symptoms after they used urea formaldehyde insulation in their home renovation. As soon as it was installed, they noticed an odor. The contractor said not to worry, it would be gone in a few days. The only thing that was gone in a few days was the contractor. They phoned and phoned, but he never returned their calls.

By the end of the week the whole family had what appeared to be a bad cold, their eyes and noses streaming. The children developed skin rashes, and they all were irritable, headachy, and tired. When the "cold" didn't go away in ten days they went to the doctor, who saw their red, irritated skin and mucous membranes but no signs of infection, except for swollen neck glands. The doctor suggested they might be allergic to something. That clinched it; they knew it was the insulation. They didn't know what they could do about it. They tried toughing it out to see if the chemical would dissipate, but when the central heating came on the next month the problem actually got worse. They were beginning to be allergic to more and more things, and none of them felt well at all. Finally they decided to rip out all the insulation, no matter what it cost.

Elizabeth, Ted, and the children eventually got better, as did Natalie. With much time, effort, and money and the help of sympathetic and knowledgeable health practitioners who understand the effects of the environment and the need to detoxify and nourish the body, they regained their health. The modalities they used were pure alkaline water, fresh air, organic foods, rotation diets, sauna therapy, vitamin and mineral supplements (especially 300 mg of elemental magnesium twice a day), homeopathy, acupuncture, and a positive attitude.

Some people with environmental illness are not as fortunate as Natalie, Elizabeth, and Ted, who at least knew what was harming them almost from the start. Those who gradually build up allergies and sensitivities to environmental toxins never know they're getting sick until they've developed asthma, eczema, or even cancer. What follows is a short overview of our chemical environment and how its impact on our health can be lessened by neuroprotectants such as magnesium.

OUR CHEMICAL ENVIRONMENT

In the first edition of *The Magnesium Miracle*, I reported that toxic chemicals were being found in all foods, all bodies of water, and all humans in every study performed. In 2003 blood levels for twenty-seven chemicals in around 2,400 Americans far exceeded safe levels. You can read the transcript of a CDC telebriefing on this report.[2] Unfortunately, the number of chemicals tested for is minuscule compared with the more than 100,000 chemicals in everyday use.

In 1993, the U.S. Department of Agriculture (USDA) and the U.S. Environmental Protection Agency (EPA) pledged they would reinforce a cutback in the use of chemical pesticides. Chemical pesticide use, however, increased from 900 million pounds in 1992 to 940 million pounds in 2000, while total cropland had decreased. And the riskiest chemical pesticides, such as organophosphates and carbamates, which are probable or possible carcinogens, still account for over 40 percent of the pesticides used in U.S. agriculture.[3]

Each new series of tests that are done to assess chemicals in the population shows worsening results. The latest testing was from the years 2003–2004 and wasn't published until

2009.[4] It's called "The CDC Fourth National Report on Human Exposure to Environmental Chemicals." The report includes data on the U.S. population's exposure to 212 chemicals. Seventy-five of these chemicals were measured for the first time. You can access the 2009 report at the CDC government website, CDC.gov/ExposureReport, where there are updated tables from February 2015, but no new reports. The 2009 report is a hefty 1,095 pages long; the length of this paper and the contents remind me that the CDC is just interested in reporting data and is not offering solutions.

After you read the "Fourth Report" you will have to patiently wait for the "Fifth Report," which is not yet available, but it will tell you the same thing—we are being increasingly poisoned by our environment.

What is the origin of all this toxic waste? The average American household generates fifteen to twenty-two pounds of household hazardous waste each year, according to the Texas Natural Resource Conservation Commission. "Our homes contain an average of three to eight gallons of hazardous materials in kitchens, bathrooms, garages and basements," the government agency reports.[5]

And what is the consequence of all these chemicals in our home environment? In a California study the number of people with sensitivities to one or more common chemicals is "surprisingly large," according to researchers. Just over 6 percent of the subjects reported having a diagnosis of multiple chemical sensitivities or environmental illness, and nearly 16 percent reported being allergic or unusually sensitive to everyday chemicals.[6]

Dr. Samuel Epstein, a medical doctor and professor emeritus of environmental and occupational health at the University of Illinois, Chicago School of Public Health, is an internationally recognized authority on the toxic and carcinogenic effects of environmental pollutants in air, water, and the workplace. His research was key to banning DDT and other problematic ingredients and contaminants found in consumer products—food, cosmetics, and household products. In his keynote address to a Health Canada–sponsored cancer conference, he reported that all of us now carry more than 500 different chemical compounds in our cells, none of which existed before 1920, and that "there is no safe dose for any of them."[7] With this information, activists have been demanding more use of safe alternatives to chemicals. But government and industry are still not listening.

Chemicals can destroy or paralyze different enzymes that protect us from external toxins. Thus, being exposed to chemicals prevents the body from protecting us from those very chemicals.

METALS AND MAGNESIUM

Mercury pervades our environment through industrial exposure, but the major source of elemental mercury in the general North American population is mercury vapor released from dental amalgams.[8, 9, 10, 11] These amalgams are, on average, 50 percent mercury, and they off-gas, or vaporize, into your body's cells every time you chew, brush your teeth, or eat anything hot or acidic. There is a significant positive correlation between the number of amalgams in the mouth and the mercury content of human tissues, including the brain.[12]

Mercury drastically increases the excretion of magnesium and calcium from the kidneys, which may be the cause of the kidney damage seen in mercury poisoning.[13] Such mineral losses impair cell production, the storage and utilization of energy, and cellular repair and replication. Sufficient magnesium supplementation can undo some of this damage and can also prevent certain types of heavy metal toxicity.[14, 15]

Long-term fetal exposure during pregnancy to even low concentrations of mercury can lead to irreversible developmental disorders.[16] The concentration of magnesium in the placental and fetal tissues normally must increase during pregnancy.[17] Unfortunately, the demand for magnesium usually exceeds its supply, and thus anything that further lowers magnesium levels, such as mercury, puts the unborn child at risk.

Lead and cadmium have a cumulative toxic effect on the kidneys and heart in particular. Magnesium appears to be a competitive inhibitor of these two polluting metals at different sites, particularly during combined intoxication.[18] A Yugoslavian research team found that increased intake of magnesium eliminates lead via the urine and may do the same with certain other heavy metals. Under experimental conditions, they found that magnesium increased excretion of cadmium via the urine.[19] Adequate magnesium levels can also help prevent the toxic effects of aluminum, which include breakdown of sugar stores and disruption in the production of ATP energy.[20] However, if magnesium levels are low, these heavy metals will stay in the body, binding to tissues in the kidneys and heart and (in the case of aluminum especially) crossing the blood-brain barrier and destroying brain cells.

TREATMENT FOR ENVIRONMENTAL ILLNESS

The hallmark of a mineral-deficient person is one who takes vitamins without minerals and feels worse or does well for a short while but then deteriorates.[21] Magnesium is necessary for energy production, but if it is deficient, certain areas of the body may be overstimulated by vitamin supplements, while other areas can't respond. Therefore, if you suffer severe environmental illness, it is important to have a knowledgeable health care practitioner monitor your supplement intake and to begin with magnesium as one of your first supplements.

The treatment for environmental illness must be individualized. Since allopathic medicine does not recognize environmental disease, treatment protocols have not been established, and even those limited protocols that do exist use medications instead of nutrients. According to environmental experts, magnesium is essential to build up the body's energy stores and fully utilize its detoxification systems. The source of environmental toxins, however, must be eliminated or avoided; otherwise it is like bailing out a sinking boat with your bare hands. You first have to be aware of the chemicals in your environment, avoid them like the plague, and work diligently with natural therapies to clean out your body.

The lowly dry-cleaning chemicals, the mercury in dental fillings, and the cleaning products under the kitchen sink all build up in our bodies and cause chronic disease. Air purifying machines, water filters, organic food, organic vitamins, well absorbed minerals, and natural alternatives to chemicals provide the foundation of environmental health therapies.

DIET, HYDRATION, AND SAUNAS

- The key to treating environmental illness is to eat organic, free-range, unprocessed, unadulterated foods. The pesticides added to the soil and the antibiotics used on poultry and beef sicken the animals and the people who eat them. Diseases in cattle for which they are fed tons of antibiotics are likely related to the low quality of their feed, the drugs they are given to fatten them up, and the gallons of chemicals sprayed on them to treat pests and parasites. Unfortunately, even organic farms are subjected to acid rain, contaminated groundwater, and polluted air, which means that all of us should take an active role in detoxifying our bodies of suspected chemicals.

- Drink one-half your body weight in ounces of water daily. To each liter of your drinking water add ¼ tsp of unrefined sea salt, pink Himalayan salt, or Celtic sea salt. Chemicals in our environment that are water-soluble are eliminated through the kidneys and colon, especially if you drink enough pure water. Use a water filter that has a pore size of less than 0.5 micron and guarantees the elimination of many chemicals as well as parasites.
- To help excrete fat-soluble chemicals such as pesticides and herbicides, which can become even more toxic when they are broken down by the liver, use sauna therapy (dry or far infrared).
- Fasting is not recommended to eliminate toxins when someone has chemical sensitivities. Fat-soluble chemicals are stored in fat cells, which keeps them out of circulation. When you try to fast or diet, your fat stores are broken down for energy, and out come the chemicals. Headaches, nausea, light-headedness, and irritability are not just from lack of food but also from poisons flooding your bloodstream. While fasting, I've tasted and felt the numbing effect of dental anesthetics from decades before. If you are already feeling ill, fasting and dieting are going to be very unpleasant experiences.

Dry Sauna

Numerous cultures use sweat lodges, steam baths, or saunas for cleansing and purification. Many health clubs and apartment complexes have saunas and steam baths, and more and more people are building saunas in their own homes. Low-to-moderate-temperature saunas are one of the most important ways to detoxify from pesticide exposure. Head-to-toe perspiration through the skin, the largest organ of elimination, releases stored toxins and opens the pores.

Fat that is close to the skin is heated, mobilized, and broken down, releasing toxins and breaking up cellulite. The heat increases metabolism, burns off calories, and gives the heart and circulation a workout. This is a boon if you don't have the energy to exercise. It is well known in medicine that a fever is the body's way of burning off an infection and stimulating the immune system. Fever therapy and sauna therapy are employed at alternative medicine healing centers to do just that. The controlled temperature in a sauna is excellent for relaxing muscular aches and pains and relieving sinus congestion. The only way I made it through my medical internship was by having regular saunas in the nurses' residence to reduce my daily stress.

Far-Infrared Saunas

Far-infrared (FIR) saunas are inexpensive, convenient, and highly effective. Detox expert Dr. Sherry Rogers says that FIR saunas are a proven and efficacious way of eliminating stored environmental toxins, and she thinks everyone should use them. There are one-person sauna domes that you lie under or more elaborate sauna boxes that seat several people.

Far infrared provides a heat that increases the body temperature but the surrounding air is not overly heated. One advantage of the dome is that your head remains outside, which most people find more comfortable and less confining. Sweating begins within minutes of entering the dome and can be continued for thirty to sixty minutes. Besides the hundreds of toxins that can be removed through simple sweating, saunas create a mild "heat shock," which researchers feel acts as a stimulus for the body's cells to work more efficiently.

The outward sign of an effective sauna is the production of sweat, which is the body's attempt to decrease the body temperature, but there is much more going on. Further research on sauna therapy is destined to make it an important medical therapy.

SUPPLEMENTS FOR ENVIRONMENTAL ILLNESS

If you have environmental illness, you feel as though you are sensitive or allergic to everything. When it comes to taking supplements, you may feel you are unable to tolerate anything, but you might also be deficient in everything. Being sensitive to supplements does not necessarily mean that you are allergic; rather, when you take a supplement, your body responds by increasing some metabolic processes, which results in the body throwing off waste products that make you feel nauseated or headachy. That is why an organic diet, saunas, and exercise should be slowly implemented before taking supplements, because even those measures can cause detox symptoms.

For environmental illness, the first supplement to add is magnesium.

- To make it a very safe and gradual process, you can take Epsom salts baths, or use transdermal ReMag (from a spray bottle).
- Later, you can begin ¼ tsp (75 mg) of ReMag or 100 mg of elemental magnesium from magnesium citrate, increasing every three days. If magnesium citrate causes loose stools, just take the non-laxative ReMag.
- "Green drinks" are the next food supplement to add. They are made from a variety of organic land and sea vegetables, and the better ones are flavored with stevia or noth-

ing at all. Green drinks can be combined with whey, rice, or pea protein (or a combination of all three found in ReStructure) and make a good cleansing drink along with a meal replacement.

By now you should be feeling much better and able to add some more supplements to help boost your immune system and provide necessary building blocks for health. But please try to do this under the guidance of a knowledgeable practitioner. The supplements I recommend adding after ReMag are ReMyte (a multiple-mineral supplement), and ReAline, a gentle detoxifier. Environmental illness does not require high-dose supplementation. In fact, since most megavitamins and minerals are derived synthetically, it is a far better approach to use low-potency, well-absorbed minerals and food-based vitamins from organic sources.

14

Asthma, Cystic Fibrosis

THREE THINGS YOU NEED TO KNOW ABOUT MAGNESIUM AND ASTHMA

1. Research shows that many patients with asthma and other bronchial diseases have low magnesium.
2. Many drugs used in the treatment of asthma cause a loss of magnesium, only making symptoms worse.
3. Patients treated with simple magnesium supplementation report marked improvement in their symptoms.

As a child, Gerry had eczema. Every possible skin cream and lotion was tried, to no avail, but finally, after many years, the last patch disappeared on its own. It was followed almost immediately, however, by his first asthma attack. In his early thirties, Gerry was suffering attacks of wheezing and coughing when he exercised and when he was around cats, dogs, horses, dust, flowers, and chemical smells. Various inhalers helped initially, but after a year or two they would stop working. He wasn't satisfied with them, anyway; one gave him heart palpitations, and another contained steroids, which made him gain weight and retain fluid. Then one day a vitamin newsletter came in the mail. He almost threw it out, but a headline caught his attention: "Magnesium Halts Asthma Spasms."

Asthma is characterized by bronchial spasm, swelling of the mucous membranes of the lung, excessive mucus production, and an inability to fully empty the lungs of air. Asthma finds its easiest victims in children under ten and is twice as common in boys and men, although it affects about 3 percent of the general population. Tabulating all the triggers of an asthma attack is a daunting task; there seems to be a variety of stimuli, including lung infection, exercise, emotional upset, food sensitivities, inhalation of cold air or irritating substances (smoke, gas fumes, paint fumes, chemical fumes), and reactions to specific allergens, such as pollens.

Bronchial spasms occur in both extrinsic asthma (an allergic reaction to external substances such as mold, dust, animal hair, pollens, and chemicals) and intrinsic asthma (from exercise, infection, and emotional upset). The allergic triggers, called allergens, initiate the release of histamines in your body, which try to eliminate the allergens by stimulating lots of mucus to mop up the allergens and push them out through sneezing, coughing, and watery eyes. One of the side effects of too much histamine is tightening of the bronchial tubes, which go into spasm. Such spasms can initiate episodic wheezing, coughing, and shortness of breath, which quickly lead to rapid breathing, difficulty exhaling, anxiety, and dehydration. The anxiety of an asthma attack can create a gripping fear that tenses up the whole body and is hard to shake off. Bronchial spasms are worse in magnesium-deficient patients because there is not enough magnesium to relax the smooth muscles of the bronchial tubes.

There is much more to histamine than its action on bronchial tissue. It appears that mast cells (that produce histamine) increase in number, and histamine becomes elevated in the midst of magnesium deficiency. So the more magnesium-deficient you are, the more allergic reactions you may experience. Antihistamine enzymes in the body usually control the overproduction of histamine, however they require magnesium, copper, and vitamin B_6 for them to work properly.

Gerry really identified with what he read about asthma and magnesium in the newsletter. He realized that his whole body was tense. He decided to try some magnesium supplements under his doctor's supervision, and with them he was able to greatly decrease his medications. Further in the article he read that many asthma inhalers are fluoride compounds and the fluoride may bind with magnesium, making it unavailable to the body. Gerry was more convinced than ever to try magnesium for his symptoms.

MAGNESIUM TREATS ASTHMA

Magnesium is an excellent treatment for asthma because it is a bronchodilator and an antihistamine, naturally reducing histamine levels in the body. It has a calming and dilating effect on the muscles of the bronchial tubes that go into spasm during an asthma attack. It can actually calm the whole body. Certainly, drug therapy for asthma can often be lifesaving; drugs, however, are not curative and side effects are cumulative if they are used chronically.

You have to eliminate the underlying cause of asthma and replace magnesium to fully treat this condition. Without magnesium, asthma can become chronic, especially if the various triggers are not eliminated; even the fear of an attack can magnify the emotional component and escalate the physical symptoms. Conventional allergy shots have been used for decades to try to trick the body into accepting irritating allergens, but they often do not work, especially when the condition is due to a nutrient deficiency.

According to Dr. Mildred Seelig, the drug treatment of

asthma consists of magnesium-wasters such as beta-blockers, corticosteroids, and Ventolin (albuterol). The side effects of these drugs include severe magnesium deficiency, which can result in arrhythmia and sudden death.[1] Taking theophylline (aminophylline) can cause loss of magnesium and suppression of vitamin B_6 activity, which assists magnesium function. Prednisone wastes magnesium, causes sodium retention and fluid retention, suppresses vitamin D, and promotes increased urinary excretion of zinc, vitamin K, and vitamin C.[2] Advair, an asthma inhaler, is a fluoride drug with the potential to irreversibly bind magnesium.

CHILDHOOD ASTHMA

Childhood asthma can be life-threatening, but safe methods of treating this condition are available and can be used together with medications. In a European study, a group of children who had deteriorated in spite of conventional drug therapy were given magnesium sulfate intravenously. Comparing the magnesium group with the placebo group, the magnesium group had lower clinical asthma scores and a significantly greater improvement in lung function over a ninety-minute period. No significant side effects were observed.[3]

Dr. Lydia Ciarallo in the Department of Pediatrics, Brown University School of Medicine, treated thirty-one asthma patients ages six to eighteen who were deteriorating on conventional treatments. One group was given magnesium sulfate and another group was given saline solution, both intravenously. At fifty minutes the magnesium group had a significantly greater percentage of improvement in lung function, and more magnesium patients than placebo patients were discharged from the emergency department and did not need hospitalization.[4]

ADULT ASTHMA

A clinical trial showed a correlation between intracellular magnesium levels and airway spasm.[5] The investigators found that patients who had low cellular magnesium levels had increased bronchial spasm. This finding confirmed not only that magnesium was useful in the treatment of asthma by dilating the bronchial tubes but also that lack of magnesium was probably causing this condition.

A team of researchers identified magnesium deficiency as surprisingly common, finding it in 65 percent of an intensive-care population of asthmatics and in 11 percent of an outpatient asthma population. They supported the use of magnesium to help prevent asthma attacks. The blood test used in this study was serum magnesium. If the more definitive ionized magnesium test had been used, there likely would have been a higher percentage of asthmatics with evidence of low magnesium. Magnesium has several antiasthmatic actions beyond being an antihistamine and bronchodilator. It also reduces airway inflammation, inhibits chemicals that cause spasm, and increases anti-inflammatory substances such as nitric oxide.[6]

The same study established that a lower dietary magnesium intake was associated with impaired lung function, bronchial hyperreactivity, and an increased risk of wheezing. The study included 2,633 randomly selected adults ages eighteen to seventy. Dietary magnesium intake was calculated by a food frequency questionnaire, and lung function and allergic tendency were evaluated. The investigators concluded that low magnesium intake may be involved in the development of both asthma and chronic obstructive airway disease.

In a very thorough literature review, fourteen studies comprising 2,313 people with acute asthma were treated with IV magnesium sulfate and their results tabulated.[7] The reviewers concluded that "a single infusion of 1.2 g or 2 g IV $MgSO_4$ over 15 to 30 minutes reduces hospital admissions and improves lung function in adults with acute asthma who have not responded sufficiently to oxygen, nebulized short-acting beta2-agonists and IV corticosteroids." Since IV magnesium will be out of the reach of many asthma sufferers, please read Dana's story in Chapter 18 to see how ReMag may simply and inexpensively replace IV magnesium and improve serum magnesium levels.

DIET ADVICE FOR ASTHMA

Any mention of what to eat and what not to eat when you have a chronic health condition is fraught with inconsistencies and inaccuracies. My general diet recommendations for asthma are as follows:

- Eliminate alcohol, coffee, white sugar, white flour, gluten, fried foods, and trans fatty acids (found in margarine and in baked, fried, and processed foods made with partially hydrogenated fats).
- Limit red meat and dairy, which contain chemicals that increase inflammation in the body.
- If you eat animal protein, choose organically raised grass-fed beef, free-range chicken and eggs, and fish (especially wild-caught salmon).
- For vegetarian protein, choose fermented dairy, lactose-free cheese, and ReStructure Meal Replacement (it has no casein, very-low-lactose whey protein, pea protein, and rice protein).
- Vegan protein choices include legumes, gluten-free grains, nuts, and seeds.
- Healthy carbs include raw, cooked, and fermented vegetables: increase yellow vegetables and green leafy vegetables,

which contain substances that inhibit inflammation. Eat two or three pieces of fruit a day. The skins of grapes (choose organic) contain quercetin, which prevents histamine release and inhibits inflammatory products.

- Include magnesium-rich foods listed in Appendix A and calcium-rich foods listed in Appendix B.
- For fats and oils, choose butter, olive oil, sesame oil, and coconut oil.
- For anti-inflammatory purposes, increase the intake of fish oils, seed and nut oils, cold-water fish (herring, sardines, salmon), flaxseed oil, and walnuts.
- Try a modified fast to decrease inflammation: use a whey, rice, or pea protein powder such as ReStructure, a green drink, and/or fresh organic juices plus fiber for three days, followed by a vegetarian diet for four days.
- Get out of the rut of eating the same foods every day. To eliminate possible food allergies, avoid your top three favorite foods (people often crave foods they are sensitive to). Eggs, shellfish, and peanuts usually cause immediate sensitivity reactions; milk, chocolate, wheat, citrus, and food colorings cause delayed food reactions.
- Carefully check labels in the grocery store and speak up in restaurants to avoid even small amounts of potential allergic triggers such as MSG, aspartame, and sulfites.

Other health measures that relate to asthma include:

- Avoid aspirin and nonsteroidal anti-inflammatories (e.g., ibuprofen), which can cause allergic reactions.
- Clean out environmental allergens.
- If you can part with them, find other homes for cats and dogs.
- Remove wall-to-wall carpeting, wall hangings, and feather pillows.

- Frequently replace or clean air filters for heating and cooling systems.
- Obtain environmentally sound cleaning products.
- Use a vacuum cleaner specifically for allergies. Research HEPA air cleaners for your home.
- Since yeast overgrowth may be related to asthma, see #18 under the heading "Dr. Dean's Personal Recommendations" in the Resources section.

SUPPLEMENTS FOR ASTHMA

First line of treatment:

- **ReMag:** With picometer, stabilized ionic magnesium you can reach therapeutic amounts without laxative effects. Start with ¼ tsp (75 mg) and work up to 2–3 tsp (600–900 mg) per day. Add ReMag to a liter of water and sip all day to achieve full absorption.
- **ReMyte:** Picometer twelve-mineral solution. Take ½ tsp three times a day, or add 1½ tsp to a liter of water with ReMag and sip throughout the day.
- **ReAline:** B vitamin complex plus amino acids. Take 1 capsule twice per day. Contains food-based B_1 and four methylated B vitamins (B_2, B_6, methylfolate, and B_{12}), plus L-methionine (precursor to glutathione) and L-taurine (which supports the heart and weight loss).
- **Vitamin C complex:** 200 mg twice a day, from a food-based source, or make your own liposomal vitamin C (see Appendix D for a liposomal vitamin C recipe), and ascorbic acid, 1,000 mg twice a day.

Second line of treatment to be added to the above if necessary:

- **Pantothenic acid:** 500 mg daily.
- **Vitamin E, as mixed tocopherols:** 400 IU daily.
- **Flaxseed oil:** 1–2 tbsp daily (keep the bottle in the freezer between uses).
- **Betaine HCl:** Take one or two 650 mg capsules in the middle or at the end of meals, to help fully digest your food.
- **Probiotics:** Prescript-Assist, one or two capsules per day, taken thirty minutes before or after food.

CYSTIC FIBROSIS

A review of twenty-five studies on magnesium and cystic fibrosis (CF) found the following:[8]

- Hypomagnesemia affects more than half of the CF patients with advanced disease.
- Magnesium in the blood decreases with age in CF.
- Aminoglycoside antimicrobials used for CF lung infections frequently induce both acute and chronic renal magnesium-wasting.
- Magnesium concentration in sweat was normal in CF patients.
- Limited data suggest the existence of an impaired intestinal magnesium balance in CF.
- Observations suggest that magnesium supplements might achieve an improvement in respiratory muscle strength and mucolytic activity.

The researchers concluded that "the potential of supplementation with this cation deserves more attention." I would conclude that magnesium deserves more than just attention; people with cystic fibrosis deserve treatment with therapeutic levels of magnesium.

Aging, Alzheimer's, Parkinson's, Dementia

THREE THINGS YOU NEED TO KNOW ABOUT MAGNESIUM AND AGING

1. Aging itself is a risk factor for magnesium deficiency; as we get older we become more deficient in magnesium and therefore require more in our diet and in supplement form.
2. Magnesium is deficient in people who have Alzheimer's disease and Parkinson's disease.
3. Telomeres, the deciding factor in aging, are protected by magnesium.

Three hundred years ago, people did not live as long as we do today. Conditions back then were so unsanitary that simple scrapes and cuts became mortal wounds. Bathing was looked upon with suspicion. Tuberculosis, fostered by extremely close quarters, little sun exposure, dampness, and lack of fresh vegetables, was highly contagious and struck down many in their prime. Indoor fires without adequate ventilation caused chronic bronchitis and emphysema, if the people even lived long enough to develop these conditions.

When we implemented universal sanitation, the infectious diseases began to recede. The land was still fertile, and plants soaked up vital nutrients. Farm animals ate the plants, and humans absorbed the nutrients from eating fresh meat and fresh produce. The industrial revolution, however, harmed our health in a new way, with factories belching smoke and chemical poisons. Industrial farming techniques began poisoning the soil with pesticides, herbicides, and nitrogen fertilizers. The soil became lifeless.

We may think we are better off in this century with our drugs and medical technology, but as we've seen, they have also become toxic and undermined our health, especially in a polluted environment where our basic nutrition is impaired. Popping antiaging pills and megavitamins, however, does not add years to your life. An excellent diet that provides optimal nutrition, exercise, an outgoing and optimistic attitude, and therapeutic nutrients are the true keys to longevity.

AGING EQUALS CALCIFICATION

Aging in industrialized societies is associated with an increasing prevalence of hypertension, heart disease, reduced insulin sensitivity, and type 2 diabetes. Aging in general also means altered calcium and magnesium ion levels, indistinguishable from those observed in hypertension and diabetes.[1] As noted in the introduction to Part Three, French magnesium researcher Dr. Pierre Delbet, who practiced in the early 1900s, was convinced that the aging body's tissues have three times more calcium than magnesium. He knew that calcium precipitates out into tissues that are deficient in magnesium. He observed the toxicity of excess calcium in the testicles, brain, and other tissues and concluded almost a century ago that magnesium deficiency plays a role in senility.

In Chapter 8, I talked about insulin resistance and its

role in exacerbating hypertension, heart disease, and diabetes. Insulin-resistant states, as well as what is often thought of as "normal" aging, are characterized by the accumulation of calcium and depletion of magnesium in the cells. With this in mind, clinical researchers are finally suggesting that an imbalance of calcium and magnesium ions might be the missing link responsible for the frequent clinical coexistence of hypertension, atherosclerosis, and metabolic disorders in aging.[2]

As is evident from animal experiments and epidemiological studies, magnesium deficiency and calcium excess may increase our susceptibility to cardiovascular disease as well as accelerate aging.[3] In a study of nursing home residents, low magnesium levels were significantly associated with two conditions that plague the elderly, calf cramps and diabetes.[4] Centenarians (individuals reaching 100 years of age) have higher total body magnesium and lower calcium levels than most elderly people.[5]

"Smart drugs" such as piracetam, oxiracetam, pramiracetam, and aniracetam are thought to enhance learning, facilitate the flow of information between the two hemispheres of the brain, help the brain resist physical and chemical injuries, and be relatively free of side effects. Magnesium fits all the above criteria for "smart drugs," but it is much less costly and has no side effects.

LONGEVITY

In 1993, Dr. Jean Durlach, a preeminent magnesium expert in France, summed up the existing research on magnesium and aging with the following seven points.[6]

1. Chronic marginal magnesium deficiency reduces life span in rats.

2. Magnesium deficiency accelerates aging through its various effects on the neuromuscular, cardiovascular, and endocrine apparatus; kidneys and bones; and immune, antistress, and antioxidant systems.

3. In developed countries, magnesium intake is marginal throughout the entire population regardless of age: around 4 mg/kg/day instead of the minimum of 6 mg/kg/day recommended to maintain balance. However, diseases, handicaps, and physical or psychological impairments expose elderly individuals to more severe nutritional deficiencies and higher requirements.

4. Around the age of seventy, magnesium absorption is two-thirds of what it is at age thirty.

5. Various mechanisms of deficiency include intestinal malabsorption; reduced bone uptake and mobilization (osteoporosis); increased urinary losses; chronic stress; insulin resistance leading to diabetes with severe magnesium loss in the urine; lack of response to adrenal stimulation; loss caused by medication, especially diuretics; alcohol addiction; and cigarette smoking.

6. Magnesium deficiency symptoms in the elderly include central nervous system symptoms that seem largely "neurotic": anxiety, excessive emotionality, fatigue, headaches, insomnia, light-headedness, dizziness, nervous fits, sensation of a lump in the throat, and impaired breathing.

   Peripheral nervous system signs are common: pins and needles of the extremities, cramps, muscle pains.

   Functional disorders include chest pain, shortness of breath, chest pressure, palpitations, extra systoles (occasional heart thumps from an isolated extra beat), abnormal heart rhythm, and Raynaud's syndrome.

   Autonomic nervous system disturbances involve both the sympathetic and parasympathetic nervous systems, causing hypotension on rising quickly or borderline hypertension. In elderly patients, excessive emotionality, tremor, weakness, sleep disorders, amnesia, and cognitive disturbances are particularly important aspects of magnesium deficiency.

7. A trial of oral magnesium supplementation is the best diagnostic tool for establishing the importance of magnesium.

MORTALITY IN MAGNESIUM DEFICIENCY

In 2006, the journal *Epidemiology* reported that there is a 40 percent lower risk of dying from all types of cancer and cardiovascular disease in men whose magnesium levels were highest compared to the group that had the lowest levels.[7] A study published in 2014 documented a 34 percent lower risk of all causes of death in men and women with a higher intake of magnesium.[8]

The converse is seen in the 2014 study "Hypomagnesaemia in Patients Hospitalised in Internal Medicine Is Associated with Increased Mortality."[9] In this study, the researchers concluded that "the prevalence of hypomagnesaemia in internal medicine is very high. It is associated with higher mortality and longer hospital stay in our population. It can be a useful tool in predicting morbidity and mortality. Although no causal role can be defined for it at present, the low cost and minimal discomfort of measuring magnesium justifies its routine measurement and replacement in patients hospitalised in internal medicine." Unfortunately, the measurement that will be used is the highly inaccurate serum magnesium test.

FREE RADICALS, ANTIOXIDANTS, AND AGING

A free radical is an unstable molecule that is the product of normal body metabolism. It is formed when molecules within our own cells react with oxygen, causing an oxidation reaction. A free radical has an unpaired electron that tries to steal a stabilizing electron from another molecule and, as a consequence, can produce harmful effects. External sources of free radicals include chemicals (pesticides, industrial pollution, auto exhaust, cigarette smoke), heavy metals (dental amalgam, lead, cadmium), most infections (viruses, bacteria, parasites, fungi), X-rays, alcohol, allergens, stress, and even excessive exercise.

Antioxidants are vitamins and minerals, such as magnesium, selenium, vitamin C, and vitamin E, that turn off free radicals. The greater the amount of other antioxidants in the body, the more magnesium is spared from acting as an antioxidant and is free to perform its many other functions. This means that taking supplemental antioxidants protects the level of magnesium in the body; this prevents elevation of calcium, and prevents vascular muscle spasm.[10] If there are not enough antioxidants available, overabundant free radicals begin to damage and destroy normal, healthy cells.

Free radicals are necessary and normal products of metabolism, but uncontrolled free radical production plays a major role in the development of degenerative disease, since free radicals can damage any body structure: proteins, enzymes, fats, even DNA. Free radicals are implicated in more than sixty different health conditions, including heart disease, autoimmune disease, and cancer.

According to current research, low magnesium levels not only magnify free radical damage but also can hasten the production of free radicals.[11] One study utilizing cultures of skin cells found that low magnesium doubled the levels of free radicals.[12] In addition, cells grown without magnesium were twice as susceptible to free radical damage as were cells grown in normal amounts of magnesium. Another study showed that red blood cells from hamsters fed low-magnesium diets were deficient in magnesium and consequently more susceptible to free radical damage.

One study found that low magnesium levels are associated with increased oxidative stress and decreased cell proliferation.[13] Another found that after several months in incubation, magnesium-depleted human fibroblasts exhibited characteristics of cells many times their age.[14]

It appears that low magnesium levels can compromise cell membrane integrity, damaging the vital fatty layer in the cell membrane, making it more susceptible to destruction, and allowing leakage through the membrane.[15] This particular finding, which implicates magnesium deficiency as one of the causes of leaky cell membranes, or leaky gut, is extremely important because disruption of this type can be fatal to cells and cause widespread problems that ultimately manifest in dozens of symptoms and conditions, including aging.

A 2015 review on the mechanisms of aging noted that the prevalence of cardiovascular and cerebrovascular diseases rises with age and classified the molecular pathways of aging associated with these diseases.[16] The investigators identified increased oxidative stress produced in the mitochondria and cytosol (free fluid inside the cell) of the heart and brain as a common denominator to almost all cardiovascular and cerebrovascular diseases. They found a particular mitochondrial protein and family of enzymes that regulate the aging process and determine lifespan of many species and are involved in cardiovascular diseases. They focused on the latest scientific advances as well as delineating potential novel therapeutic targets derived from aging research for cardiovascular and cerebrovascular diseases.

Using this review as a guide, I think the best way to reduce oxidative stress in the mitochondria, heart, and brain and to ensure efficient mitochondrial function is to saturate the body with therapeutic levels of magnesium. I've mentioned several times in this book that six of the eight steps in the mitochrondrial Krebs cycle require magnesium in order to make ATP energy molecules. In Chapter 2, I quote Dr. Guy Abraham, who said that in order to protect the fluid inside the cell from becoming saturated with calcium, there is a magnesium-dependent mechanism that shunts calcium in and out of the mitochondria. But if calcium goes in and doesn't come out, because there isn't enough magnesium to maintain that shunt, mitochondrial calcification occurs and eventually results in cell death. This research makes me wonder if calcium excess and magnesium deficiency could be the underlying reason for the recent upsurge in mitochondrial dysfunction.

MEMORY

It's much easier to view the tangible, structural benefits of magnesium—the bones, the proteins, and even the energy it produces—but much more difficult to contemplate its effects on the brain. Research at MIT, however, produced a study in 2004 that elevates magnesium to the position of memory enhancer.[17]

Particular brain receptors important for learning and memory depend on magnesium for their regulation. The researchers describe magnesium as an absolutely necessary component of the cerebrospinal fluid in order to keep these learning and memory receptors active. The term they use for this activity, interactivity, and changeability is *plasticity*. You might not think a plastic brain is a good thing to have, but it's the loss of plasticity in the region of the brain responsible for storing short-term memories that causes forgetfulness in the elderly.

Magnesium is instrumental in opening brain receptors to important information while at the same time allowing them to ignore background noise. The MIT researchers were quite struck by their findings and concluded, "As predicted by our theory, increasing the concentration of magnesium and reducing the background level of noise led to the largest increases of plasticity ever reported in scientific literature."

A 2011 study, "Effects of Elevation of Brain Magnesium on Fear Conditioning, Fear Extinction, and Synaptic Plasticity in the Infralimbic Prefrontal Cortex and Lateral Amygdala," concludes that "elevation of brain magnesium might be a novel approach for enhancing synaptic plasticity in a regional-specific manner leading to enhancing the efficacy of extinction without enhancing or impairing fear memory formation."[18] In English, that statement simply means that magnesium reduces the physical reaction to fear, which can only be a good thing!

TREATING TELOMERES

What's a telomere? A telomere is an essential part of chromosomes that affects how our cells age. Telomeres are the caps at the ends of chromosomes that protect them from unraveling or getting attached to another chromosome. They are like the plastic cap at the end of a shoelace or the knot at the end of a string to keep it from unraveling. Here's another analogy: it's like the many extra stitches you put at the end of a line of sewing to prevent the thread from pulling free. Those extra stitches represent redundant sequences of nucleotides—the building blocks of DNA. They don't have a function other than protecting chromosomes.

The current research on aging is firmly tied up with telomeres. As we baby boomers age, we're desperately trying to find ways to stay younger. Antiaging research is a multibillion-dollar industry. And besides facelifts and Botox, finding a way to protect our telomeres has become the holy grail of longevity research.

It should come as no surprise that magnesium is closely associated with telomeres. But the real shock is how few researchers are focusing on the miracle of magnesium in keeping telomeres from unraveling. Instead they are looking for drugs or formulating expensive supplements to save the telomeres—ignoring the solution that's right before their eyes.

Aging is documented in our DNA: year by year, greater numbers of redundant telomere segments at the end of our chromosomes are nibbled away, eventually leaving the chromosome exposed. Telomere segments keep genes stable but shorten over time as cell division becomes less efficient, especially if the enzyme telomerase reverse transcriptase is deficient or not working properly. You don't have to guess at what mineral this enzyme depends upon—magnesium, of course.

THE ALTURAS' TELOMERE RESEARCH

Shortened telomeres correspond with many conditions associated with aging, including heart disease. Heart disease is often a product of magnesium deficiency. Two brilliant magnesium researchers, Drs. Burton and Bella Altura, who wrote the foreword to this book, have published well over 1,000 scientific articles, most of them on magnesium. In 2014 the Alturas participated in a groundbreaking study on magnesium and the enzyme telomerase.[19]

Please Google the title "Short-Term Magnesium Deficiency Downregulates Telomerase, Upregulates Neutral Sphingomyelinase and Induces Oxidative DNA Damage in Cardiovascular Tissues: Relevance to Atherogenesis, Cardiovascular Diseases and Aging," and read the paper online in its entirety. In it the Alturas review twenty-five years of their research that prefigures this present study. The paper's discussion section is especially important, showing how telomeres are damaged by a host of environmental factors and how this damage is treatable and preventable by therapeutic levels of magnesium. The paper is supported with 142 references, and it is so brilliant that I'm quite beside myself with excitement and want to quote every word of it for you. Instead, I will try to summarize this extraordinary achievement of the Alturas.

Let me first report the findings of the study and then present excerpts from the paper itself. In this animal study, healthy rats were tested for their magnesium levels. The animals were then divided into two groups. One group ate rat chow with standard amounts of magnesium; the other group was given chow with reduced magnesium. After twenty-one days, telomerase levels had dropped a significant 70–88 percent in the low-magnesium group. Telomerase measured specifically in heart cells was similarly reduced. Markers for free radical damage to DNA were increased; free radicals shorten telomeres.

The title of the paper says "short-term" to indicate that it only took twenty-one days for this extensive damage to occur. In my clinical experience, most people who approach me with magnesium deficiency symptoms have suffered years or even decades of magnesium deficiency.

In their conclusion, the Alturas say, "We believe in view of the current report, and other works recently published by our labs, prolonged magnesium deficiency should be categorized as another epigenetic mechanism." By epigenetic mechanism, they mean that telomerase is being affected not by some factor inherent in our genes and chromosomes but rather by an outside "switch." That outside switch is magnesium. Epigenetics is the study of cellular or genetic variations that result from external or environmental factors that switch genes on and off and affect how cells express genes. It's great news that magnesium has the ability to positively affect our genes and keep our telomeres where they belong, at the end of chromosomes.

The following overview of the Alturas' paper may sound complex and scientific, but I want you to understand the incredible value of magnesium in all tissues, in all cells, in all our mitochondria, and in the production of our RNA and DNA. It also summarizes many aspects of magnesium research.

Aging and Magnesium Deficiency
It's common knowledge that over the age of sixty-five, many people show metabolic decline, with the appearance of atherosclerosis, hypertension, cardiovascular diseases, and type 2 diabetes, culminating in congestive heart failure. All of the attributes of aging have been associated clinically and experimentally with magnesium deficiency. The authors make the following very important observation: "The aging process is also associated with an increase in the levels of proinflammatory cytokines in tissues and cells all present in Mg-deficient animals, tissues, and different cell types."

Oxidative Stress, Telomerase, and the Heart
Certain markers of oxidative stress appear in cardiovascular tissues and DNA with an accompanying

decrease in ionized magnesium levels. This indicates that magnesium deficiency could lead to multiple mutations in the genomes of multiple cell lines. The Alturas' study shows that magnesium deficiency shaves off the ends of telomeres, which can be equated with aging and cardiovascular changes including hypertension, decreased ejection fraction, and cardiac failure.

Magnesium Deficiency and Endothelial Damage

Studies by the Alturas in the late 1980s demonstrated changes in the endothelial lining of blood vessels due to magnesium deficiency. The Alturas say that magnesium's importance in controlling microcirculation and in lipid buildup in the arterial walls is still being overlooked by the next generation of researchers.

Magnesium Deficiency and Chronic Stress

Recent studies confirm that short-term magnesium deficiency causes marked reduction in heart cellular glutathione and in cells activating nitric oxide synthases that protect DNA. These findings support the theory that magnesium deficiency can cause mutations in many types of cells.

Magnesium Deficiency and Heart Failure

All studies to date have confirmed, experimentally and clinically, that congestive heart failure is an inevitability by age seventy-five to eighty-five for people in magnesium-deficient states.

Magnesium and Cell Signaling for the Heart

In the mid-1990s, the Alturas theorized that magnesium ions function as extracellular signals in the pathobiology of cardiovascular disease. A total of forty-two studies now support that theory. Magnesium has a critical role in the regulation of cardiac hemodynamics; vascular tone and reactivity; endothelial functions; carbohydrate, nucleotide, and lipid metabolism; prevention of free radical formation; and stabilization of the genome. Another seventeen studies find that magnesium has a crucial role in control of calcium uptake, subcellular content, and subcellular distribution in smooth muscle cells, endothelial cells, and cardiac muscle cells.

Magnesium Deficiency and Genotoxicity

Summing up the role of magnesium in our genes, the Alturas point out that magnesium deficiency can induce cell cycle arrest (and senescence), can initiate programmed cell death, and is associated with DNA damage (genotoxic events). These magnesium-deficiency-related changes can occur in multiple cell types, including cardiac and vascular smooth muscle cells. Of note is that atherosclerotic plaque in the arterial walls of hypertensive patients shows considerable DNA damage, activation of DNA repair pathways, increased expression of p53 (a tumor suppressor protein), oxidation, apoptosis, and increased levels of ceramide (a waxy lipid).

TELOMERES IN SPACE

A fascinating paper published in 2012 jumps on the telomere bandwagon and describes what happens to humans as they develop magnesium deficiency in the unique environment of space.[20] What follows are several excerpts from this paper, which is called "Correcting Magnesium Deficiency May Prolong Life."

The International Space Station provides an extraordinary facility to study the accelerated aging process in microgravity, which could be triggered by significant reductions in magnesium (Mg) ion levels with, in turn, elevations of catecholamines and vicious cycles between the two.

With space flight there are significant reductions of serum Mg that have been shown in large studies of astronauts and cosmonauts. The loss of the functional capacity of the cardiovascular system with space flight is over ten times faster than the course of aging on Earth.

Magnesium is an antioxidant and calcium blocker and in space there is oxidative stress, insulin resistance, and inflammatory conditions with evidence in experimental animals of significant endothelial injuries and damage to mitochondria.

The aging process is associated with progressive shortening of telomeres, repetitive DNA sequences, and proteins that cap and protect the ends of chromosomes. Telomerase can elongate pre-existing telomeres to maintain length and chromosome stability. Low telomerase triggers increased catecholamines while the sensitivity of telomere synthesis to Mg ions is primarily seen for the longer elongation products. Mg stabilizes DNA and promotes DNA replication and transcription, whereas low Mg might accelerate cellular senescence by reducing DNA stability, protein synthesis, and function of mitochondria. Telomerase, in binding to short DNAs, is Mg dependent.

ALZHEIMER'S AND PARKINSON'S

These two conditions are included in the chapter on aging because they are often regarded as diseases of aging. There is evidence that magnesium deficiency can trigger or worsen Alzheimer's disease and Parkinson's disease.[21] These conditions are the neurological equivalent of heart disease. After all, both heart and brain are excitable tissues that give off electrical energy, and both must have magnesium.

ALZHEIMER'S DISEASE

In North America, approximately 10 percent of the population over sixty-five and 50 percent over eighty-five suffer from Alzheimer's. It is associated with severe memory loss, impaired cognitive function, and inability to carry out activities of daily life.

Alzheimer's disease should be diagnosed only when all the other identifiable brain conditions have been ruled out (e.g., brain tumor, alcoholism, vitamin B_{12} deficiency, vitamin and mineral deficiency, mercury amalgam poisoning, depression, hypothyroidism, Parkinson's, stroke, excessive prescription drug use, malnutrition, and dehydration). In truth, it is only at autopsy that a definitive diagnosis can be made, as the brain will show the identifying characteristics of Alzheimer's—plaques and tangles in the nerve fibers, particularly in the cerebral cortex and hippocampal area.

Dr. Abram Hoffer, the founder of orthomolecular medicine (along with Linus Pauling), cautions that almost half the cases of what is assumed to be Alzheimer's may in fact be dementias caused by such treatable conditions as simple dehydration, prescription drug intoxication, severe cerebral allergic reactions to foods or chemicals, or chronic nutrient deficiencies. I would place magnesium deficiency high on that list. Allopathic medicine ignores these treatable causes and searches for a drug to "cure" the disease. Drugs that can worsen Alzheimer's include chlorpromazine, antihistamines, barbiturates, psychotropic drugs, and diuretics, with more being added to the list every day. In fact, since prescription drug intoxication is on the list of causes, why would we use drugs that may worsen the condition?

NOTE: Some cases of Alzheimer's are so extreme—the behavior of some patients may even be violent—that medication becomes necessary.

Chemicals and toxic metals, particularly mercury and aluminum, are associated with Alzheimer's disease. The Alzheimer's/mercury connection has been made by Dr. Boyd Haley, a professor of chemistry and chair of that department at the University of Kentucky. Dr. Haley proved that the tangles and plaques in the Alzheimer's brain are identical to those produced by mercury poisoning. Mercury can be absorbed in the brain from dental amalgams, be acquired by taking flu shots (which are preserved with mercury), or come from habitually eating fish contaminated with mercury. Magnesium, when it is available in the body, will help detoxify heavy metals, even ones as poisonous as mercury.

Many Americans are exposed to aluminum through aluminum pots, aluminum cans, aluminum-containing antacids and antiperspirants, aluminum foil, and tap water that may be high in aluminum.[22, 23] Considerable research has proven that brain neurons affected in Alzheimer's disease have significantly higher levels of aluminum than normal neurons. The damage is compounded because Alzheimer's patients also have consistently low magnesium levels within the hippocampus, the area of the brain most affected by Alzheimer's.[24] Furthermore, aluminum is able to replace magnesium in certain enzyme systems in the body, disrupting their function and causing harm.[25] Aluminum can also become a substitute for magnesium in the brain, which leaves calcium channels in the brain nerve cells wide open, allowing calcium to flood in, causing certain cell death.[26]

William Grant, the atmospheric scientist I quoted in Chapter 2, had a personal interest in Alzheimer's because of a strong family history. Grant already knew that people with Alzheimer's typically have elevated concentrations of aluminum in their brains. He put that piece of information together with the fact that acid rain increases the levels of aluminum in trees and makes trees age prematurely. Grant theorized that the diets of Alzheimer's patients might be very acidic, leaching calcium and magnesium from the body. He found that people with Alzheimer's have elevated amounts of aluminum, iron, and zinc and have reduced amounts of alkaline metals such as magnesium, calcium, and potassium, which neutralize the acidity in the diet. A typical Western diet—high in protein, fat, and sugar—is acid-forming and may be an additional factor in creating aluminum overload in Alzheimer's.

Neurosurgeon Dr. Russell Blaylock reports that when scientists study the soil of regions that have a high incidence of neurological diseases, they find high levels of aluminum and low levels of magnesium and calcium. The neurons from victims of the disease also show high levels of aluminum and low levels of magnesium. On the island of Guam the areas with the lowest levels of magnesium and calcium in the soil are also the areas of highest incidence for all neurological diseases. Fortunately, magnesium plays a vital role in protecting neurons from the lethal effects of aluminum.[27]

A study published in *Magnesium Research* that used ionized magnesium testing found alterations in magnesium levels in patients with mild to moderate Alzheimer's.[28] Similar findings were reported in the PATH Through Life Project, which published "Dietary Mineral Intake and Risk of Mild Cognitive Impairment."[29] A report on autopsy studies of brain tissue concluded, "Magnesium values are found to be

significantly decreased in brain regions of Alzheimer's patients compared to controls."[30] Animal research shows that magnesium is a positive agent in the treatment of Alzheimer's by protecting cognitive functions and synaptic plasticity.[31, 32]

PARKINSON'S DISEASE

Parkinson's is a progressive nervous system disease evidenced by a visible tremor, muscular rigidity, and slow, imprecise shuffling or stuttering movements, chiefly affecting middle-aged and elderly people. It is associated with degeneration of the basal ganglia of the brain and a deficiency of the neurotransmitter dopamine. Statistically, it is estimated that 7 to 10 million people worldwide are living with Parkinson's disease. Only about 4 percent of people with Parkinson's are diagnosed before the age of fifty. Men are 1.5 times more likely to have Parkinson's than women.

There is very little human research on magnesium and Parkinson's, but there has been a flurry of animal research. In the 2015 review "Magnesium in Man: Implications for Health and Disease" the authors state, "Parkinson's patients have low Mg^{2+} concentrations in cortex, white matter, basal ganglia, and brain stem."[33] According to the writer, "rats with chronic low Mg^{2+} intake exhibit a significant loss of dopaminergic neurons." They also showed that "in this experimental model, mitochondrial Mg^{2+} concentrations were decreased." Several other significant findings allowed them to conclude, "Mg^{2+} supplementation may be beneficial for patients suffering from Parkinson's disease."

As with Alzheimer's, aluminum can be a contributing factor in Parkinson's. In one autopsy study, calcium and aluminum were elevated in the brains of victims of Parkinson's disease as compared to people with normal brains.[34] When I hear that excess calcium is involved, as in this study, I know magnesium therapy should be considered. In another study, magnesium was lower in the brain cortex than in the white matter of Parkinson's brains.[35]

Research indicates that ample magnesium can protect brain cells from the damaging effects of aluminum, beryllium, cadmium, lead, mercury, and nickel. We also know that low levels of brain magnesium contribute to the deposition of heavy metals in the brain that heralds Parkinson's and Alzheimer's. It appears that the metals compete with magnesium for entry into the brain cells. If magnesium is low in the brain, heavy metals gain access much more readily.

Heavy metals such as cadmium, aluminum, and lead attach themselves to certain enzyme systems in the body. Enzymes function when they have access to the proper cofactors, which are mostly minerals and vitamins, especially magnesium, selenium, vitamin C, vitamin B_6, and vitamin E. Displacing minerals such as magnesium either prevents normal enzyme activity or creates abnormal activity leading to cell destruction. I've mentioned that magnesium is necessary in as many as 800 enzyme systems in the body. If the body is already magnesium deficient, enzyme systems that require magnesium but are not filled with magnesium will be most vulnerable to heavy metal infiltration.

There is also competition in the small intestine for absorption of minerals and heavy metals. If there is enough magnesium, aluminum won't be absorbed. When monkeys are fed diets low in calcium and magnesium but high in aluminum, for instance, they become apathetic and begin to lose weight. When their spinal cords are examined under the microscope, they show swelling of the anterior motor cells (movement centers), plus accumulation of calcium and aluminum in these cells.[36]

If you eat from aluminum pots, use aluminum-containing

antiperspirants, wrap your food in aluminum foil, and drink tap water with high aluminum content, the levels could overwhelm the magnesium in your gut, and aluminum will be absorbed instead. This has consequences for the amount of magnesium in your brain and may allow the buildup of aluminum associated with Alzheimer's and Parkinson's disease.

A number of reports have identified pesticides as another possible cause of Parkinson's disease, with in-home exposure to insecticides carrying the highest risk.[37] Glutathione, which I talk about in the introduction to Part Three under "The Magnesome," is a naturally occurring antioxidant made in all the cells of the body, including neurons. Glutathione acts to detoxify the body of certain chemicals and heavy metals.

Cells grown in magnesium-deficient conditions, however, have lower glutathione levels. Adding free radicals to a low-magnesium cell culture causes the level of glutathione to fall rapidly as it is used up, making the cells much more susceptible to free radical damage. Neurosurgeon Dr. Russell Blaylock tells us that a fall in cellular glutathione within part of the brain called the substantia nigra appears to be one of the earliest findings in Parkinson's disease.[38] I support the body's glutathione with ReAline, which contains the amino acid precursor to glutathione, L-methionine, as well as four methylated B vitamins, all of which greatly assist the detoxification of heavy metals and chemicals.

DOPAMINE AND MAGNESIUM

The website for *Psychology Today* features the following description of dopamine:[39]

> Dopamine is a neurotransmitter that helps control the brain's reward and pleasure centers. Dopamine also helps regulate movement and emotional responses, and it en-

ables us not only to see rewards but to take action to move toward them. Dopamine deficiency results in Parkinson's Disease, and people with low dopamine activity may be more prone to addiction. The presence of a certain kind of dopamine receptor is also associated with sensation-seeking people, more commonly known as "risk takers."

Several steps on the pathway leading to production of dopamine require magnesium as a necessary cofactor. You don't have to wait for researchers to complete further studies; you can take magnesium and do your own personal research.

MAGNESIUM-DEFICIENCY DEMENTIA

Dementia may be caused by magnesium depletion alone.[40] Several studies show that severe neurological syndromes can result when conditions cause extremely low levels of brain magnesium. One situation in which this can occur is with the chronic use of diuretics, which millions of people take to control high blood pressure. These neurological conditions can present as seizures, delirium, coma, or psychosis, which are quickly reversed by administering large doses of intravenous magnesium.

The body's ability to absorb magnesium declines with age, so at particular risk are elderly people who do not eat an adequate diet and who use drugs that deplete the body's magnesium. Studies show that senior citizens take on average six to eight medications regularly, and there is no research to show what deficiencies and side effects are created by this blind polypharmacy. Add to that the effects of over-the-counter antacids, which many elderly people take to cover up symptoms caused by a bad diet. Antacids suppress normal stomach acid and can lead to incompletely digested food, which causes gas, bloating, and constipation. As previously noted, another hidden danger is the use of aluminum in most antacids.

Aspartame and MSG (glutamate) are regularly used as sweeteners and flavor enhancers. As taste buds decline, the elderly gravitate to more sugar and spice to stimulate their appetite. However, aspartame and MSG are neurotoxins, and we don't know how much is too much, especially in an elderly, vulnerable brain. Therefore, I recommend that they be entirely avoided since they can cause brain irritability that is magnified in magnesium deficiency.

TREATMENT BEYOND MAGNESIUM

Management of Alzheimer's Aluminum Toxicity

- Use only filtered water, and ensure that the filter guarantees removal of aluminum.
- Stay hydrated. Drink half your body weight (in pounds) in ounces of water. If you weigh 150 pounds, you will drink 75 ounces. Add unrefined sea salt, pink Himalayan salt, or Celtic sea salt, ¼–½ tsp to every liter of drinking water.
- Check labels and avoid antacids containing aluminum.
- Use natural antiperspirants without aluminum.
- Avoid cooking in aluminum pots.
- Do not drink fruit juice or soft drinks stored in aluminum containers.
- Get checked for thyroid disease and treat appropriately. Investigate ReMyte, which provides the nine minerals required for thyroid hormone production.
- Check for heavy metal toxicity (aluminum, mercury, copper, lead, and iron) through urine testing or hair analysis.
- Pursue gentle detoxification of heavy metals. I recommend ReAline, which provides precursors to glutathione and methylated B vitamins.

- Avoid mercury fillings or have them replaced by a practitioner who has been trained in their safe removal, as improper removal can result in more mercury being released into the tissues (see Resources).
- Clean out all the chemicals in your home and immediate environment.
- Eat organic food.
- Exercise.
- Take regular saunas.

DIET ADVICE FOR LONGEVITY

My general diet recommendations for health and longevity are as follows:

- Eliminate alcohol, coffee, white sugar, white flour, gluten, fried foods, and trans fatty acids (found in margarine and in baked, fried, and processed foods made with partially hydrogenated fats).
- If you eat animal protein, choose organically raised grass-fed beef, free-range chicken and eggs, and fish (especially wild-caught salmon).
- For vegetarian protein, choose fermented dairy, lactose-free cheese, and ReStructure Meal Replacement (it has no casein, very-low-lactose whey protein, and pea and rice proteins).
- Vegan protein choices include legumes, gluten-free grains, nuts, and seeds.
- Eat healthy carbs such as a variety of raw, cooked, and fermented vegetables, two or three pieces of fruit a day, and gluten-free grains.
- Include magnesium-rich foods listed in Appendix A and calcium-rich foods listed in Appendix B.
- For fats and oils, choose butter, olive oil, flaxseed oil, sesame oil, and coconut oil.

- Therapeutic foods include cilantro, garlic, onions, seaweed, and ginger, which help bind and excrete heavy metals.

SUPPLEMENTS FOR LONGEVITY

- **ReMag:** With picometer, stabilized ionic magnesium you can reach therapeutic amounts without laxative effects. Start with ¼ tsp (75 mg) and work up to 2–3 tsp (600–900 mg) per day. Add ReMag to a liter of water and sip all day to achieve full absorption.
- **ReMyte:** Picometer twelve-mineral solution. Take ½ tsp three times a day, or add 1½ tsp to a liter of water with ReMag and sip throughout the day.
- **ReCalcia:** Picometer, stabilized ionic calcium, boron, vanadium. Take 1–2 tsp per day (1 tsp provides 300 mg calcium) if you don't obtain enough calcium from your diet. It can be taken with ReMag and ReMyte.
- **ReAline:** B vitamin complex plus amino acids. Take 1 capsule twice per day. Contains food-based B_1 and four methylated B vitamins (B_2, B_6, methylfolate, and B_{12}), plus L-methionine (precursor to glutathione) and L-taurine (which supports the heart and weight loss).
- **Vitamin E, as mixed tocopherols:** 400 IU daily.
- **Vitamin C complex:** 200 mg twice a day, from a food-based source, or make your own liposomal vitamin C (see Appendix D for a liposomal vitamin C recipe).
- **Vitamin D_3:** 1,000 IU or 20 minutes in the sun daily; Blue Ice Royal (from fermented cod liver oil and butter oil), for vitamins A, D, and K_2, 1 capsule twice per day.
- **Ginkgo biloba and gotu kola** are two herbs that can improve cerebral circulation but may not be necessary with the above nutrients.

PART FOUR

Determining Your Needs and Deciding What to Take

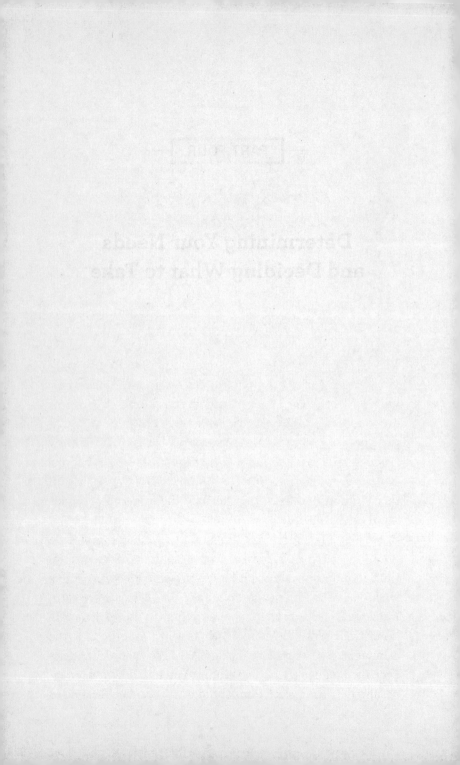

Magnesium Testing and Recommended Intake

MAGNESIUM TESTING

You've heard the saying "To err is human, to forgive is divine"? In the medical world, to err is human, to test is divine. I'm not a huge fan of laboratory tests because the results are compared to average values in our unhealthy population, not to optimal values. And errors can occur. I tell my readers that lab testing should be used to confirm what our senses and intuition tell us. But all too often doctors place all their faith in tests and only glance at the results, looking for numbers above or below normal.

When it comes to supplementing with magnesium, I do not think that the majority of people require testing. Magnesium is extremely safe, and it does produce a laxative effect when you take too much at one time or when you are saturated with magnesium after several months of supplementation. Even with ReMag, which is fully absorbed at the cellular level, when cell saturation is reached you will experience the laxative effect. I encourage you to follow your magnesium deficiency symptoms and the "100 Factors Related to

Magnesium Deficiency," in Chapter 1, as guides to how much magnesium you should take.

Since most people are deficient and magnesium is one of the safest nutrients, I tell people to just start taking it and keep track of symptoms, and you will see for yourself how it's working for you. This process is called an oral clinical trial.

THE ORAL CLINICAL TRIAL

For the average individual, one way to diagnose magnesium deficiency is simply to begin supplementing. First, run through the "100 Factors Related to Magnesium Deficiency" in Chapter 1 and tick off the ones that apply to you. Then for one to three months take magnesium while recording all changes in your physical and mental health. You may do this trial under the guidance of a health professional who knows about magnesium therapy, especially if you are on medications or have an existing medical condition. Personally, I don't think that's necessary for most people. We have long been our own caretakers, and that right should not be taken away from us.

The alleviation of symptoms after thirty to ninety days constitutes the best proof that you had a magnesium deficiency and you are treating it. If you reach the laxative effect before you obtain relief from your magnesium-deficiency symptoms, don't give up, as many people do. Switch to a well-absorbed magnesium such as ReMag to avoid the laxative effect and reach therapeutic levels.

MAGNESIUM RBC TESTING

The magnesium RBC test is more accurate than the serum magnesium test, but it's not as accurate as the ionized magnesium test, which is only available in research labs. Since it's not highly accurate, please don't just let the numbers be the gauge of how you are doing; you must also keep track of your magnesium deficiency symptoms and assess whether they are improving as you treat yourself with magnesium.

Your doctor or your local lab may not even know about the magnesium RBC test. Don't worry; the test can be obtained easily online if your doctor can't or won't write you a requisition for it. Go to www.RequestATest.com or www .DirectLabs.com and type in "magnesium RBC." You will be asked for your zip code and sent to a local lab for a blood draw. You will receive your results within seventy-two hours. The test only costs about $49, which may be less than the copay for an office visit so your doctor can write you a lab order. (Note: This type of testing is not available in all states.)

Be aware that lab values for magnesium don't give you an optimum or a therapeutic range. The lab just measures the magnesium level of people that walk in the door and charts them on a bell curve. The current magnesium range for most labs is 4.2–6.8 mg/dL, but recently I've seen some labs go even lower, to 3.5–6.0 mg/dL, as the population gets more and more deficient! About 80 percent of the population is deficient in magnesium, so I tell people that for optimal health, we want to be at the high end of the range, at or above the 80th percentile, or about 6.0–6.5 mg/dL.

You can repeat the test every three to six months and use it as a guide for the form of magnesium you should take and how much. However, you may find that the second test after three months produces a result that is the same as the first test or even lower, yet you are feeling better. That's because the 700–800 enzyme systems that require magnesium are getting all revved up and using more and more magnesium, so the levels can dip down in the beginning of treatment. Then at the six- and nine-month stages, your levels will be higher as you become more saturated. It can take a year or more for you to reach full saturation and begin to need less magnesium. Read "How Much Magnesium Should I Take?"

in the Introduction and "What Magnesium Should I Take?" in Chapter 18 for more guidance.

A huge caveat in lab testing is that doctors only look at "red-flagged" results, those that are out of range, so if they do your magnesium RBC test and the result is 3.8 mg/dL, you will be told that your magnesium is normal. But you're really at the bottom rung of magnesium and probably experiencing many magnesium deficiency symptoms. If you want to pull yourself out of that heap and eliminate your symptoms, you want to take enough magnesium to reach a level of 6.0–6.5 mg/dL.

Another reason the magnesium RBC test is still not the perfect test is because there are no mitochondria in red blood cells. There are mitochondria in all the cells of the body except red blood cells. Each liver cell has between 1,000 and 2,000 mitochondria, for example. Mitochondria are the energy factories inside cells. Six of the eight steps to make ATP (the energy molecule) in the mitochondrial Krebs cycle require magnesium. Therefore, there will be a lot more magnesium in cells that contain mitochondria than in red blood cells. The superior test is the ionized magnesium test, which does not measure the magnesium in cells but measures the ionized magnesium in the blood, which is the type of magnesium that is readily absorbed into the cell. But this test is not available outside of research settings.

Below are the normal ranges for magnesium RBC testing using the three different measurements that are commonly used worldwide. If your test results come back in mmol/L, multiply that result by 2.433 to give you the result in mg/dL. Remember that you want your magnesium RBC levels to be optimal, about 6.0–6.5 mg/dL. You want to be above the 80th percentile of the population, as 80 percent of people are deficient in magnesium.

Magnesium Test	mg/dL	mmol/L	mEq/L
Mg RBC	4.2–6.8	2.4–2.57	3.37–5.77

Note: Do not take magnesium for at least 12 hours before your test.

CLINICAL MAGNESIUM DEFICIENCY TESTS

There are two clinical tests that can be done in a doctor's office, the results of which can indicate both calcium deficiency and magnesium deficiency.

1. Chvostek's sign (a contraction of the facial muscles caused by tapping lightly on the facial nerve located in front of the ear)
2. Trousseau's sign (a spasm of the hand muscles caused by applying a tourniquet or blood pressure cuff to the forearm below the elbow for three minutes)

Since neither test distinguishes calcium deficiency from magnesium deficiency, doctors use the tests only to diagnose and treat calcium deficiency. As a result, if calcium supplements are recommended based on either of these tests, magnesium levels are driven even lower, causing more magnesium-deficiency symptoms.

BLOOD IONIZED MAGNESIUM TEST

Over the years, lab testing for minerals evolved from measurements done on whole blood to isolating minerals inside cells. The present state of the art lies in testing mineral ions, which are the active component of minerals working at the cellular level. The blood ionized magnesium test, pioneered and tested extensively at the State University of New York Downstate Medical Center in Brooklyn by magnesium researchers Bella and Burton Altura, is the most accurate and reliable magnesium blood test available, but presently it is limited to research use. The Alturas have researched the health effects of magnesium since the 1960s and did the original research for the test in 1987.[1, 2, 3, 4, 5, 6]

The ionized magnesium test is a very refined procedure, backed up by results on many thousands of patients with over twenty-two different disease states and published in dozens of journals, including five papers in *Science* and papers in the prestigious *Scandinavian Journal of Clinical Laboratory Investigation* and *Scientific American.*[7]

To determine the efficacy and efficiency of the new test, research included a comparison of magnesium levels found with the Alturas' ionized magnesium test to levels found in various body tissues using expensive and sensitive digital imaging microscopy, atomic absorption spectroscopy, and the magnesium fluorescent probe. The ionized magnesium test proved itself to be a highly sensitive, convenient, and relatively inexpensive means of determining magnesium status in healthy or ill subjects.

Here's how it works. Magnesium exists in the body either as active magnesium ions or as inactive magnesium complexes (such as magnesium chloride) in which the magnesium is bound to proteins or other substances. A magnesium ion is an atom that is missing two electrons, which makes it want to attach to another substance that will replace its missing electrons. Magnesium ions constitute the physiologically active fraction of magnesium in the body; they are not attached to other substances and are free to join in biochemical body processes.[8] But they are very unstable and bind as soon as they can to other atoms. The reason ReMag is so well tolerated is because its magnesium ions are stabilized using a proprietary process, which allows it to be completely absorbed at the cellular level.

Most clinical laboratories assess only total serum magnesium, which includes both active and inactive types. Only 1 percent of the body's magnesium circulates in the blood, which means the serum magnesium test can only sample that 1 percent. With the blood ionized magnesium test, you can directly measure the levels of magnesium ions in the blood using ion-selective electrodes that give an accurate accounting of the actual magnesium ions at work in the body.[9]

In 85 to 90 percent of all patients tested, low magnesium ion levels match tissue levels of free magnesium and accurately diagnose magnesium deficiency found in asthma, brain trauma, coronary artery disease, diabetes (both type 1 and type 2), gestational diabetes, eclampsia and preeclampsia, heart disease, elevated homocysteine, hypertension, tension headaches, posttraumatic headaches, ischemic heart disease, liver transplant, renal transplant, polycystic ovarian disease, stroke, and syndrome X. In many of these conditions, low magnesium ion levels exist in spite of normal serum magnesium levels, making the ionized magnesium test more reliable for diagnosing magnesium deficiency.[10, 11, 12, 13, 14, 15, 16, 17, 18, 19] In one study, ionized magnesium testing on 3,000 migraine patients shows that 90 percent of those with low magnesium ion levels improve with magnesium therapy.

Because laboratories are slow to acquire new equipment, at present the FDA-approved ionized magnesium test is unfortunately mainly limited to only about fifty university laboratories and used mostly for research purposes. In the past, the Alturas have provided this test to doctors who sent in their patients' blood, but that avenue is no longer available and few other labs are offering the test.

SERUM (BLOOD) MAGNESIUM TEST

As mentioned previously, most magnesium research studies follow magnesium levels using the serum magnesium blood test. There are very few studies that compare serum magnesium testing with ionized magnesium testing. Drs. Burton and Bella Altura tried their best to champion the superior ionized magnesium test, but allopathic medicine is still firmly locked into the highly inaccurate serum magnesium test.

Less than 1 percent of our body's total magnesium can be measured in blood serum; the rest is busily occupied in the cells and tissues or is holding our bones together. Therefore, it is virtually impossible to make an accurate assessment of the level of magnesium in various body tissue cells using a routine serum magnesium test. Magnesium in the blood does not correlate with the amount of magnesium in other parts of your body. The active magnesium in your cells is ionized magnesium.

If you are under the stress of various ailments, your body pumps magnesium out of the cells and into the blood, giving the mistaken appearance of normality on serum magnesium testing in spite of body-wide depletion. Unfortunately, most magnesium evaluations done in hospitals and in laboratories use the antiquated serum magnesium test.

A serum magnesium test is actually worse than ineffective, because a test result that is within normal limits lends a false sense of security about the status of the mineral in the body. It also explains why doctors don't recognize magnesium deficiency: they assume serum magnesium levels are an accurate measure of all the magnesium in the body.

A research group published a study titled "The Underestimated Problem of Using Serum Magnesium Measurements to Exclude Magnesium Deficiency in Adults."[20] The investigators issued a health warning in their conclusion that I wish doctors would heed: "The perception that 'normal' serum magnesium excludes deficiency is common among clinicians. This perception is probably enforced by the common laboratory practice of highlighting only abnormal results. A health warning is therefore warranted regarding potential misuse of 'normal' serum magnesium because restoration of magnesium stores in deficient patients is simple, tolerable, inexpensive and can be clinically beneficial."

Magnesium must remain at an effective level in the blood to maintain certain vital functions, like keeping the heart beating effectively. To maintain this crucial balance, when serum magnesium levels drop, magnesium is pulled out of bone and muscle to top up the tank. Since doctors don't recognize this feedback mechanism, they think that serum magnesium is always normal, so they usually don't even bother testing for it on an electrolyte panel; instead they only look at sodium, potassium, calcium, and chloride.

For this reason, I offer a list of "100 Factors Related to Magnesium Deficiency" in order to help people judge their level of deficiency. You can find that list in Chapter 1. These factors contribute to your magnesium burn rate. Or you can use your clinical symptoms of magnesium deficiency along with the magnesium RBC test, knowing that you want to achieve the optimal level of 6.0–6.5 mg/dL.

RED AND WHITE BLOOD CELL MAGNESIUM TESTS

All body cells, including red and white blood cells, contain magnesium—up to 40 percent of the body's total. Because red blood cells are 500 times more abundant in blood than white blood cells, they are the preferred test material. But, as I've noted above, because red blood cells do not contain mitochondria, they hold less magnesium. White blood cells do have mitochondria and therefore will hold more magnesium than red blood cells.

Many studies show that red blood cell magnesium is a much more accurate measure of total body magnesium than the serum magnesium test. One study in childhood asthmatics compared serum magnesium levels to total white blood cell magnesium levels. While serum magnesium became elevated on the first day of an asthma attack, the white blood cell magnesium levels dropped dramatically, indicating the real state of affairs. As mentioned above, under stress, magnesium is released from the cells, depleting the cells as it floods into the bloodstream, making serum magnesium look higher.[21]

SPECTRACELL MICRONUTRIENT TESTING ON WHITE BLOOD CELLS

I'm not a big fan of doing a lot of blood testing because I think nutrient values shift from day to day. And if you are just looking for an accurate magnesium test, SpectraCell Micronutrient Testing is overkill.[22] The test is done using white blood cells from a blood sample. Considering that white blood cells do have mitochondria, where most of the magnesium in the cell is located, this is a more accurate test than magnesium RBC. Red blood cells do not have mitochondria and therefore have less magnesium than other cells, including muscle cells.

I have not ordered this test, but I've had patients and customers who have had this test done and shown me the results. According to company information, available on their website, "SpectraCell's Micronutrient tests measure the function of 35 nutritional components including vitamins, antioxidants, minerals and amino acids within our white blood cells. Scientific evidence shows us that analyzing the white blood cells gives us the most accurate analysis of a body's deficiencies."

The test costs $390. The company says that Medicare covers most of the test, as does private insurance. It appears that you can order the test yourself online or through a practitioner.

THE BUCCAL CELL SMEAR TEST (EXA TEST)

Using cells gently scraped from an area in the mouth between the bottom teeth and the back of the tongue provides an accurate means of measuring the amount of magnesium in the tissue cells of the body.[23] Measuring cellular magnesium in this way is a reflection of the amount of magnesium in other tissue cells such as heart and muscle cells, the two major body tissues affected by magnesium deficiency.

The buccal cell smear test can be used to sample many substances contained in cells. IntraCellular Diagnostics has developed a testing procedure called EXA Test specifically to identify the amounts of certain minerals in the cell. The company sends sampling kits to your doctor's office, where a simple procedure, which takes about sixty seconds, is performed.

Your doctor uses a small wooden spatula, like a tongue depressor, to scrape off superficial layers of cells under your tongue. The scrapings are carefully placed on a microscope slide and sent back to the lab. A special electron microscope then measures the amount of magnesium and other minerals in the sample on the slide. The results are sent back to your doctor. The test is expensive but it is covered by insurance; you still have to pay your doctor's fees.

For those who are curious about the details of the testing, an analytical scanning electron microscope with high-tech, computerized elemental X-ray analysis (EXA) bombards the specimen with high-energy electrons, whereupon energy is released in the form of wavelengths that are distinct and unique to each mineral element. A computer measures the wavelengths and calculates what is called a "spectral finger-print" for each patient that identifies the mineral levels and ratios within the cell. (See Resources.)

THE MAGNESIUM CHALLENGE TEST

This test, also called the magnesium loading test, is time-consuming and cumbersome but necessary for people who may be magnesium-wasters or who have a genetic magne-sium deficiency disease. A magnesium-waster is someone whose magnesium blood levels are consistently low in spite of supplementing with oral or IV magnesium.

The magnesium challenge test requires twenty-four-hour urine collections on two separate occasions. The first urine collection is done when you are taking your normal supple-ments. Then, in the doctor's office, a dose of 0.2 meq/kg of magnesium chloride or magnesium sulfate is given intrave-nously, infused over a four-hour period. A second urine col-lection begins after the IV, and every urine sample is collected for twenty-four hours.

Magnesium deficiency is diagnosed when the body ex-hibits an excessive need for magnesium by holding on to more than 25 percent of the magnesium given. A decade ago, the magnesium challenge test was the best method of determining body stores.[24] Today, comparison studies using magnesium challenge testing and ionized magnesium test-ing indicate that ionized magnesium testing appears to be a better indicator and is more easily done—except it's only available in research settings![25]

Magnesium-wasting is diagnosed if more than 75 per-cent of the magnesium given in the IV test is excreted. You could also assume that you have enough magnesium and are not deficient if you lose more than 75 percent. However, if a clinical assessment is made that you have magnesium deficiency symptoms and you lose most of the magnesium given by IV, then magnesium-wasting is the probable diagnosis. The treatment for magnesium-wasting is to take regular IV magnesium treatments or use ReMag.

There are genetic causes of magnesium-wasting, where the kidneys just can't seem to hold on to this vital mineral, but they are very rare. I was surprised when at a recent seminar a doctor came up and thanked me for my talk on magnesium and said he suffered from magnesium-wasting. He reported that in spite of having a good diet, taking supplements, and being on no magnesium-wasting drugs such as diuretics or digitalis, he still had slightly high blood pressure, moderately high cholesterol, and leg cramping. When he read the first edition of *The Magnesium Miracle* he realized his problem might be magnesium deficiency. But even when he took more magnesium, he still had some symptoms. That's when he decided to do a magnesium challenge test and found out he was not retaining enough magnesium.

The doctor began taking regular IV treatments of magnesium. However, using ReMag orally and spraying ReMag transdermally is an effective treatment for people who need high amounts of magnesium and want to avoid the dangers, expense, and inconvenience of IV magnesium. Read Dana's story of his transition from IV magnesium to ReMag in Chapter 18 under the heading "ReMag: Therapeutic Magnesium."

GOVERNMENT MAGNESIUM GUIDELINES

Feel free to skip this next section, which is an overview of government nutrient guidelines. It's confusing enough trying to determine your individual needs for magnesium without having to wade through the alphabet soup of guidelines set by government agencies.

Nutrient guidelines include the DRI, RDA, RDI, AI, UL, and EAR. In 1997, the Food and Nutrition Board of the National Academy of Sciences created the Dietary Reference Intakes (DRIs), which added another set of guidelines apart from the Recommended Dietary Allowances (RDAs) that were the standard from 1941 to 1989. Most people just talk about the RDAs because they have been around the longest. In my experience, all the guidelines fall far short of the amount of magnesium that people really need to stay healthy. I think the magnesium levels are set very low in order to avoid the "side effect" of diarrhea.

In one government meeting, I was told point-blank that the guidelines for nutrients were simply to prevent frank vitamin and mineral deficiencies, not to prevent or treat illness. In fact, the definition of a drug is a substance used to prevent or treat illness, so if a mineral is said to treat a disease, then it must, by definition, be called a drug!

Numerical analysis of diets for the amounts of certain nutrients is necessary for the planning of menus to meet the nutrient needs of different age groups. They are also used to evaluate food consumption patterns and to create guidelines for nutrition labeling, all with an eye to preventing nutrient deficient diseases. Let me repeat this important point: the RDA nutrient intake guidelines do not recommend levels for optimal health and vitality but only tell you how much vitamin C to take so you won't get scurvy, or how much vitamin B_3 to take, so you won't get pellagra.

The DRIs are a compilation of four different reference values: the Estimated Average Requirement (EAR), the Recommended Dietary Allowance (RDA), the Adequate Intake (AI), and the Tolerable Upper Intake Level (UL). The UL recommends higher intake of nutrients than the RDA in an inept attempt to reduce the risk of chronic diseases such as osteoporosis, cancer, and cardiovascular disease. However, in the case of osteoporosis, the recommendation was to increase calcium intake without a similar increase in magnesium.

Implementation of the DRIs was done in stages from 1997 to 2005. Focusing on the prevention of osteoporosis, the first report, published in 1997, was "Dietary Reference Intakes for Calcium, Phosphorus, Magnesium, Vitamin D and Fluoride." Four additional reports have covered folate and other B vitamins, dietary antioxidants (vitamins C and E, selenium, and the carotenoids), micronutrients (vitamins A and K, and trace elements such as iron, iodine, etc.), macronutrients (such as dietary fat and fatty acids, protein and amino acids, carbohydrates, sugars, and dietary fiber, as well as energy intake and expenditure), electrolytes and water, bioactive compounds (such as phytoestrogens and phytochemicals), and the role of alcohol in health and disease.

While the DRIs are used mainly by academic research scientists and nutritionists and are not a household word, doctors who focus on nutrition, such as myself, appreciate having the information in these reports. The confusing part in the magnesium report is that two different values are given for dietary magnesium and for supplemental magnesium. There is no total requirement and no acknowledgment that the intake of magnesium in the average diet is less than the RDA.

In 1997, the RDA of magnesium was raised 15 percent, from 350 mg/day to 420 for men and from 280 mg/day to 320 for women. However, the same 1997 report on the safe upper limit of dietary magnesium for adults states that "because magnesium has not been shown to produce any toxic effects when ingested as a naturally occurring substance in foods, a UL cannot be established for dietary magnesium at this time." The report also noted, "no specific toxicity data exist on which to establish a UL [for dietary magnesium] for infants, toddlers, and children."

Looking at supplemental magnesium, the committee set what some consider to be a very low UL for pregnant and breast-feeding women, despite their high magnesium needs and despite saying there is no upper limit for dietary magnesium. Even though the report states that "no evidence suggests increased susceptibility to adverse effects of supplemental magnesium during pregnancy and lactation," they set the UL for this group at 350 mg (14.6 mmol) per day. This is the same UL for supplemental magnesium in adults who are not pregnant or lactating. Setting such a low UL is harmful to pregnant women and can result in high blood pressure, fluid retention, and seizures such as seen in preeclampsia and eclampsia. The report also states that it would not factor in the high amounts of IV magnesium used in eclampsia and preeclampsia in their determination of the UL for pregnancy. This means they know full well that magnesium is used successfully in these life threatening conditions, yet, oddly, they won't give women more magnesium to prevent these conditions from occurring in the first place.

The report parrots the old line that "individuals with impaired renal function are at greater risk of magnesium toxicity." I thoroughly debate the notion that impaired renal function can result in magnesium toxicity in Chapter 11. About kidney disease patients they say, "Magnesium levels obtained from food are insufficient to cause adverse reactions even in these individuals." That's quite true since an average diet has less than the RDA, so where are these patients going to get even the minimum amount of magnesium? They do concede that "patients with certain clinical conditions (for example, neonatal tetany, hyperuricemia, hyperlipidemia, lithium toxicity, hyperthyroidism, pancreatitis, hepatitis, phlebitis, coronary artery disease, arrhythmia, and digitalis intoxication . . .) may benefit from the prescribed use of magnesium in quantities exceeding the UL in the clinical setting." However, I don't know who they expect to administer this magnesium, since doctors learn nothing about magnesium therapy in medical school.

MAGNESIUM RDA

As noted, the Recommended Daily Allowance for nutrients is set at the minimum level to stave off frank deficiency symptoms, not at the optimum that ensures good health. But even with the RDA set so low, most Americans are still deficient in magnesium, with men obtaining only about 80 percent of the RDA and women averaging only 70 percent.

The following table shows the RDAs for magnesium in children and adults.

Children 1 to 3 years: 80 mg
Children 4 to 8 years: 130 mg
Children 9 to 13 years: 240 mg

Life Stage	Men	Women	Pregnancy	Lactation
Age 14–18	410 mg	360 mg	400 mg	360 mg
Age 19–30	400 mg	310 mg	350 mg	310 mg
Age 31+	420 mg	320 mg	360 mg	320 mg

The RDA for magnesium is also expressed in mg/kg and is roughly 6 mg per kg (2.2 lb) of body weight. This standard helps to determine the magnesium requirements for someone who is overweight; a fifty-year-old who weighs 300 pounds needs more magnesium than a fifty-year-old who weighs 100 pounds. In my clinical experience, the RDA is set far too low and people with magnesium deficiency conditions may require 10–15 mg/kg per day.

The higher amounts are often necessary in people who are on magnesium-depleting medications, who are under severe stress, before and after surgery, or in those who are exposed to fluoride. As your body becomes saturated with magnesium, you will need to take less. This is the opposite of many drugs, where people need more over time as the body becomes drug-resistant or drug-dependent.

Many magnesium experts feel that the RDA of magnesium should be increased. Twenty years of research shows that under ideal conditions approximately 300 mg of magnesium is required merely to offset daily losses. If you are under mild to moderate stress caused by a physical or psychological disease, physical injury, athletic exertion, intake of medications, exposure to fluoride, chlorine, heavy metals, or emotional upheaval, your requirements for magnesium escalate.[26, 27]

Dr. Mildred Seelig wrote that active adolescent boys and girls may need 7–10 mg/kg/day and pregnancy requirements should be a minimum of 450 mg a day or up to 15 mg/kg/day.[28] I agree with Dr. Seelig and think that both women and men of all ages would benefit from a higher daily intake of at least 7–10 mg/kg of magnesium. Every day I speak with people who require double and triple the RDA of magnesium. I personally required 20 mg/kg/day when I was first overcoming my magnesium-deficiency symptoms of heart palpitations and leg cramps and building up my magnesium stores. Now, depending on my workload, exercise, and stress levels, I only need 10 mg/kg/day. The RDA of 6 mg/kg/day would only give me about 300 mg of magnesium and would bring back my magnesium deficiency symptoms.

Let me expand this conversation about magnesium requirements. Please reread the sections "When Magnesium Makes Me Worse" in the Introduction and "Causes of Magnesium Deficiency: The Magnesium Burn Rate" and "100 Factors Related to Magnesium Deficiency," both in Chapter 1, to understand the magnesium-deficiency epidemic and the many ways you can burn off your magnesium leaving you without magnesium reserves and vulnerable to magnesium deficiency diseases.

An average good diet may supply about 120 mg of magnesium per 1,000 calories, for an estimated daily intake of about 250 mg.[29, 30] Since at best the body is actually absorbing only half of what is taken in, researchers feel that most people would benefit from magnesium supplementation. Otherwise, body tissue must be broken down to supply vital areas of the body with essential magnesium.[31, 32]

I've been invited to high-level magnesium meetings with a dozen top magnesium research scientists and policy makers, and it appears their hands are tied when it comes to increasing the RDA, removing the serum magnesium test as the medically accepted method of measuring magnesium, or banning magnesium oxide and recommending better-absorbed magnesium supplements.

Government officials are in a double bind regarding magnesium requirements and recommendations. Most magnesium research has been done on magnesium oxide; however, magnesium oxide is very laxative. So the people on the panel deciding nutrient levels feel they have to keep the RDA down to a level low enough that less than 10 percent of the population has an adverse reaction such as diarrhea. Codex Alimentarius (mentioned in the Introduction) also follows the directive that nutrients should not interfere with prescription drugs, and they advise a very low minimum daily dosage.

The breakthrough that I bring to the table is the discovery of a unique magnesium that can be taken without the laxative effect. Thus, instead of limiting magnesium intake to 350 mg of a poorly absorbed form and only getting a few milligrams into the cells, you can take picometer, stabilized ionic magnesium in the form of liquid ReMag and absorb the therapeutic amount you require to eliminate your symptoms and elevate your magnesium RBC levels to 6.0–6.5 mg/dL.

To sum up: the magnesium RDA is far too low, most people require two or three times the RDA, and in order to get that amount without causing a laxative effect, I recommend you look into ReMag—a picometer, stabilized ionic form of magnesium. See Chapter 18 and Resources for more information.

A Magnesium Eating Plan

Good nutrition creates a solid structural foundation of tissue and bone as well as nutrients for making hormones and neurotransmitters. The basis of good nutrition is the consumption of protein, minerals, trace minerals, vitamins, amino acids, and essential fatty acids. Clearly there is more to life than magnesium, but life can't exist without it. Just as important as magnesium is calcium, and the Magnesium Eating Plan will also focus on how much calcium you need in your diet and in your supplement bottle.

The present American diet is heavily biased toward refined flour, sugar, and unhealthy fats. Over one-quarter of our diet may consist of what are in essence nonfoods that don't contain even a smattering of healthy nutrients. Magnesium is banished during food processing and never replaced, as some nutrients are, in fortified foods.

George Eby, whose foundation provided funds to educate members of Congress about magnesium and presented them with copies of *The Magnesium Miracle,* has a personal interest in magnesium, having suffered from magnesium deficiency for many years. He is convinced that magnesium deficiency causes 50 to 70 percent of all our chronic illnesses and accounts for a huge share of medical and hospital expenses. He's also concerned that because most of us have grown up in a society with widespread magnesium deficiency, which began about 100 years ago with the large-scale refining of grain, we are unable to recognize that we are deficient. Eby says that white flour should be called not "refined" wheat but "depleted" wheat, and points to the November 2002 issue of the *Harvard Heart Letter,* which shows that only 16 percent of the magnesium remains after wheat is refined.

Eby reminds us that refining also depletes other critical nutrients, such as vitamins E and B_6, vital for proper absorption of magnesium. However, magnesium is the main nutrient that is not adequately obtained by eating other foods. He says we are too fond of foods made with depleted wheat, such as pancakes, waffles, biscuits, tortillas, bread, cake, cookies, and doughnuts. These products take up a large amount of shelf space in grocery and convenience stores, mirroring our insatiable appetite for them. Clearly, he says, people love these foods—although a better verb would be *crave,* because people feel empty after eating depleted wheat, and keep eating more, perhaps searching for magnesium and other nutrients necessary for the body to function properly.

To obtain enough magnesium from the diet takes special care, knowledge of magnesium-rich foods, and a knowledge of whether or not the soil in which the plants are grown is fertilized with minerals. Even so, we still need to supplement with magnesium. In 2005, Eby produced a DVD showing a long list of foods with the amounts necessary to deliver 400 mg of magnesium. Imagine 1.8 ounces of rice bran, which provides 400 mg of magnesium, beside 54.25 ounces of doughnuts, which is the quantity you have to eat to obtain the same amount of magnesium. Or visualize a few ounces of nuts compared to 25 ounces of white bread. Such a picture, showing the nutrient deficiency of refined foods, is worth a thousand words.

FOODS CONTAINING 400 MG OF MAGNESIUM
PER SERVING IN OUNCES*

Food	Portion (in ounces) containing 400 mg
Rice bran, crude	1.8
Wheat bran, crude	2.3
Cocoa, dry powder	2.65
Pumpkin seeds	2.65
Brazil nuts	3.9
Peanut butter	3.9
Kellogg's All-Bran	3.9
Cashew nuts	4.80
Almonds	5.1
Rolled oats	5.1
Unsweetened chocolate	5.2
Molasses	5.3
Buckwheat flour	5.65
Oat bran	5.9
Wheat germ	5.9
Peanuts	8.0
Tortilla chips	14.5
Dinner rolls	16.6
Whole-wheat bread	17.3
English muffins	20
Potatoes	21.7
Spaghetti	22.0
Macaroni	22.0
Tortillas	22.0
Potato flour	22
Crackers	22.75
Melba toast	25
White bread	25
Potato chips	26
Brown sugar	48
Doughnuts	54.25

* Statistics from USDA data

WHAT ABOUT CALCIUM?

As you can see from the list "Calcium Content of Common Foods" in Appendix B, calcium is plentiful in nuts, seeds, whole grains, and leafy green vegetables, just like magnesium, but only if the minerals are already in the soil. In theory, when you eat these foods you are getting a balanced amount of calcium and magnesium.

Calcium is much higher in dairy compared to magnesium. So if you eat dairy you shift the balance of calcium and magnesium in favor of calcium. Another important aspect of dietary calcium and magnesium is the effect of processing and cooking on these minerals. More magnesium than calcium is lost in food processing and cooking, so once again, more calcium is found in the diet than magnesium. Calcium, thought to be so deficient in our population, is also fortified in many foods—even orange juice.

All these reasons strengthen the case for taking magnesium in supplement form in equal amounts with dietary calcium. Yes, you should be able to get enough calcium in your food if you eat calcium-rich foods, especially dairy products— just consult the calcium food list. If you don't eat dairy, then you can make or purchase bone broth and focus on all the other calcium-rich foods, or do what I do and take ReCalcia, a picometer, stabilized ionic calcium formula.

ORGANIC FOOD

Many people would say that organic food should be higher in magnesium than the offerings from Big Agriculture, but that may not be the case. If your organic farmer does not remineralize the land with minerals in the form of rock dust, the plants will be as magnesium-deficient as plants from any other farmland.

Seek out organic farmers who are educated about crop rotation, who test regularly for mineral deficiencies in the soil, and who use mineral-rich fertilizers. The smart way to be assured of quality organic food is to join a community-sponsored agriculture (CSA) cooperative and buy a share in a local organic farm every year, which means you may be able to have a say in what the farm produces and make recommendations. (See Resources for CSA information.)

USDA FINDINGS

United States Department of Agriculture (USDA) surveys of women's diet find that:

1. Approximately 25 percent of their magnesium is supplied by grain products. This means you should try to include a variety of whole grains and avoid white bread and pasta, which are devoid of minerals. If you crave bread (and sugar), you may be feeding yeast in your intestines and should try to limit your intake to achieve weight loss and blood sugar balance. Or you may be craving nutrients that your body knows are absent from refined grains—you eat more carbs, but the empty calories don't seem to satisfy a deeper need. You have to eat a pound and a half of white bread to get the RDA of magnesium.

2. Another 25 percent of women's magnesium intake comes from fruits and vegetables.

3. The high-protein foods—meat, poultry, and fish—provide only about 18 percent of total magnesium intake. Since high-protein diets are now becoming more popular, you must make sure to increase your magnesium when on such a diet.

4. Fats, sweets, and beverages supply only 14 percent of the

total magnesium intake. These foods, especially refined
fats and sweets, should be limited because they contain
empty calories devoid of nutrients. Also, sugar causes
a big drain on magnesium, which is required in high
amounts to metabolize it.
5. Nuts and seeds and their butters are the richest sources
of magnesium, but they are not even mentioned in most
food surveys.

THE MAGNESIUM DIET GUIDELINES

According to top French magnesium experts, highly effective heart- and blood-vessel-protective diets that reduce saturated fats, increase monounsaturated fat and omega-3 fatty
acids (from fish and flaxseed), limit the consumption of alcohol, and increase the intake of cereals, fruits, vegetables, fish,
and low-fat dairy products are rich in magnesium. They
stress that among several protective nutrients, magnesium
should be given particular consideration because of the very
frequent occurrence of chronic primary magnesium deficiency, which acts as a cardiovascular risk factor.[1] I agree
with the French dietary recommendations except I do encourage the use of healthy saturated fats as noted below and
in the recommendations throughout this book.

- Eat a wide variety of vegetables daily. Always include
greens such as kale, collards, spinach, and curly-leaf let-
tuce, and magnesium-rich herbs such as dandelion, chickweed, and nettles.
- Enjoy starchy vegetables three or four times a week, such
as red-skinned potatoes, winter squash, corn on the cob,
lima beans, and burdock root.
- Eat fruits moderately.

- Include a variety of whole grains: buckwheat, millet, rye, oats, amaranth, and quinoa.
- Fish, shellfish, organic chicken, meat, turkey, or free-range eggs can be eaten once a day as rich animal protein sources.
- Have beans, tempeh, nuts, seeds, and legumes as a vegetarian source of protein daily.
- Cook with fresh and dry herbs and include lots of garlic.
- Use organic cold-pressed oils for your cooking: extra-virgin olive oil, coconut oil, and sesame oil.
- Enjoy organic butter in moderation.
- Take 1–2 tbsp of flaxseed oil daily.
- Eat whole-grain breads and pasta.
- For a sweetener, use stevia.
- Drink natural spring or filtered water.
- Enjoy organic herbal teas.
- Eat sea vegetables: dulse, nori, arame, wakame, kombu, and hijiki. All are exceedingly high in magnesium.
- Use natural raw, unheated nuts, seeds, and nut and seed butters, all rich magnesium sources.
- Use a high-quality mineral-rich sea salt.

FOODS TO AVOID (READ LABELS)

- All refined and processed foods of any kind, such as cookies, cakes, doughnuts, bagels, white bread, luncheon meats, and soy protein powder.
- All refined and processed sugars, including fructose or corn syrup and diet products with artificial sweeteners such as aspartame and sucralose (NutraSweet and Splenda).
- Dairy products except organic butter, unsweetened yogurt, and kefir.

- Regular and decaffeinated coffee or black tea.
- Any foods containing hydrogenated or partially hydroge-nated oils or trans fatty acids.
- All alcoholic beverages.
- Pasteurized fruit juices and sodas.
- Foods containing MSG, hydrolyzed vegetable protein, and chemical preservatives.
- Commercial iodized salt.

A MAGNESIUM EATING PLAN

Upon rising: Juice of ½–1 fresh lemon in warm water. Sweeten with stevia.

BREAKFAST

CROCKPOT CEREAL

- Choose two grains, one nut, and one seed from the follow-ing: organic buckwheat, millet, rye, oats, amaranth, qui-noa, sunflower seeds, pumpkin seeds, almonds, cashews, filberts, walnuts, pecans.
- Dress with flaxseed oil and organic fresh or frozen blue-berries, cherries, strawberries, raspberries, banana, peach, or pear.

DIRECTIONS:

For one person, put 2 oz of dry mixture, including nuts and seeds, and 5 oz of water in a 1-quart crockpot. Cook overnight. In the morning place in a bowl, add 2–4 oz of fruit, mix, and add 2 tbsp flaxseed oil or 1 tbsp butter (organic) or 2 tbsp ground flaxseeds (ground fresh in a coffee grinder).

You may add rice milk, almond milk, or coconut milk as desired. For extra magnesium, sprinkle on wheat germ (kept in the freezer).

SUBSTITUTIONS:

1. Instead of using a crockpot, you can soak 2 oz of grain mixture overnight in 5 oz of water, with or without 2 tbsp of plain yogurt or kefir. In the morning bring to a boil and let simmer on the lowest setting for 20 minutes. You may have to add more water to avoid dryness. Serve with 2 tbsp ground flaxseeds (ground fresh in a coffee grinder).
2. Instead of soaking overnight, cook 2 oz of grain mixture in 6 oz of water. Bring to a boil and let simmer for 30 minutes.

LUNCH *(Choose one)*

1. Brown rice and vegetables, cooked with 2 oz dulse or other sea vegetables
2. Leafy green salad, soup with added sea vegetables, and Essene sprouted bread or Ezekiel bread
3. Fish, greens (collards, spinach, Swiss chard), and salad
4. Egg omelet with sautéed vegetables
5. Chicken with vegetables

DINNER *(Choose one)*

1. Soup (with sea vegetables) and salad
2. Stir-fried grains (leftover grains from breakfast) and vegetables
3. Roasted vegetables with wild rice
4. Salad with cooked organic legumes (kidney beans, lentils, black beans, pinto beans, chickpeas)
5. Wheat-free pasta (rice, spelt, kamut) with pesto, tomato sauce, and green vegetables
6. Mixed salad with avocado

SNACKS

1. Raw vegetables
2. Dried fruit (prunes and figs)
3. Shelled nuts and seeds (raw, not processed or salted)
4. Baked blue corn chips
5. Popcorn
6. Chocolate Frozana (see recipe in Chapter 9)

DRINKS

1. Pure, clean water
2. Green tea
3. Freshly squeezed lemon juice and water
4. Cranberry juice sweetened with stevia
5. Kukicha (roasted twig tea)
6. Bone broth (see recipe in Appendix C)

Kukicha twig tea, also known as bancha twig tea, is a Japanese blend of green tea made of roasted stems, stalks, and twigs of the tea plant, *Camellia sinensis*. It has a mildly nutty and slightly creamy sweet flavor. There are many variations of how to brew kukicha tea, depending on the taste you want. Stir 1 to 3 tsp in 6–8 oz of boiling water and steep for 1–6 minutes. This tea is said to be high in calcium, but I could not find any laboratory data to confirm.

FOODS RICH IN MAGNESIUM

In Appendix A you will find a complete list of foods with their magnesium content. Below is a short list of the richest sources of magnesium.[2] The quality of the soil from which these sources were assayed is unknown. Therefore, use these figures as a rough guide to making wise food choices.

MAGNESIUM CONTENT OF SELECTED FOODS

Food	Magnesium (mg) per 3½ oz (100 g)
Kelp	760
Wheat bran	490
Wheat germ	336
Almonds	270
Cashews	267
Molasses	258
Brewer's yeast	231
Buckwheat	229
Brazil nuts	225
Dulse	220
Filberts	184
Peanuts	175
Wheat grain	160
Millet	162
Pecans	142
English walnuts	131
Rye	115
Tofu	111

HERB SOURCES OF MAGNESIUM

Green plants, including most herbs such as purslane and cilantro, are loaded with magnesium, according to authors Wood, Weed, Duke, and Chevallier.[3, 4, 5, 6] Here are some other commonly used magnesium-rich herbs recommended by these authors that you can introduce into your diet. Herbs have the added advantage of often being organic or picked wild, so they usually don't contain pesticides and herbicides and may be grown on mineral-rich soil. It is when they are commercially harvested that the soil becomes depleted.

Burdock root (*Arctium lappa*), 537 mg magnesium per 100 g

Master herbalist Matthew Wood describes burdock root as a natural diuretic useful for flushing out very small kidney stones, an excellent blood cleanser, and a liver detoxifier. It can be grated into salads or cooked like potato and eaten several times per week.

Chickweed (*Stellaria media*), 529 mg magnesium per 100 g

Herbalist Susun Weed describes chickweed as a perfect food with "optimum nutrition." Chickweed encourages absorption of minerals and nutrients and is also naturally high in magnesium. Used several times a week in salads, it provides an excellent source of dietary magnesium.

Dandelion (*Taraxacum officinale*), 157 mg magnesium per 100 g

This amazing herb has been vilified as a nuisance weed, but its healing properties are legion. According to Andrew Chevallier, an experienced medical herbalist, it is used as a safe, natural diuretic to treat high blood pressure, and as a detoxifier to remove waste products from the gallbladder and the kidneys, thereby ameliorating many conditions such as gallstones, constipation, acne, eczema, arthritis, and gout. No doubt it owes some of its actions to the properties of magnesium. Dandelion leaves, used in salads, add a necessary bitter property that stimulates the bile. The root can be cooked or grated raw into salads.

Dulse (*Palmaria palmata*), 220 mg magnesium per 100 g

Dulse is a type of seaweed, of which there are many kinds; all dietary seaweeds are very nutritious. They are very high in digestible protein, around 25 percent by weight. Iodine to support the thyroid gland is their most notable benefit. They are high in most minerals as well as vitamins. Dulse can be introduced several times a week in soups and stews, and don't forget vegetarian sushi rolls, which are wrapped in seaweed.

Nettles (*Urtica dioica*), 860 mg magnesium per 100 g

Nettles are used to soften gallstones or kidney stones in the body. Susun Weed has some excellent recipes for nettles in her book *Healing Wise*. When nettles are lightly steamed they lose their stinging properties and make an excellent vegetable addition to any meal.

MAGNESIUM SALT SUBSTITUTES

Most doctors tell patients with high blood pressure to avoid salt, but they mean refined table salt. Salt from the sea and salt high in magnesium not only are safe but also can be therapeutic for someone with heart disease. They do contain sodium, however, so be sure to read labels. But we all require some sodium, so do not try to eliminate it entirely.

Sea salt is all the rage and available in gourmet food shops and health food stores, and it should be in your kitchen and dining room as well. However, it's big business now, so be careful to buy a good-quality unrefined sea salt, pink Himalayan salt, or Celtic sea salt. Make sure there is some color to the salt; if it's pure white, it's been overly refined and lost some of its mineral advantage. Sea salt in Maui is copper-colored!

Salt from evaporated seawater is relatively high in magnesium and is a wonderful way to get extra magnesium—about 20 mg in a teaspoon. However, the sodium content is still high. A lot of people have questions about sodium intake, since doctors tell people it's bad for high blood pressure. But there is more to sea salt with its seventy-two minerals than just sodium. Read the sections in Chapter 6 about diuretics, edema, and dehydration to understand the relationship between water, minerals, and cellular hydration.

Smart Salt is just that—a smart way to stock up on magnesium and cut back on sodium for those who must. Smart Salt is a product of the United States, produced by evaporation from Utah's Great Salt Lake. It has the following levels of minerals in 3 tsp: 626 mg of magnesium, 865 mg of potassium, and only 1,596 mg of sodium. (A similar amount of table salt contains about 5,000 mg of sodium.)

Cardia Salt also offers a healthy combination of salt, potassium, and magnesium that tastes just like regular salt. It produced a reduction in blood pressure in a double-blind placebo-controlled study carried out in 1997 on 233 hypertensive patients on medication. Another half dozen studies have confirmed its safety and effectiveness. Researchers comment that the product works because it reduces the amount of sodium by 54 percent and raises potassium and magnesium levels. For every teaspoon of salt you net about 40 mg of magnesium. The average amount of salt used per day is about 3 tsp, which means a significant 120 mg of magnesium per day. But in 3 tsp there would be 3,487 mg of sodium, which is more than twice as much as Smart Salt. (See Resources.)

MINERAL WATER AND MAGNESIUM

One of the natural sources of our minerals should be from water in the natural cycle of ice and snow from the mountains melting in the spring and scraping along the rocks to create mineral-rich waters that flood the plains where we grow our crops. That's not happening anymore—the rivers are dammed, floodplains are where we build houses, and water is chlorinated and run through lead, copper, or rusty iron pipes. We've polluted our water to such an extent that we feel the need to filter it, which removes minerals as well as pollutants.

Researchers have been aware of the importance of magnesium in our drinking water, but one research group was concerned that epidemiological studies demonstrated inconsistent associations between levels of magnesium in drinking water and risk of mortality from coronary heart disease (CHD).[7] To sort out these inconsistencies, they performed a meta-analysis. They tabulated 77,821 cases of patients with CHD and published their results in the journal *Nutrients*. They concluded once and for all that drinking water high in magnesium is significantly associated with lower CHD mortality.

An important source of magnesium, popular in Europe, is magnesium-rich mineral water. We have magnesium-rich water sources in the United States too, but not many people know about them. These local waters that have high magnesium levels could help to reduce magnesium deficiency in the population.

When choosing bottled water, be careful to consider the calcium content in relation to magnesium. A close reading of mineral water labels tells us that the calcium and sodium content are usually much higher than magnesium. Therefore, choose water with equal parts calcium and magnesium. This will ensure that you are getting enough of both minerals. If, however, you know you have a magnesium deficiency, by your symptoms or from medical or naturopathic diagnosis, choose water with high magnesium and low calcium content. Be aware that even though a label says "mineral water," the mineral content may be minuscule and not worth the price you pay.[8]

MAGNESIUM IN WATER[9]

Water Name	Country of Origin	Magnesium (mg/L)	Calcium (mg/L)	Sodium (mg/L)
Adobe Springs	USA	96	3.3	5
Santa Ynez	USA	87	19	—
San Pellegrino	Italy	57	203	46
Penafiel	Mexico	41	131	159
Vittel	France	38	181	3.7
Evian	France	24	78	5
Naya	Canada	22	38	6
Volvic	France	7	10	10.7
Saratoga	USA	7	64	9
Perrier	France	5	143	15.2
Alhambra	USA	5	9.5	5.4
Arrowhead	USA	5	20	3
Sparkletts	USA	5	4.6	15.2
Calistoga	USA	2	8	163
Cobb Mountain	USA	2	5.6	4.6
Poland Spring	USA	2	13.2	8.9
Sante	USA	1	4.2	160
Black Mountain	USA	1	25	8.3
Crystal Geyser	USA	1	1.5	30

Magnesium Supplementation and Homeopathic Use

WHAT MAGNESIUM SHOULD I TAKE?

In my decades of experience with magnesium, I've found that the best forms to take are:

1. ReMag: picometer, stabilized ionic magnesium from magnesium chloride
2. Natural Calm: magnesium citrate powder
3. Epsom salts: magnesium sulfate for your bath

In an Amazon review of *The Magnesium Miracle,* someone remarked that my exhaustive list of magnesium products in the first edition was much too confusing and time-consuming for her to research. She just wanted to know the best forms of magnesium to take, based on my research and experience. So that's what I'm providing in this edition. I'll also list some of the other forms of magnesium and give my reasons for not using them. If you want to take magnesium in pill form, I recommend capsules instead of solid tablets because capsules dissolve faster. The best capsule form of magnesium is

ReMag capsules, which have the same picometer, stabilized ionic magnesium found in ReMag liquid.

REMAG: THERAPEUTIC MAGNESIUM

The best form of magnesium is picometer, stabilized ionic magnesium in liquid and capsule form (from magnesium chloride), called ReMag. I don't say it's the best just because I created it; I say that because it is fully absorbed and assimilated at the cellular level. The magnesium ions in ReMag are stabilized with a unique proprietary process, which allows them to be completely absorbed into the cells that depend on these important ions for as many as 800 metabolic processes.

Since all the magnesium in ReMag is absorbed into the cells, this means you can take therapeutic amounts without reaching the bowels to create a laxative effect. There is little to none left over to reach the intestines. The ability to reach therapeutic levels of magnesium in the cells is unprecedented. Other magnesium products seem to cause diarrhea well before therapeutic levels are reached.

The application of therapeutic magnesium is the single biggest discovery I've made in the nearly twenty years that I've been actively researching this important mineral. Being able to take enough magnesium to fully treat health conditions without the laxative effect represents a major medical breakthrough.

Any health book or website about magnesium will tell you that magnesium treatment is limited by the laxative effect. Most medical references say you should only take 200–250 mg of magnesium per day. That's a far cry from the 600–1,200 mg of elemental magnesium that many people really need to treat their severe magnesium deficiency conditions.

In the creation of ReMag, magnesium chloride is broken down into picometer-size particles and delivered in an ionic form. A proprietary process stabilizes the very reactive magnesium ions from magnesium chloride, making them "stand still" for long enough to be fully absorbed into cells. Lack of hydrochloric acid in the stomach, a leaky gut, a sensitive bowel, IBS, yeast overgrowth, weight loss surgery, intestinal surgery, a history of diarrhea, Crohn's, colitis, or microscopic colitis—none of these conditions hamper the complete absorption of ReMag. This is another amazing breakthrough because I've heard practitioners say that you shouldn't even bother taking supplements until your gut is healed because a leaky gut means you can't absorb nutrients! It's actually an absurd statement because you need nutrients in order to heal a leaky gut. In fact, magnesium deficiency is a cause of leaky cell membranes.

In my discussion under the heading "Free Radicals, Antioxidants, and Aging" in Chapter 15, I cite a study that says low magnesium levels can compromise cell membrane integrity, damaging the vital fatty layer in the cell membrane, making it more susceptible to destruction, and allowing leakage through the membrane.[1] This study helps me convince people who are told they have leaky gut that magnesium is a necessary part of their healing. Since many people with leaky gut can get the laxative effect from magnesium, I assure them that ReMag, taken very slowly and increased gradually, can help heal damaged cell membranes.

When I first wrote *The Magnesium Miracle*, I was mainly interested in educating people about magnesium itself. It was before I even realized the extent of my own magnesium deficiency, which was causing daily heart palpitations and nightly leg cramps. Initially I believed that magnesium supplements were much alike, and I was committed to researching an exhaustive list of magnesium supplements and comparing their effectiveness. I quickly learned that absorption of supplements varies greatly. Magnesium oxide, for example, is only 4 percent absorbed. Even so, most magnesium research is done using magnesium oxide.

I was told that, back in the day, a magnesium oxide supplement company, in order to promote their products, gave truckloads of free magnesium oxide to researchers for their clinical trials. That's why magnesium oxide was, and still is, a doctor's first recommendation, because it shows up in all the research studies. It wasn't until many years later that magnesium oxide was found to be only 4 percent absorbed; the other 96 percent that isn't absorbed flushes through the intestines, causing diarrhea. Yet investigators consistently reported beneficial results in all their magnesium oxide studies, showing the importance of even a small amount of magnesium. However, the studies always mention the distressing "side effect" of diarrhea.

That was precisely my problem with magnesium—no matter what form I took, I would get the laxative effect. One time I started a new multiple vitamin and mineral supplement and didn't realize it contained a few milligrams of magnesium oxide. I lost 10 pounds from chronic diarrhea before I realized the cause. After that stressful experience, I spent almost ten years trying to convince several mineral companies to formulate a non-laxative magnesium. They deemed it too expensive to research and formulate and said it would require too much consumer education to market. But I was willing to spend the money and take the time to educate people because I knew that a certain percentage of the population was suffering like me.

With the creation of ReMag, everything we knew or thought we knew about magnesium therapy changed overnight. We never really understood how far we could go with magnesium therapy because people could never take enough. Now people are able to take high enough doses of magnesium to get relief from dozens of health conditions without any laxative effect. ReMag is able to meet the challenge of an increasing magnesium burn rate in our magnesium-depleted society.

The majority of magnesium products have a laxative effect at increasing doses. Even so, allopathic and alternative practitioners tell their patients that they will know when they have reached a saturation point with magnesium when they get diarrhea; at that point they should cut back by one dose. They tell patients to guide their magnesium intake by their laxative effect. In my case and that of a certain undefined and undiagnosed segment of the population, even one dose can cause the laxative effect. That means if we cut back by that one dose we would be getting no magnesium at all—and we would be very far from being saturated. Thus, the standard means of dosing magnesium fails many people.

If you get diarrhea when you take magnesium, you can end up losing most of that magnesium, which means your magnesium deficiency symptoms can get worse. If you realize your magnesium supplement is causing the diarrhea, you will stop taking it, thinking it's not doing you any good or that it's even harmful. I shudder to think how many people have tried magnesium and gotten diarrhea and never touched it again. Symptoms that are due to magnesium deficiency will then be treated, ineffectively, with drugs.

There is a lotion form of ReMag, or you can put ReMag in a spray bottle and spray it or rub ReMag on your skin to relieve pain or inflammation. Or you can spray or apply a daily dose of ReMag on your child's skin, if they won't take ReMag by mouth. These forms of ReMag are not itchy or irritating compared with magnesium oil applications.

We have reports of people mixing a teaspoon of ReMag in a gallon of water in a humidifier; putting 5–6 drops of ReMag in the ear to help with tinnitus and deafness that may be due to calcification; spraying ReMag on a toothbrush, with or without toothpaste, for oral health; or pouring ReMag in a jar of facial scrub to enhance circulation, detox, and healing. I top off my ReNew skin serum with ReMag.

One enterprising eighty-year-old puts her drops of ReMag and my multiple-mineral supplement ReMyte in empty gelatin capsules so she doesn't have to taste them.

At a time when people are losing magnesium from chronic stress and from taking drugs that deplete magnesium, and getting little magnesium from their diet, a therapeutic form of magnesium is exactly what we need. ReMag's ability to be fully absorbed at the cellular level means it will be able to detox your cells and activate all your enzyme systems, including your mitochondrial Krebs cycle, to produce lots of energy.

Before ReMag, IV magnesium used to be the only hope for severe magnesium deficiency in people who easily get the laxative effect. The following story is from Dana, who switched from IV magnesium to ReMag with great success. Dana proves that the therapeutic effectiveness of ReMag surpasses that of IV magnesium.

> January 14, 2014; Thank you, Dr. Carolyn Dean and ReMag! My name is Lynn. My husband, Dana, has hypomagnesemia. He was diagnosed with malabsorption at the Mayo Clinic. He loses magnesium through his bowels, therefore oral magnesium was never an option. We have been told by forty well-known specialists that all he could do was IV magnesium.
>
> He has had a PICC line for over seven years and required 4 grams of IV magnesium 3 times per week up until September 2013. In the past two years he has had three life-threatening events as a direct result of the PICC line (blood infection and on two different occasions blood clots). When the PICC line stopped working the next step was to put a permanent port in his chest.
>
> In September the PICC line came out for good as a result of another blood clot. We took a giant leap of faith against all of his doctors' advice and he started on

ReMag under the guidance of Dr. Dean. The results were immediate, his magnesium levels are testing higher on ReMag than they did on weekly IV infusions. We are forever grateful to Dr. Carolyn Dean and her commitment to helping others.

My husband now has a quality of life he was told was not possible! ReMag does not affect his bowels. We still do weekly labs because we have no room for error with his condition but we know we are close to backing off on labs. His lowest serum magnesium on IVs was 0.8 and now on ReMag he is running at 1.7 and higher.

Dr. Dean was the one who pointed out the obvious to us: that my husband's IV would give him highs and lows on magnesium, whereas ReMag has stabilized his levels because he can take it several times a day, and it has also gotten his labs higher than they have ever been on the IV mag.

We have paid out of pocket for a home health nurse weekly for over 7 years. Our insurance would not cover the cost unless he was homebound. We have both primary and secondary insurance; however, we still paid a small fortune annually for home health, labs, supplies, medicine, etc. But a one-hour consultation and a couple of emails with Dr. Dean forever changed the course of our lives.

The timing of all of this coming together is no coincidence either. Our phone call with Dr. Dean was one week prior to the unexpected issue with the PICC line. Had I not spoken with her on that particular day and things fallen into place like they did, my husband would have a port and be sitting in an infusion center three times a week. I still can't believe the answer was so simple. I have given Dr. Dean's book to several of his doctors. I wonder how many people are not as lucky as we are.

The PICC line was his lifeline to magnesium; however, it almost cost him his life more than once. I refused to believe that was his path and that is how I found Dr. Carolyn Dean. Dr. Dean not only gave him a better quality of life, there is no doubt that she saved his life!

NATURAL CALM

Natural Calm is the most widely recognized form of magnesium in the United States health food market, and it is my second magnesium recommendation. Natural Calm is a powdered magnesium citrate sweetened with organic stevia. If I could take enough Natural Calm to treat my heart palpitations and leg cramps, I would never have created ReMag. If I take even one dose of Natural Calm, I get the laxative effect.

I like the fact that Natural Calm is a powder that you stir into water, which means it's better absorbed than pills. However, the magnesium in Natural Calm is not isolated and stabilized, so it's not nearly as well absorbed and it can cause a laxative effect. I recommend a combination of ReMag and Natural Calm for people who have constipation. That way you can get the laxative effect of Natural Calm, plus some absorption into the cells, and then with ReMag you get complete absorption and you take care of all your magnesium deficiency needs. You can mix ReMag and Natural Calm together in water and sip throughout the day for a tasty drink. If you begin to get a laxative effect as you become more saturated with magnesium, then wean off Natural Calm.

Don't confuse the 300 mg dose of magnesium citrate in Natural Calm with the bowel-purging magnesium citrate in the drugstore. Magnesium citrate is given in doses of 12,000 mg to completely purge the bowel before bowel X-rays, barium enemas, sigmoidoscopies, and colonoscopies. That's probably why your doctor thinks magnesium is simply a laxative.

EPSOM SALTS

In the Introduction, I mentioned that magnesium was first discovered many centuries ago, and there was even a paper written in 1697 about its health benefits. Epsom salt is magnesium sulfate, and that's important because bathing in it gives you a healthy supply of sulfur along with the magnesium. Sulfur is another important mineral that we may be lacking.

Children especially benefit from baths with Epsom salts. Most kids love their baths, and adding magnesium salts just makes sense. For kids and adults, 1–2 cups in a bath is sufficient. However, I've used up to 8 cups when I've had a severe muscle spasm or injury.

Before I began to use my ReMag for my heart palpitations and leg cramps, I was taking a lot of Epsom salts baths, and they helped, but not enough. However, I recommend the baths along with ReMag for the extra boost to muscle relaxation and detoxification through the skin.

Susan, whom I introduced in Chapter 4, suffered tingling sensations on the back of her head for three years. She said the symptoms matched a condition called occipital neuralgia, which is an inflammation of the nerves from the back of the neck up into the scalp. ReMag after only a few weeks helped 75 percent of her symptoms, which included Ativan withdrawal and Neurontin withdrawal. She was still very discouraged, however, and I told her to take Epsom salts baths and immerse the back of her head in the water. She happily reported that her symptoms were now improving dramatically after only a few baths.

Epsom salts in a bath are absorbed through the skin and are known to be relaxing. I remember one patient, Arlene, as "the woman who soaked too long." She put several pounds of Epsom salts in a bath, fell asleep in the water, and found out that magnesium sulfate is indeed absorbed through the skin:

she developed diarrhea due to magnesium's laxative effect. Someone with a skin condition such as eczema might absorb magnesium even more readily. Soak for thirty minutes in a moderately hot bath and use one to two cups at a time. If you don't have a tub or can't easily get in and out of a tub, use a footbath with 1 cup of Epsom salts.

MAGNESIUM DOSAGE

Government agencies try to create uniformity in the nutrient dosage world, but that's just not the way the body works. If you go back to Chapter 1 and consult "Causes of Magnesium Deficiency: The Magnesium Burn Rate," it's obvious that a one-size-fits-all approach does not apply to magnesium dosage—there are just too many variables.

In Chapter 16, under "Government Magnesium Guidelines," I've gone over the RDA values that have been foisted on Americans. Below I've summarized what we know about magnesium dosing.[2, 3, 4, 5] All magnesium dosages are in milligrams of elemental magnesium, not the milligram weight of the whole magnesium compound. I discuss elemental magnesium in more detail below.

- The RDA is a mere 6 mg/kg/day, which would give a 120-pound woman only 325 mg of magnesium per day.
- Dr. Mildred Seelig wanted active adolescent boys and girls to have 7–10 mg/kg/day.
- Dr. Seelig wanted athletes to have 6–10 mg/kg.
- Dr. Seelig recommended that magnesium requirements during pregnancy be a minimum of 450 mg a day or up to 15 mg/kg/day.
- I think both women and men of all ages would benefit from a higher daily intake of at least 7–10 mg/kg of magnesium.

- Someone with serious magnesium deficiency symptoms may require 15–20 mg/kg of elemental magnesium (I needed 20 mg/kg/day for two years to rid myself of heart palpitations and leg cramps). Since high levels of most magnesium products cause diarrhea, I recommend ReMag for people who need this much magnesium.

Testing of magnesium RBC levels every three to six months can ensure your levels are steadily increasing to the optimal blood level of 6.0–6.5 mg/dL. (See Chapter 16 for details.) Remember that magnesium RBC is not a completely accurate test, so you must go by your clinical symptoms and how you feel rather than relying solely on a blood test.

NOTE: Be aware that in the first few months of ReMag therapy, your magnesium RBC levels may not improve or may drop even lower than your initial test because the body is so busy grabbing on to all the magnesium it can, as the nearly 800 enzyme processes in the body gear up to finally do the work they were meant to do.

When I first began taking ReMag, I was using 1,200 mg per day. After about two years my body became saturated and I would get the laxative effect with that much magnesium. For one more year I required about 600 mg per day. Now I only seem to need 300–450 mg per day, but I do try to stay at 600 mg per day so I can remain fully saturated. My magnesium needs were also reduced when I added sea salt to my drinking water and took my multiple-mineral supplement, ReMyte. I reasoned that I was using the extra ReMag to treat the symptoms of other mineral deficiencies, and when I was no longer deficient in those minerals, by taking ReMyte, I needed less magnesium.

CONTRAINDICATIONS TO MAGNESIUM THERAPY

1. **Kidney failure.** With kidney failure there is an inability to clear magnesium from the kidneys.
2. **Myasthenia gravis.** Intravenous administration could accentuate muscle relaxation and collapse the respiratory muscles.
3. **Excessively slow heart rate.** Slow heart rates can be made even slower with magnesium, as magnesium relaxes the heart. Very slow heart rates often require an artificial pacemaker.
4. **Bowel obstruction.** The main route of elimination of oral magnesium is through the bowel.

Even with these contraindications, there are many exceptions to the rule. Please read the section called "Kidneys Need Magnesium" in Chapter 11 to help understand how magnesium is actually necessary for kidney health, but it has to be a picometer, stabilized ionic form—ReMag.

As for the second contraindication, I have had people with myasthenia gravis tell me that magnesium helped them overcome their disease when it was originally caused by heavy metal poisoning and/or yeast overgrowth.

If someone has an excessively slow heart rate that's not just related to adrenal fatigue or exhaustion, they can benefit from a pacemaker and then be able to take magnesium. I encourage people to get fitted with a pacemaker if it seems medically justified and not avoid it because they are afraid of allopathic medicine. A pacemaker is one of the great benefits of modern medicine.

Someone with bowel obstruction should be hospitalized and not have access to the laxative effects of magnesium, which would just further bloat their intestines.

THE SAFETY OF MAGNESIUM SUPPLEMENTS

For the majority of the population, oral magnesium, even in high dosages, has no side effects except loose stools, which is a mechanism to release excess magnesium. Excess magnesium is also lost through the urine. Even non-laxative picometer magnesium—ReMag—will create a laxative effect when you reach saturation and take more than you require.

THE MANY FORMS OF MAGNESIUM

There is a heavy marketing campaign surrounding the sale of magnesium. Many companies have popped up claiming that the only way to get magnesium without the laxative effect is to use transdermal magnesium oils and sprays. That is no longer the case, as you can take ReMag orally. You can also put ReMag in a spray bottle to treat local aches, pains, and muscle spasms. The best way to apply it is to spray the painful area four or five times, letting the magnesium dry in between sprays for several minutes.

In addition to Epsom salts baths, I used magnesium oil transdermally before creating ReMag, and I developed skin irritation and rashes, trying to take enough for my symptoms, because the magnesium oil was too irritating on my skin. I would dilute it, but then I would get even less of the mineral. The skin irritation caused by magnesium oil is not dangerous, but if you get it, you can't use the oil on that area anymore because it can become painful.

We don't know how much magnesium is absorbed from most of the various types on the market. We do know that magnesium oxide is only 4 percent absorbed. Magnesium researchers have told me that they feel the maximum absorption of magnesium pills and powders is about 20 percent. But there really are not any proper magnesium absorption studies; they mostly focus on where magnesium is absorbed, not how much. Fortunately, now with ReMag you have a magnesium that is fully absorbed at the cellular level and doesn't require a healthy intestine for absorption.

One thing to be aware of when reading labels is how many pills you have to take to get the dosage they are advertising. Look at the serving size. It may say you have to take not one but two or three tablets to achieve the dosage on the label. It may be in small print, but read it carefully to understand exactly what each tablet contains.

I also have concerns about the quality of all the new products on the market. This is another reason I don't just give a blanket recommendation for a particular magnesium compound beyond my own ReMag and Natural Calm, which I know have superior ingredients and implement quality control. Many companies use cheap ingredients and do not follow good manufacturing practice (GMP) guidelines that call for rigorous third-party testing several times throughout the manufacturing process. Also, please read labels to make sure there are no unnecessary binders, fillers, dyes, and additives.

On the advice of neurosurgeon Dr. Russell Blaylock, I do not recommend magnesium aspartate or magnesium glutamate because they can break down into the single amino acids aspartic acid and glutamic acid, which can act like dangerous excitotoxins in the brain.

There are dozens of magnesium compounds, because an ion of magnesium is very reactive and loves to join with another ion to make a compound. That means the other ion, tagging along with magnesium, has a specific weight. For example, 1,000 mg of magnesium citrate, the most commonly used form of magnesium, offers 125 mg of elemental magnesium—the other 775 mg is the citrate component.

When reading the label, the amount of elemental magnesium is what you want.

Magnesium oxide looks like it has the most elemental magnesium, at 300 mg in 500 mg of compound. But looks can be deceiving because magnesium oxide is only 4 percent absorbed into the bloodstream, which means you only have access to 12 mg of magnesium. The other 488 mg becomes a strong bowel laxative.

A recent study obscured magnesium oxide's poor absorption when it was compared to magnesium citrate—the study reported that the oxide was better absorbed than the citrate. If you read the whole study you find that twice as much magnesium oxide was given to the test subjects compared to magnesium citrate, thus accounting for a higher amount of magnesium being absorbed.

Every month I come across a new magnesium on the market, each one claiming to be the best. See my note below on magnesium threonate.

Magnesium Salt	Amount of Elemental Magnesium per 500 mg Salt
Magnesium oxide	300 mg
Magnesium carbonate	150 mg
Dimagnesium malate	95 mg
Dolomite	75 mg
Magnesium citrate	75 mg
Magnesium malate	75 mg
Magnesium chloride	60 mg
Magnesium lactate	60 mg
Magnesium glycinate	50 mg
Magnesium sulfate	50 mg
Magnesium taurate	50 mg
Magnesium orotate	30 mg
Magnesium gluconate	25 mg

Below are the most common magnesium salts divided into inorganic and organic forms. Organic simply means that the substance binding to magnesium contains a carbon atom, which theoretically makes it better absorbed.

Inorganic salts	Organic salt chelates
Magnesium bicarbonate	Dimagnesium malate
Magnesium carbonate	Magnesium adipate
Magnesium chloride	Magnesium aspartate
Magnesium oxide	Magnesium citrate
Magnesium phosphate	Magnesium glutamate
Magnesium sulfate	Magnesium glycinate
Magnesium lysinate	
Magnesium malate	
Magnesium orotate	
Magnesium taurate	

ALL MAGNESIUMS CROSS THE BLOOD-BRAIN BARRIER

The January 28, 2010, issue of *Neuron* published a paper titled "Enhancement of Learning and Memory by Elevating Brain Magnesium."[6] This rat study concluded that "an increase in brain magnesium enhances both short-term synaptic facilitation and long-term potentiation and improves learning and memory functions." The study compares several different forms of magnesium for absorption into the cerebrospinal fluid and concluded that only the rats that received magnesium l-threonate showed an increase of magnesium in their cerebrospinal fluid, which was only 7 percent higher at day twenty-four of intake. Based on this result, promoters of magnesium l-threonate products say that theirs is the only magnesium that significantly increases the levels of magnesium in the brain.

I disagree with the above statement. Giving superpowers

to these products obscures the reality that any magnesium could produce some or all of these same effects. The treatment of migraines, seizures, strokes, head injuries, and other nervous system problems with even poorly absorbed magnesium oxide shows that all magnesiums can produce beneficial results at the neuron level, which means at least part of it gets into the brain. See the listing of the twenty-four chapters in *Magnesium in the Central Nervous System* in Chapter 5 or download the entire book from the Internet for conclusive proof.[7]

Personally, when I take magnesium l-threonate, I get the laxative effect, which means to me that it is not fully absorbed at the cellular level. Also, most capsules of magnesium l-threonate contain less than 50 mg of elemental magnesium. I would have to take about a dozen capsules a day to meet my magnesium requirements, but I would never get past 1 or 2 capsules because of the laxative effect.

ALL MAGNESIUMS HELP THE HEART

In a series of studies published since the early 1970s it appears that the amino acid taurine is important for heart health and may prevent arrhythmias and protect the heart against the damage caused by heart attacks.[8, 9] So one might think that magnesium taurate would be an especially helpful form of magnesium. But as with many other forms of magnesium, therapeutic dosage is important. Most magnesium taurate products come in a dosage of 125 mg of elemental magnesium. I know that for my heart palpitations and leg cramps, in the past I would have to take about 10 capsules a day; however, I get the laxative effect with one pill.

Knowing that taurine is important for the heart but magnesium is more important, I take ReMag so I can get therapeutic amounts of magnesium, and I also take ReAline, which has L-taurine and L-methionine along with methyl-ated B vitamins in a capsule. (ReAline is one of my products.)

WHEN TO TAKE MAGNESIUM

I used to recommend that magnesium supplements be taken two or three times a day to help reduce the laxative effect. That advice still stands. But if you are taking ReMag or Natural Calm, you can put a whole day's dose in a liter of water and sip it through the day. That way, every hour you are filling up your cells with life-giving magnesium and not wasting it, as the excess of one large dose can be lost through the urine or the bowels.

If you take your magnesium in divided doses through the day, take your first dose when you wake up in the morning and the last dose at bedtime. If you take a third dose, make it late in the afternoon. Magnesium is most deficient in the early morning and late afternoon. In the beginning of magnesium therapy, a very few people feel that magnesium is sufficiently energizing that it keeps them awake at night, but that's because magnesium is revving up hundreds of enzyme systems in their body. Most people find magnesium better than a sleeping pill to help get a good night's rest. Others, who suffer from leg cramps, restless legs, fibromyalgia, or general muscle tension, take magnesium at night and find that it diminishes pain and tension and helps them sleep. There are so many ways that magnesium can work on the body that it is important for you to decide what timing is best for you.

This would be the perfect time to remind you of the section "When Magnesium Makes Me Worse" in the Introduction. It is crucial for you to realize that when you take a well-absorbed form of magnesium like ReMag, especially in therapeutic amounts, it's going to activate the hundreds of enzyme systems under its influence, and your cells are going to wake up; they can also begin to detox.

MAGNESIUM LAXATIVES

Oral doses of magnesium sulfate (Epsom salts), magnesium hydroxide (milk of magnesia), magnesium oxide, and magnesium citrate are not fully absorbed into the blood or the cells and the excess finds its way to the intestines. Magnesium in the colon has the ability to draw water to itself and acts as an effective laxative. But it's all a matter of dose. As a laxative, 1,000–2,000 mg of milk of magnesia provides an effective dose; however, as a magnesium supplement, doses of 200–600 mg are more common. These salts are, in fact, more gentle than cascara and senna, herbs that cause muscle contraction of the intestinal wall. In *IBS for Dummies* (2005) I talk about magnesium as an excellent treatment for IBS-related constipation; it can be taken as a daily supplement to prevent constipation from occurring.

Laxatives, in general, are not recommended because you can become dependent on them and they can flush out beneficial intestinal bacteria and electrolytes. It is far better to take magnesium supplements to help relax the bowel and allow normal action. With regular consumption of ReMag, constipation is alleviated because the intestinal muscles are relaxed enough to perform their normal peristaltic function.

Magnesium laxatives are contraindicated in patients with nausea, vomiting, appendicitis, intestinal obstruction, undiagnosed abdominal pain, or kidney disease.

MAGNESIUM AND OTHER NUTRIENTS

Magnesium is extremely important for the metabolism of calcium, potassium, phosphorus, zinc, copper, iron, sodium, lead, cadmium, hydrochloric acid, acetylcholine, and nitric oxide, as well as for the activation of vitamin B_1. Therefore, magnesium is needed for a very wide spectrum of crucial body functions.[10] A shift in any one of these nutrients has an impact on magnesium levels and vice versa. It is the interwoven nature of the body's components that makes it so difficult to isolate one substance to scientifically "prove" what it can do.

Magnesium cannot be taken out of context, either in a research setting or in your body. For example, you should increase magnesium intake when you consume more vitamin D. Magnesium is necessary to convert dietary vitamin D into one of the hormones that makes efficient use of calcium in bone formation.[11, 12] Vitamin B_6 increases the amount of magnesium that can enter cells; as a result, these two nutrients are often taken together. In one experiment, serum vitamin E levels improved after magnesium supplementation.[13] We also know that magnesium and the essential fatty acids (EFAs, found in fish, nuts, seeds, and flaxseed oil) are interdependent; each works much more efficiently when the other is present in sufficient amounts.

HOMEOPATHIC MAGNESIUM: ANOTHER FORM OF MAGNESIUM

Developed by Samuel Hahneman in the early nineteenth century, homeopathy is a natural medical science that uses mostly plants and mineral extracts diluted in alcohol or water to infinitesimal amounts in order to stimulate the individual's natural healing response. Research has shown that these substances, if given in a toxic amount, can cause symptoms similar to those that the patient is experiencing, but that the infinitesimal dose can cure those symptoms. After two centuries of clinical use and observation, homeopathy is now more successful than the tools we have available to measure how it works. Although skeptics often attribute its success to the placebo effect, in which a patient's belief in an outcome produces that outcome, the millions who have benefited from homeopathy include infants and animals, two groups that are clearly not susceptible to the placebo effect.

Nonetheless, in America homeopathy continues to be marginalized in favor of pharmaceutical drugs, even in the face of such early evidence as the influenza epidemic of 1919, in which the homeopathic hospitals in England and the United States showed a greater cure rate than conventional hospitals. In Europe, both homeopathic medicine and herbal medicine enjoy a respected place in the health care system.

Homeopathic remedies typically come in dosages of 6, 12, or 30 X (10) or C (100) potency—the higher the number, the greater the dilution and the more potent the remedy. Usually you take three pellets or four drops of a remedy several times a day. For a very acute, painful symptom, a dose can be taken every fifteen minutes. However, if after taking five or six doses of a remedy there is no change in symptoms, the remedy is probably ineffective and you should seek a new one. Be assured that taking an inappropriate or ineffective remedy a half dozen times does not cause any negative side effects.

In homeopathy, magnesium is used primarily for acute muscle spasms or chronic complaints.[14] Please consult a homeopath for a more detailed evaluation of your case.

Magnesia phosphorica (magnesium phosphate, or mag phos) is a great antispasmodic remedy and the most commonly used magnesium homeopathic remedy. It readily treats cramping of all muscles, including hiccups, leg cramps, writer's cramp, abdominal colic, heart pain, lung pain, menstrual pain accompanied by radiating pains, neuralgic pains, and all sorts of tics and tremors including twitching of the eyelids. It works especially well in debilitated subjects who are both mentally and physically tired.

Dr. Margery Mullins, an internist and acupuncturist, told me about the success she has had recommending magnesium phosphate for muscle spasms to her patients. She said patients would get instant relief and then didn't seem to need the remedy after their magnesium deficiency was corrected with diet and supplements. One of her young patients, a nine-year-old girl, was having such severe muscle spasms that she was referred to a pediatric neurologist. In the interim, Dr. Mullins gave her Magnesia phosphorica 6X, and by the time of her appointment with the specialist the child no longer had the problem. Dr. Mullins noted that the girl's mother had had toxemia (eclampsia) during her pregnancy, requiring intravenous magnesium, which means the daughter was likely born with magnesium deficiency, setting the stage for her present symptoms.

APPENDIXES

Appendix A

MAGNESIUM CONTENT OF COMMON FOODS

Food	Magnesium (mg) per 3½ oz (100g) serving
Kelp	760
Wheat bran	490
Wheat germ	336
Almonds	270
Cashews	267
Molasses	258
Brewer's yeast	231
Buckwheat	229
Brazil nuts	225
Dulse	220
Filberts	184
Peanuts	175
Millet	162
Wheat grain	160
Pecans	142
English walnuts	131
Rye	115
Tofu	111
Coconut meat, dried	90
Brown rice	88
Soybeans, cooked	88
Figs, dried	71

Food	Magnesium (mg) per 3½ oz (100g) serving
Apricots	62
Dates	58
Collard greens	57
Shrimp	51
Corn, sweet	48
Avocado	45
Cheddar cheese	45
Parsley	41
Prunes, dried	40
Sunflower seeds	38
Barley	37
Beans, cooked	37
Dandelion greens	36
Garlic	36
Raisins	35
Green peas, fresh	35
Potato with skin	34
Crab	34
Banana	33
Sweet potato	31
Blackberry	30
Beets	25
Broccoli	24
Cauliflower	24
Carrot	23
Celery	22
Beef	21
Asparagus	20
Chicken	19
Green pepper	18
Winter squash	17
Cantaloupe	16
Eggplant	16
Tomato	14
Milk	13

Appendix B

CALCIUM CONTENT OF COMMON FOODS

Food	Mg Calcium
VEGETABLES	
½ cup cooked spinach	88
1 cup cooked dried beans (white, kidney, soy, and so on)	95–110
½ cup cooked kale	103
½ cup cooked collards	110
1 cup cooked turnip greens	126
½ cup cooked dandelion greens	147
½ cup cooked beet greens	157
1 medium stalk broccoli	158
1 cup bok choy (Chinese cabbage)	252
BAKED GOODS AND INGREDIENTS	
1 slice whole-wheat bread	50
1 medium waffle	76
1 medium corn muffin	96
½ cup soy flour	132
1 tablespoon blackstrap molasses	140
SEAFOOD	
¾ 8-oz can clams	62
6 scallops	115

Food	Mg Calcium
½ 7-oz can salmon with bones	284
20 medium oysters	300
7 sardines with bones	393
NUTS AND SEEDS	
½ cup sesame seeds	76
½ cup Brazil nuts	128
½ cup almonds	175
FRUIT	
½ cup cooked rhubarb	200
DAIRY	
Yogurt, plain, low-fat, 8 ounces	415
Mozzarella, part skim, 1.5 ounces	333
Yogurt, fruit, low-fat, 8 ounces	350
Cheddar cheese, 1.5 ounces	307
Milk, nonfat, 8 ounces	299
Soy milk, calcium-fortified, 8 ounces	299
Milk, reduced-fat (2% milkfat), 8 ounces	293
Milk, buttermilk, low-fat, 8 ounces	284
Milk, whole (3.25% milkfat), 8 ounces	276
Cottage cheese, 1% milkfat, 1 cup	138
Frozen yogurt, vanilla, soft-serve, ½ cup	103
Ice cream, vanilla, ½ cup	84
Sour cream, reduced fat, 2 tablespoons	31
Cream cheese, regular, 1 tablespoon	14

Appendix C

BONE BROTH RECIPE

Drink 1 cup a day on the days you need to increase your calcium intake.

- 2 pounds (or more) of organic bones (beef, chicken, fish)
- 1 onion
- 2 carrots
- 2 stalks of celery
- 2 tablespoons apple cider vinegar (this is mandatory)
- Enough water to cover the bones

Optional: 1 tbsp sea salt, herbs or spices to taste, 2 cloves of garlic, and several sprigs of parsley in the final 30 minutes.

Bring to a boil and simmer:

- Beef broth/stock: 48 hours
- Chicken or poultry broth/stock: 24 hours
- Fish broth: 8 hours

Remove from heat and let cool. Use a fine metal strainer to remove all bone and vegetable. When cool enough, store in the fridge for up to 5 days, or freeze for later use.

Appendix D

LIPOSOMAL VITAMIN C RECIPE

Make your own liposomal vitamin C at home.

INGREDIENTS

Rose hips powder and/or camu camu powder
Lecithin granules (most are soy lecithin, but you can find
    non-soy sources)
Distilled water
Ultrasonic jewelry cleaner (here is the one I used, which
    I purchased from Amazon: iSonic P4810 Commercial
    Ultrasonic Cleaner, 2.1Qt/2L)

DIRECTIONS

Put 3 tablespoons lecithin granules in 1 cup of distilled
water.

Put 2 tablespoons of rose hips powder or camu camu
powder in ½ cup distilled water (I use 1 tablespoon of each).

Let the ingredients dissolve in their respective containers for several hours on the counter, or covered in the
refrigerator overnight.

After soaking, pour the lecithin solution together with

the rose hips or camu camu solution in a blender and blend on low for a minute or two.

Pour into your ultrasonic cleaner and run through however many cycles you need to get to 30 minutes, stirring the entire time with a wooden spoon.

Put in a covered glass container in the fridge.

Use 2–4 tbsp per day.

It will keep for several weeks in the fridge.

Appendix E

POTASSIUM BROTH

To 2 quarts of water add:

2 large potatoes, chopped into ½-inch cubes
1 cup sliced or shredded carrots
1 cup chopped celery, leaves and all
1 handful beet tops
1 handful turnip tops
1 handful parsley
1 medium onion
Herbs for seasoning: garlic, thyme, sage, rosemary

Optional: 1 teaspoon miso or beef bouillon after straining
off the liquid, for extra flavor and extra sodium

DIRECTIONS

Combine all ingredients (except the miso or beef bouillon, if using) in a stainless steel, glass, or earthenware pot.
Cover and cook slowly for about ½ hour.

Strain the broth off. Add the miso or beef bouillon to
the broth, if using. Cool.

Serve the broth warm or cold. Keep refrigerated.

This is the type of broth favored in fasting clinics. It's a mineral-rich, alkalizing, cleansing broth.

Resources

I often marvel at the extensive resource lists at the back of health books. I wonder, how can a writer recommend resources without knowing all the participants? After fifty years of reading and studying health and medicine topics, I have created an extensive list of resources and recommendations, mostly related to my own work, that you can trust. I am a generalist, not a specialist, which means I always look at the whole picture. This worldview allowed me to see the big picture with magnesium and how the lack of it can cause so much disability.

I will also list various holistic dental and medical organizations, but I do not know the practitioners in these organizations and cannot vouch for their abilities. It is important to work with a knowledgeable health care practitioner, but it's you who must be in charge. And don't simply replace an allopathic doctor with a "green allopath," which is what I call naturopaths or holistic doctors who simply match your symptoms with supplements. They may not be giving you drugs, but you end up with dozens of costly products, yet you still don't feel well.

DR. DEAN'S PERSONAL RECOMMENDATIONS

The following is a list of print, audio, and video educational materials and products that will give you enough information and resources to take responsibility for your own health and healing.

1. Wellness Tips from the Future: Sign up for my free online newsletter at www.drcarolyndean.com.
2. Completement Now! My 2-Year Online Wellness Coaching Program is a lifestyle approach to health and prevention, not a focus on disease. Sign up for the program at www.drcarolyndean.com.
3. Listen to or call in to my two-hour weekly radio show on www.AchieveRadio.com every Monday at 4:00 P.M. PST. Phone or Skype 602-666-6027, or listen online. Archived shows are under "Blog" at www.RnAReSet, where you can search for the conditions you want to research.
4. Walk through the Dr. Dean Health Library with a thousand entries: audio, video, and print, located at www.RnAReSet, under "Blog."
5. Many health questions are dealt with in a general manner on my *Future Health* blog. Sign up at www.drcarolyndean.com.
6. If there is a specific topic that you would like my opinion on, just Google that topic and my name and something often comes up in one of the thousand blog entries, articles, videos, audios, and interviews that I've done.
7. I have written 33 print books and 113 Kindle books. You can find links to them at www.drcarolyndean.com under "Books." My favorites are *The Magnesium Miracle, Future Health Now Encyclopedia, Atrial Fibrillation: Remineralize Your Heart, IBS for Dummies,* and *Death by Modern Medicine: Seeking Safe Solutions.*

8. *Future Health Now Encyclopedia* covers 138 health conditions and gives detailed information on how to treat those conditions using a combination of diet, supplements, homeopathy, herbs, and common sense.

9. The URL http://bit.ly/mg-miracle-gift provides you with a shortcut to obtain four free modules of my Completement Now! Online Wellness Program, and several free ebooks: *Invisible Minerals Part I: Magnesium—ReMag; Invisible Minerals Part II: Multiple Minerals—ReMyte; Atrial Fibrillation: ReMineralize Your Heart; Magnesium Deficient Anxiety; ReStructure: A Completement Formula to ReSet Your Body;* and *ReMineralize Your Thyroid.*

10. I used to mainly reach out to people through the written or spoken word, but in the past few years, with more people demanding to know what supplements are safe and effective, I have taken the next step and provided a handful of products that are safe, effective, and beneficial for everyone. These products are the basis of my Total Body ReSet protocol using my Completement Formulas: ReMag, ReMag Lotion, ReMyte, ReAline, RnA Drops, ReCalcia, ReStructure, and ReNew, located at www.RnAReSet.com.

11. Free books: *Invisible Minerals Part I—Magnesium; Invisible Minerals Part II—Multiple Minerals; Atrial Fibrillation: Remineralize Your Heart; ReStructure: A Completement Formula to ReSet Your Body,* available at www.RnAReSet.com under "Books."

12. Regarding magnesium: I do think ReMag is the best magnesium available on the market. It's the only one I know that is fully absorbed at the cellular level, has no laxative effects, and is at a high enough concentration to be therapeutic. Most people need twice the RDA, a total of 700–800 mg a day, and most people can take ReMag without any side effects. Some people's symptoms disappear within days, while some tougher symptoms—like atrial fibrillation—

can take months, especially if you are still taking medications. Reread the section "When Magnesium Makes Me Worse" in this book to understand why you should begin your magnesium slowly and increase gradually.

13. ReMyte is a multimineral product that helps remineralize the body to support the treatment of hypothyroidism, osteoporosis, diabetes, inflammation, toxicity, arthritis, and dozens of other conditions that have been created by chronic mineral deficiency. The combination of ReMag and ReMyte is designed to help treat all chronic conditions, including chronic fatigue syndrome and fibromyalgia.

14. ReAline is a detox antioxidant that makes glutathione from L-methionine in the body and supplies sulfur groups along with another sulfur-based amino acid, L-taurine. ReAline also contains methylated B vitamins, with B_2, B_6, folate, B_{12}, and food-based B_1 to assist liver detoxification, to support the adrenal glands, and the nervous system.

15. RnA Drops and ReNew are made from the newly created iCell, which works via RNA through chromosome 14 to help perfect fading DNA code, restore telomeres, and create perfect cells.

16. ReCalcia is a calcium, boron, and vanadium supplement for bones and more! I created ReCalcia to meet the needs of people who don't eat dairy and therefore can't get enough dietary calcium. What is extremely important and unique about ReCalcia is its picometer, stabilized ionic form. This makes ReCalcia 100 percent absorbed at the cellular level. It will not suffer the same fate as other calcium supplements and cause constipation or build up in your tissues, slowly calcifying your vital body organs, including your arteries. ReCalcia, being fully absorbed at the cellular level, taken along with equal amounts of ReMag, creates the perfect synergistic balance of those two minerals to enhance body function.

17. ReStructure is a third-generation protein powder that I've been enjoying since it was first formulated in 1990. In 2015, the owners of the second-generation product retired, so I decided to take it on and add something very unique to this, its third generation—RnA Drops powder. ReStructure is primarily made from whey protein powder that is casein-free and very low in lactose. Beyond the whey, it's a balanced protein, carb, and fat meal replacement containing rice bran, rice protein, potato fiber, pea protein, flaxseed, marine algae oil, and extra lysine, as well as the RnA Drops powder. Each ingredient is important in the total makeup of ReStructure to provide you with a delicious, easy-to-digest, high-fiber, low-calorie, and low-glycemic-index food formula that helps control weight and maintain lower blood sugar levels. ReStructure is also the perfect protein powder meal replacement for a yeast-free diet. In fact, ReStructure is a unique protein powder, because it contains RnA Drops powder.

18. After magnesium and mineral deficiency, another huge area of concern that I have is yeast overgrowth. I think the key to balancing yeast in the body is to stop feeding yeast with lactose sugar from dairy, glucose from the breakdown of grains, and foods made with table sugar. Several of my Completement Formulas help balance yeast in the body. ReStructure makes an excellent addition to a yeast-free diet since it has only 1 gram of sugar. You will digest ReStructure so well that you won't feed yeast with undigested food. ReStructure will also help you digest food in your regular diet. Several ingredients in ReStructure are prebiotics. ReMag helps heal a leaky gut, which is common in yeast overgrowth. RnA Drops have probiotic properties. ReAline helps eliminate yeast toxins. For the most up-to-date yeast treatment you can check the "Resources" link at www.drcarolyndean.com.

MAGNESIUM TESTING

MAGNESIUM RBC TESTING

Doctors don't learn about the inaccuracy of serum magnesium testing and don't know about the magnesium RBC blood test; however, you can obtain it over the Internet without a doctor's prescription. Go to www.RequestATest.com or www.DirectLabs.com and type in "magnesium RBC." The cost at RequestATest is $49, which may be less than your copay for a visit to the doctor. You will be asked for your zip code and sent to a local lab for a blood draw. You will receive your results within seventy-two hours. When you receive your test results, remember that upward of 80 percent of the population is deficient in magnesium, so you want your magnesium level to be above the 80th percentile. That's why, when the reference range is 4.2–6.8 mg/dL, you want your magnesium levels to be around 6.0–6.5 mg/dL. Don't make the mistake of thinking your magnesium levels are good if your results are at the low end of this range.

EXA TEST

The EXA Test, produced by IntraCellular Diagnostics, is an expensive mineral test usually run in chiropractic and naturopathic offices, but it is covered by some insurances.

IntraCellular Diagnostics, Inc.
Medford Medical Labs
945 Town Center Drive, Suite A
Medford, OR 97504-6190
(541) 245-3212
www.exatest.com

IONIZED MAGNESIUM TESTING

Nova Biomedical Corporation makes ionized magnesium
sensors to perform the ionized magnesium test, but the test is
still only used by research laboratories associated with universities.

200 Prospect Street
Waltham, MA 02254-9141
(781) 894-0800
www.novabiomedical.com

RELOX PROCEDURE FOR STROKE

Dr. Bruce Rind
800 South Frederick Avenue, #212
Gaithersburg, MD 20877
301-921-HEAL (4325)
www.drrind.com
chhteam@drrindchh.com

MAGNESIUM SALT SUBSTITUTES

If you can't tolerate sea salt on your food or in your drinking
water, use the following salt substitutes.

CardiaSalt
Nutrition 21
4 Manhattanville Road
Purchase, NY 10577
(800) 699-3533
http://nutrition21.com/item/other-products

Smart Salt
Mineral Resources International
2720 Wadman Drive
Ogden, UT 84401
(800) 731-7866
www.mineralresourcesint.com

ACCESS TO ORGANIC FOOD

Join a CSA (community-supported agriculture) program.
Become a member in a local organic farm and receive regular delivery of farm-fresh produce.
www.localharvest.org/csa/

HOLISTIC AND BIOLOGICAL DENTISTRY

The International Academy of Oral Medicine and Toxicology (IAOMT) has a page of guidelines on safe mercury
amalgam removal and a list of dentists who provide this service.

International Academy of Oral Medicine and Toxicology
8297 Champions Gate Boulevard, #193
Champions Gate, FL 33896
(863) 420-6373
www.iaomt.org

Holistic Dental Association
1825 Ponce de Leon, #148
Coral Gables, FL 33134
(305) 356-7338
www.holisticdental.org

HOLISTIC MEDICAL ORGANIZATIONS

The American College for Advancement in Medicine
(ACAM)
380 Ice Center Lane, Suite C
Bozeman, MT 59718
(800) 532-3688
www.acam.org

American Academy of Environmental Medicine
6505 East Central, #296
Wichita, KS 67206
www.aaem.com

Academy of Integrative Pain Management
975 Morning Star Drive, Suite A
Sonora, CA 95370
www.aapainmanage.org

American Holistic Health Association (AHHA)
P.O. Box 17400
Anaheim, CA 92817
(714) 779-6152
www.AHHA.org

American College of Preventive Medicine
455 Massachusetts Avenue NW, Suite 200
Washington, DC 20001
www.acpm.org

The Foundation for the Advancement of Innovative
Medicine (FAIM)
P.O. Box 2860
Loveland, CO 80539
www.faim.org

International Society for Orthomolecular Medicine
16 Florence Avenue
Toronto, Ontario, Canada M2N 1E9
www.ionhealth.ca

American Association of Naturopathic Physicians
818 18th Street NW, Suite 250
Washington, DC 20006
(202) 237-8150
Toll-free (866) 538-2267
Fax (202) 237-8152
www.naturopathic.org
Email member.service@naturopathic.org

International and American Associations of Clinical
Nutritionists
15280 Addison Road, Suite 130
Addison, TX 75001
(972) 407-9089
Fax (972) 250-0233
www.iaacn.org
Email ddc@clinicalnutrition.com

American Holistic Nurses Association
2900 SW Plass Court
Topeka, KS 66611-1980
(785) 234-1712
(800) 278-2462
www.ahna.org

NATURAL TREATMENT FOR DEPRESSION
AND BIPOLAR DISORDER

Although I've received wonderful reports of depression being alleviated with my Completement Formulas, I also recommend EMPowerplus Advanced, available at www.TrueHope .com. It's a mega multiple vitamin, mineral, and amino acid compound. The product has been studied in nineteen major universities, including Harvard, and thirty articles published in peer-reviewed medical journals have shown its safety and an effectiveness rate of over 80 percent. Drugs for depression and bipolar disorder are only about 40 percent effective. What makes TrueHope unique and important in the treatment of depression is its team of health counselors who work with customers by phone and email to help support them through their use of EMPowerplus Advanced, and to help them wean off medications, if they desire.

Notes

Introduction

1. Crossen C, *Tainted Truth: The Manipulation of Fact.* Simon & Schuster, New York, 1995.
2. Cohn M, "Industry funds six times more clinical trials than feds, research shows." *Baltimore Sun,* Dec. 15, 2015.
3. Teo KK et al., "Effects of intravenous magnesium in suspected acute myocardial infarction: overview of randomized trials." *Brit Med J,* vol. 303, pp. 1499–1503, 1991.
4. Teo KK, Yusuf S, "Role of magnesium in reducing mortality in acute myocardial infarction. A review of the evidence." *Drugs,* vol. 46, pp. 347–359, 1993.
5. Altura BM, "Sudden-death ischemic heart disease and dietary magnesium intake: is the target site coronary vascular smooth muscle?" *Med Hypotheses,* vol. 5, no. 8, pp. 843–848, 1979.
6. Altura BM, "Introduction: Importance of Mg in physiology and medicine and the need for ion selective electrodes." *Scand J Clin Lab Invest Suppl,* vol. 217, pp. 5–9, 1994.
7. Mauskop A, Fox B, *What Your Doctor May Not Tell You About Migraines.* Warner Books, New York, 2001.
8. Mauskop A et al., "Deficiency in serum ionized magnesium but not total magnesium in patients with migraines. Possible role of ICa2/IMg2 ratio." *Headache,* vol. 33, no. 3, pp. 135–138, 1993.
9. Mauskop A et al., "Intravenous magnesium sulphate relieves migraine attacks in patients with low serum ionized magnesium levels: a pilot study." *Clin Sci (Colch),* vol. 89, no. 6, pp. 633–636, 1995.
10. Seelig MS, "The requirement of magnesium by the normal adult." *Am J Clin Nutr,* vol. 14, pp. 342–390, 1964.
11. Seelig MS, "Cardiovascular reactions to stress intensified by magnesium deficit in consequences of magnesium deficiency on the enhancement of

stress reactions; preventive and therapeutic implications: a review." *J Am Coll Nutr,* vol. 13, no. 5, pp. 429–446, 1994.

12. Durlach J, *Magnesium in Clinical Practice.* Libbey, London, 1988.

13. Durlach J, "Diverse applications of magnesium therapy." In *Handbook of Metal-Ligand Interactions in Biological Fluids—Bioinorganic Medicine,* vol. 2, Marcel Dekker, New York, 1995.

14. http://articles.mercola.com/sites/articles/archive/2003/11/26/death -by-medicine-part-one.aspx.

15. http://drcarolyndean.com/natural-health-books-by-dr-dean.

16. Starfield B, "Is US health really the best in the world?" *JAMA,* vol. 284, no. 4, pp. 483–485, 2000.

17. www.anh-usa.org/stop-codex.

18. Shlezinger M et al., "Desalinated seawater supply and all-cause mortality in hospitalized acute myocardial infarction patients from the Acute Coronary Syndrome Israeli Survey 2002–2013." *Int J Cardiol,* vol. 220, pp. 544–550, 2016.

19. Fox C et al., "Magnesium: its proven and potential clinical significance." *South Med J,* vol. 94, no. 12, pp. 1195–1201, 2001.

20. Grober U, Schmidt J, Kisters K, "Magnesium in prevention and therapy." *Nutrients* vol. 7, no. 9, pp. 8199–8226, 2015.

21. Blaylock RL, *Excitotoxins: The Taste That Kills.* Health Press, Sante Fe, NM, 1997.

22. Volpe SL, "Magnesium in disease prevention and overall health." *Adv Nutr,* vol. 4, no. 3, pp. 378S–383S, 2013.

23. Volpe SL, "Magnesium and the athlete." *Curr Sports Med Rep,* vol. 14, no. 4, pp. 279–283, 2015.

24. Shah NC et al., "Short-term magnesium deficiency downregulates telomerase, upregulates neutral sphingomyelinase and induces oxidative DNA damage in cardiovascular tissues: relevance to atherogenesis, cardiovascular diseases and aging." *Int J Clin Exp Med,* vol. 7, no. 3, pp. 497–514, 2014.

25. Long S, Romani AM, "Role of cellular magnesium in human diseases." *Austin J Nutr Food Sci,* vol. 2, no. 10, 2014.

26. Glasdam SM et al., "The importance of magnesium in the human body: a systematic literature review." *Adv Clin Chem,* vol. 73, pp. 169–193, 2016.

27. de Baaij JHF et al., "Magnesium in man: implications for health and disease," *Physiol Rev,* vol. 95, no. 1, pp. 1–46, 2015.

28. Rosanoff A, "The essential nutrient magnesium—key to mitochondrial atp production and much more." 2009. www.prohealth.com/library/ print.cfm?libid=14606.

29. Golshani-Hebroni S, "Mg++ requirement for MtHK binding, and Mg++ stabilization of mitochondrial membranes via activation of MtHK & MtCK and promotion of mitochondrial permeability transi-

tion pore closure: a hypothesis on mechanisms underlying Mg++'s antioxidant and cytoprotective effects." *Gene*, vol. 581, pp. 1–13, 2015.

30. Jahnen-Dechent W, Ketteler M, "Magnesium basics." *Clin Kidney J*, vol. 5, suppl. 1, pp. i3–i14, 2012.

31. Rosanoff A et al., "Suboptimal magnesium status in the United States: are the health consequences underestimated?" *Nutr Rev*, vol. 70, no. 3, pp. 153–164, 2012.

32. Alhosaini M et al., "Magnesium and dialysis: the neglected cation." *Am J Kidney Dis*, vol. 66, no. 3, pp. 523–531, 2015.

33. Geiger H, Wanner C., "Magnesium in disease." *Clin Kidney J*, vol. 5, suppl. 1, pp. i25–i38, 2012.

34. www.adelaide.edu.au/press/titles/magnesium.

Chapter 1

1. Altura BM, Altura BT, "Cardiovascular risk factors and magnesium: relationships to atherosclerosis, ischemic heart disease and hypertension." *Magnes Trace Elem*, vol. 92, no. 10, pp. 182–192, 1991.

2. Eisenberg MJ, "Magnesium deficiency and sudden death." *Amer Heart J*, vol. 124, no. 2, pp. 544–549, 1992.

3. Turlapaty PD, Altura BM, "Magnesium deficiency produces spasms of coronary arteries: relationship to etiology of sudden death ischemic heart disease." *Science*, vol. 208, no. 4440, pp. 198–200, 1980.

4. Altura BM, "Sudden-death ischemic heart disease and dietary magnesium intake: is the target site coronary vascular smooth muscle?" *Med Hypotheses*, vol. 5, no. 8, pp. 843–848, 1979.

5. Karppanen H et al., "Minerals, coronary heart disease and sudden coronary death." *Adv Cardiol*, vol. 25, pp. 9–24, 1978.

6. Rogers SA, *Depression Cured at Last*. SK Publishing, Sarasota, FL, 2000.

7. Henrotte JG, "Type A behavior and magnesium metabolism." *Magnesium*, vol. 5, pp. 201–210, 1986.

8. Cernak I et al., "Alterations in magnesium and oxidative status during chronic emotional stress." *Magnes Res*, vol. 13, no. 1, pp. 29–36, 2000.

9. Cernak I et al., "Alterations in magnesium and oxidative status during chronic emotional stress." *Magnes Res*, vol. 13, no. 1, pp. 29–36, 2000.

10. www.adelaide.edu.au/press/titles/magnesium.

11. Rosanoff A, Seelig MS, "Comparison of mechanism and functional effects of magnesium and statin pharmaceuticals." *J Am Coll Nutr*, vol. 23, no. 5, pp. 501S–505S, 2004.

12. Weglicki WB, Phillips TM, "Pathobiology of magnesium deficiency: a cytokine/neurogenic inflammation hypothesis." *Am J Physiol*, vol. 263, no. 3, part 2, pp. R734–R737, 1992.

13. Dean CFA, Wheeler LC, *IBS for Dummies*. Wiley, Hoboken, NJ, 2005.

14. "Nearly 7 in 10 Americans are on prescription drugs." *Science News*, June 19, 2013.

15. Rodale JR, *Magnesium: The Nutrient That Could Change Your Life.* Rodale Press, Emmaus, PA 1971. Full text available at www.mgwater.com/rodtitle.shtml.

16. Hartwig A, "Role of magnesium in genomic stability." *Mutat Research,* vol. 18, no. 475 (1–2), pp. 113–121, 2001.

17. El-Charabaty E, Saifan C, Abdallah M et al., "Effects of proton pump inhibitors and electrolyte disturbances on arrhythmias." *Int J Gen Med,* vol. 6, pp. 515–518, 2013.

18. Janett S, Camozzi P, Peeters GGAM et al., "Hypomagnesemia induced by long-term treatment with proton-pump inhibitors." *Gastroenterol Res Pract,* vol. 2015, article ID 951768.

19. Shah NH et al., "Proton pump inhibitor usage and the risk of myocardial infarction in the general population." *PLoS One,* vol. 10, no. 6, 2015.

20. Wills MR, "Magnesium and potassium inter-relationships in cardiac disorders." *Drugs,* vol. 31, suppl. 4, pp. 121–131, 1986.

21. Feskanich D et al., "Calcium, vitamin D, milk consumption, and hip fractures: a prospective study among postmenopausal women." *Am J Clin Nutr,* vol. 77, no. 2, pp. 504–511, 2003.

22. Machoy-Mokrzynska A, "Fluoride-magnesium interaction." *Fluoride,* vol. 28, no. 4, pp. 175–177, 1995.

23. "Toxicological profile for fluorides, hydrogen fluoride, and fluorine." U.S. Department of Health and Human Services, Public Health Service, Agency for Toxic Substances and Disease Registry. Sept 2003. www.atsdr.cdc.gov/ToxProfiles/TP.asp?id=212&tid=38.

24. Deng X et al., "Magnesium, vitamin D status and mortality: results from US National Health and Nutrition Examination Survey (NHANES) 2001 to 2006 and NHANES III." *BMC Medicine,* vol. 11, p. 187, 2013.

25. Mursu J et al., "The association between serum 25-hydroxyvitamin D_3 concentration and risk of disease death in men: modification by magnesium intake." *Eur J Epidemiol,* vol. 30, no. 4, pp. 343–347, 2015.

26. Rosanoff A et al., "Essential nutrient interactions: does low or suboptimal magnesium status interact with vitamin D and/or calcium status?" *Adv Nutr,* vol. 7, no. 1, pp. 25–43, 2016.

Chapter 2

1. Aikawa JK, *Magnesium: Its Biologic Significance.* CRC Press, Boca Raton, FL, 1981.

2. McArdle WD, Katch FI, Katch VL, *Essentials of Exercise Physiology.* 2nd ed. Lippincott Williams & Wilkins, Philadelphia, 2000.

3. Levine BS, Coburn JW, "Magnesium, the mimic/antagonist of calcium." *N Engl J Med,* vol. 310, pp. 1253–1255, 1984.

4. Iseri LT, French JH, "Magnesium: nature's physiologic calcium blocker." *Am Heart J,* vol. 108, pp. 188–193, 1984.

5. Seelig MS, "Cardiovascular reactions to stress intensified by magnesium

deficit in consequences of magnesium deficiency on the enhancement of stress reactions; preventive and therapeutic implications: a review." *J Am Coll Nutr*, vol. 13, no. 5, pp. 429–446, 1994.

6. Rodale JR, *Magnesium: The Nutrient That Could Change Your Life.* Rodale Press, Emmaus, PA, 1971. Full text available at www.mgwater.com/rodtitle.shtml.

7. Hartwig A, "Role of magnesium in genomic stability." *Mutat Research*, vol. 18, no. 475 (1–2), pp. 113–121, 2001.

8. Yang L et al., "Critical role of magnesium ions in DNA polymerase beta's closing and active site assembly," *J Am Chem Soc*, vol. 126, no. 27, pp. 8441–8453, 2004.

9. Tao MH et al., "Associations of intakes of magnesium and calcium and survival among women with breast cancer: results from Western New York Exposures and Breast Cancer (WEB) Study." *Am J Cancer Res*, vol. 6, no. 1, pp. 105–113, 2015.

10. Walker GM, "Biotechnological implications of the interactions between magnesium and calcium." *Magnes Res*, vol. 12, no. 4, pp. 303–309, 1999.

11. Louvet L et al., "Characterisation of calcium phosphate crystals on calcified human aortic vascular smooth muscle cells and potential role of magnesium." *PLoS One*, vol. 10, no. 1, p. e0115342, 2015.

12. Teo KK et al., "Effects of intravenous magnesium in suspected acute myocardial infarction: overview of randomized trials." *Brit Med J*, vol. 303, pp. 1499–1503, 1991.

13. Eades M, Eades MD, *The Protein Power Lifeplan.* Warner Books, New York, 1999.

14. Feskanich D et al., "Calcium, vitamin D, milk consumption, and hip fractures: a prospective study among postmenopausal women." *Am J Clin Nutr*, vol. 77, no. 2, pp. 504–511, 2003.

15. Bolland MJ et al., "Vascular events in healthy older women receiving calcium supplementation: randomised controlled trial." *BMJ*, vol. 336, p. 336, 2008.

16. Bolland MJ et al., "Effect of calcium supplements on risk of myocardial infarction and cardiovascular events: meta-analysis." *BMJ*, vol. 341, 2010.

17. Bolland MJ et al., "Calcium supplements with or without vitamin D and risk of cardiovascular events: reanalysis of the Women's Health Initiative Limited Access Dataset and Meta-Analysis." *BMJ*, vol. 342, p. d2040, 2011.

18. Bolland MJ et al., "Calcium supplements and cardiovascular risk: 5 years on." *Ther Adv Drug Saf*, vol. 4, no. 5, pp. 199–210, 2013.

19. Bolland MJ et al., "Calcium intake and risk of fracture: systematic review." *BMJ*, vol. 351, p. H4580, 2015.

20. Anderson JJB et al., "Calcium intake from diet and supplements and the risk of coronary artery calcification and its progression among older

adults: 10-year follow-up of the Multi-Ethnic Study of Atherosclerosis (MESA)." *JAMA*, vol 5, no. 10.

21. Abraham GE, "The Calcium Controversy." *J Applied Nutr*, vol. 34, no. 2, 1982.

22. Kakigi CLM et al., "Self-reported calcium supplementation and age-related macular degeneration." *JAMA Ophthalmol*, vol. 133, no. 7, pp. 746–754, 2015.

23. Durlach J, "Recommended Dietary Amounts of magnesium: Mg RDA." *Magnes Res*, vol. 2, no. 3, pp. 195–203, 1989.

24. Grober U, Schmidt J, Kisters K, "Magnesium in prevention and therapy." *Nutrients*, vol. 7, no. 9, pp. 8199–8226, 2015.

25. Abood A, Vestergaard P, "Increasing incidence of primary hyperpara-thyroidism in Denmark." *Dan Med J*, vol. 60, no. 2, pp. A4567, 2013.

26. McCarthy JT, Kumar R, "Divalent cation metabolism: magnesium." In Schrier R (series ed.), *The Atlas of Diseases of the Kidney*, Blackwell, Oxfordshire, 1999.

27. Heaton FW, "Role of magnesium in enzyme systems," in Siegel H (ed.), *Metal Ions in Biologic Systems*, Marcel Dekker, New York, 1990.

28. Abraham GE, Flechas JD, "Management of fibromyalgia: rationale for the use of magnesium and malic acid." *J Nutr Med*, vol. 3, pp. 49–59, 1992.

29. Andrea Rosanoff, www.prohealth.com/library/print.cfm?libid=14606.

30. de Baaij JHF et al, "Magnesium in man: implications for health and disease." *Physiol Rev*, vol. 95, no. 1, pp. 1–46, 2015.

31. Shi J et al., "Mechanism of magnesium activation of calcium-activated potassium channels." *Nature*, vol. 418, no. 6900, pp. 876–880, 2002.

32. Kant AK, "Consumption of energy-dense, nutrient-poor foods by adult Americans: nutritional and health implications. The third National Health and Nutrition Examination Survey, 1988–1994." *Am J Clin Nutr*, vol. 72, no. 4, pp. 929–936, 2000.

33. "Junk food makes up quarter of US diet." NBC News, July 2004. http://tinyurl.com/ntr6aus.

34. *Marketplace*, March 2013. http://tinyurl.com/ovjht7q.

35. Institute of Medicine, *Dietary Reference Intake for Calcium, Phosphorus, Magnesium, Vitamin D, and Fluoride*. National Academy Press, Washington DC, 1997.

36. Sale K, "Lessons from the Luddites: setting limits on technology." *Nation*, June 5, 1995.

37. Samsel A, Seneff S, "Glyphosate, pathways to modern diseases II: celiac sprue and gluten intolerance." *Interdisc Toxicol*, vol. 6, no. 4, pp. 159–184, 2013.

38. http://soilandhealth.org/wp-content/uploads/01aglibrary/010106voisin/010106gttoc.html.

39. www.mgwater.com/leaching.shtml.

40. www.sunarc.org/JAD97.pdf.

41. Grober U, Schmidt J, Kisters K, "Magnesium in prevention and therapy." *Nutrients*, vol. 7, no. 9, pp. 8199–8226, 2015.

42. Institute of Medicine, *Dietary Reference Intake for Calcium, Phosphorus, Magnesium, Vitamin D, and Fluoride*. National Academies Press, Washington DC, 1997.

43. https://ods.od.nih.gov/factsheets/Magnesium-HealthProfessional/#h4.

44. Eades M, Eades MD, *The Protein Power Lifeplan*. Warner Books, New York, 1999.

45. Campbell-McBride N, *Gut and Psychology Syndrome*. Medinform, Cambridge, UK, 2010.

46. https://www.youtube.com/watch?v=dBnniua6-oM.

47. Werbach MR, *Nutritional Influences on Illness*. Thorstons Publishing Group, Wellingborough, Northamptonshire, 1989.

48. Werbach MR, *Nutritional Influences on Illness*. Thorstons Publishing Group, Wellingborough, Northamptonshire, 1989.

49. Graham L, Caesar J, Burger A, "Gastrointestinal absorption and excretion of Mg." *Metabolism*, vol. 9, 1960.

50. Disch G et al., "Interactions between magnesium and iron. In vitro studies." *Arzneimittel-Forschung*, vol. 44, no. 5, pp. 647–650, 1994.

51. Dean CFA, Wheeler LC, *IBS for Dummies*. Wiley, Hoboken, NJ, 2005.

52. Crook W, Dean CFA, *The Yeast Connection and Women's Health*. Square One, Garden City Park, NY, 2007.

53. Laires MJ et al., "Role of cellular magnesium in health and human disease." *Front Biosci*, vol. 9, pp. 262–276, 2004.

54. Eades M, Eades MD, *The Protein Power Lifeplan*. Warner Books, New York, 1999.

55. Freitag J, Hruska K, "Pathophysiology of Nephrolithiasis." In *The Kidney and Body Fluids in Health and Disease*, ed. S. Klahr, p. 550. Springer, New York, 2013.

56. Eades M, Eades MD, *The Protein Power Lifeplan*. Warner Books, New York, 1999.

57. Linderman RD, "Influence of various nutrients and hormones on urinary divalent cation excretion." *Ann NY Acad Sci*, vol. 162, pp. 802–809, 1969.

58. Lemann J et al., "Evidence that glucose ingestion inhibits net renal tubular reabsorption of calcium and magnesium in man." *J Lab Clin Medicine*, vol. 75, pp. 578–585, 1970.

Chapter 3

1. Michiel RR, "Sudden death in a patient on a liquid protein diet." *New Engl J Med*, vol. 298, pp. 1005–1007, 1978.

2. Werbach MR, "Nutritional influences on aggressive behavior." *J Orthomolec Medicine*, vol. 7, no. 1, 1995.

3. Boyle NB, Lawton CL, Dye L, "The effects of magnesium supplementation on subjective anxiety." *Magnes Res* 2016, Nov. 17.

4. Rogers SA, *Depression Cured at Last*. SK Publishing, Sarasota, FL, 2000.

5. Durlach J, "Diverse applications of magnesium therapy." In *Handbook of Metal-Ligand Interactions in Biological Fluids—Bioinorganic Medicine*, vol. 2, Marcel Dekker, New York, 1995.

6. Mocci F, Canalis P, Tomasi PA, Casu F, Pettinato S, "The effect of noise on serum and urinary magnesium and catecholamines in humans." *Occup Med (Lond)*, vol. 51, no. 1, pp. 56–61, 2001.

7. Penland JG, "Quantitative analysis of EEG effects following experimental marginal magnesium and boron deprivation." *Magnes Res*, vol. 8, no. 4, pp. 341–358, 1995.

8. Seelig MS, "Mechanisms of interactions of stress, stress hormones and magnesium in consequences of magnesium deficiency on the enhancement of stress reactions; preventive and therapeutic implications: a review." *J Am Coll Nutr*, vol. 13, no. 5, pp. 429–446, 1994.

9. Cernak I et al., "Alterations in magnesium and oxidative status during chronic emotional stress." *Magnes Res*, vol. 13, pp. 29–36, 2000.

10. Classen HG et al., "Coping with acute stress reaction by plentiful oral magnesium supply." *Magnes Bull*, vol. 17, pp. 1–8, 1995.

11. Sartori SB et al., "Magnesium deficiency induces anxiety and HPA axis dysregulation: Modulation by therapeutic drug treatment." *Neuropharmacology*, vol. 62, no. 1, pp. 304–312, 2012.

12. Klerman GL, Weissman MM, "Increasing rates of depression." *JAMA*, vol. 261, no. 15, pp. 2229–2235, 1992.

13. Weissman MM, "Cross-national epidemiology of major depression and bipolar disorder." *JAMA*, vol. 276, no. 4, pp. 293–299, 1996.

14. Murphy JM, "A 40-year perspective on the prevalence of depression: the Stirling County Study." *Arch Gen Psychiatry*, vol. 57, no. 3, pp. 209–215, 2000.

15. Cox RH, Shealy CN, Cady RK, Veehoff D, Burnetti Awell M, Houston R, "Significant magnesium deficiency in depression." *J Neurol Orthop Med Surg*, vol. 17, pp. 7–9, 1996.

16. Teymoor Y et al., "Dietary magnesium intake and the incidence of depression: a 20-year follow-up study." *J Affect Disord*, vol. 193, pp. 94–98, 2016.

17. Jacka FN, Overland S, Stewart R, Tell GS, Bjelland I, Mykletun A, "Association between magnesium intake and depression and anxiety in community-dwelling adults: the Hordaland Health Study." *Aust N Z J Psychiatry*, vol. 43, no. 1, pp. 45–52, 2009.

18. Kaur J et al., "Role of dietary factors in psychiatry." *Delhi Psychiatry J*, vol. 17, no. 2, pp. 452–457, 2014.

19. Gottesmann C, "GABA mechanisms and sleep." *Neuroscience* vol. 111, no. 2, pp. 231–239, 2002.

20. Moykkynen T et al., "Magnesium potentiation of the function of native and recombinant GABA(A) receptors." *Neuroreport.* July 20, 2001, vol. 12, no. 10, pp. 2175–2179.

21. Poleszak E et al., "Benzodiazepine/GABA(A) receptors are involved in magnesium-induced anxiolytic-like behavior in mice." *Pharmacol Rep,* vol. 60, no. 4, pp. 483–489, 2008.

22. Held K et al., "Oral Mg(2+) supplementation reverses age-related neuroendocrine and sleep EEG changes in humans." *Pharmacopsychiatry,* vol. 35, no. 4, pp. 135–143, 2002.

23. Nielsen FH, Johnson LK, Zeng H, "Magnesium supplementation improves indicators of low magnesium status and inflammatory stress in adults older than 51 years with poor quality sleep." *Magnes Res,* vol. 23, no. 4, pp. 158–168, 2010.

24. Omiya K et al., "Heart-rate response to sympathetic nervous stimulation, exercise, and magnesium concentration in various sleep conditions." *Int J Sport Nutr Exerc Metab,* vol. 19, no. 2, pp. 127–135, 2009.

25. Takase B et al., "Effects of chronic sleep deprivation on autonomic activity by examining heart rate variability, plasma catecholamine, and intracellular magnesium levels." *Biomed Pharmacother,* vol. 58, suppl. 1, pp. S35–S39, 2004.

26. Takase B et al., "Effect of chronic stress and sleep deprivation on both flow-mediated dilation in the brachial artery and the intracellular magnesium level in humans." *Clin Cardiol,* vol. 27, no. 4, pp. 223–227, 2004.

27. Billyard AJ et al., "Dietary magnesium deficiency decreases plasma melatonin in rats." *Magnes Research,* vol. 19, no. 3, pp. 157–161, 2006.

28. "Nearly 7 in 10 Americans are on prescription drugs." *Science News,* June 19, 2013.

29. Pigeon WR, Yurcheshen M, "Behavioral sleep medicine interventions for restless legs syndrome and periodic limb movement disorder." *Sleep Medicine Clinics,* vol. 4, no. 4, pp. 487–494, 2009.

30. Hornyak M et al., "Magnesium therapy for periodic leg movements-related insomnia and restless legs syndrome: an open pilot study." *Sleep,* vol. 21, no. 5, pp. 501–505, 1998.

31. Bartell S, Zallek S, "Intravenous magnesium sulfate may relieve restless legs syndrome in pregnancy." *J Clin Sleep Med,* vol. 2, no. 2, pp. 187–188, 2006.

32. Aurora RN et al, "The treatment of restless legs syndrome and periodic limb movement disorder in adults—an update for 2012: practice parameters with an evidence-based systematic review and meta-analyses: an American Academy of Sleep Medicine Clinical Practice Guideline." *Sleep,* vol. 35, no. 8, pp. 1039–1062, 2012.

33. Rogers SA, *Depression Cured at Last.* SK Publishing, Sarasota, FL, 2000.

34. Starobrat-Hermelin B, Kozielec T, "The effects of magnesium physiological supplementation on hyperactivity in children with attention

deficit hyperactivity disorder (ADHD). Positive response to magnesium oral loading test." *Magnes Res*, vol. 10, no. 2, pp. 149–156, 1997.

35. Olfman, S. *No Child Left Different*. Praeger, Westport, CT, 2006, p. 1.

36. Galland L, Buchman D, *Superimmunity for Kids*. Dell, New York, 1988.

Chapter 4

1. Blaylock RL, *Excitotoxins: The Taste That Kills*. Health Press, Sante Fe, NM, 1997.

2. Blaylock RL, *Excitotoxins: The Taste That Kills*. Health Press, Sante Fe, NM, 1997.

3. Weaver K, "Magnesium and migraine." *Headache*, vol. 30, p. 168, 1990.

4. Mauskop A, Fox B, *What Your Doctor May Not Tell You About Migraines*. Warner Books, New York, 2001.

5. Mauskop A et al., "Deficiency in serum ionized magnesium but not total magnesium in patients with migraines. Possible role of ICa2/IMg2 ratio." *Headache*, vol. 33, no. 3, pp. 135–138, 1993.

6. Mauskop A et al., "Deficiency in serum ionized magnesium but not total magnesium in patients with migraines. Possible role of ICa2/IMg2 ratio." *Headache*, vol. 33, no. 3, pp. 135–138, 1993.

7. Mauskop A et al., "Intravenous magnesium sulphate relieves migraine attacks in patients with low serum ionized magnesium levels: a pilot study." *Clin Sci (Colch)*, vol. 89, no. 6, pp. 633–636, 1995.

8. Mauskop A, Altura BT, et al., "Intravenous magnesium sulfate rapidly alleviates headaches of various types." *Headache*, vol. 36, no. 3, pp. 154–160, 1996.

9. Mauskop A, Altura BM, "Role of magnesium in the pathogenesis and treatment of migraines." *Clin Neurosci*, vol. 83, no. 5, pp. 24–27, 1998.

10. Peikert A, Wilimzig C, et al., "Prophylaxis of migraine with oral magnesium: results from a prospective, multi-center, placebo-controlled and double-blind randomized study." *Cephalalgia*, vol. 16, no. 4, pp. 257–263, 1996.

11. Mauskop A, "Why all migraine patients should be treated with magnesium." *J Neural Transm*, vol. 119, pp. 575–579, 2012.

12. Chiu HY et al., "Effects of intravenous and oral magnesium on reducing migraine: a meta-analysis of randomized controlled trials." *Pain Physician*, vol. 19, no. 1, pp. E97–E112, 2016.

13. Assarzadegan F et al., "Serum concentration of magnesium as an independent risk factor in migraine attacks: a matched case-control study and review of the literature." *Int Clin Psychopharmacol*, vol. 31, no. 5, pp. 287–292, 2016.

14. Mauskop A, Fox B, *What Your Doctor May Not Tell You About Migraines*. Warner Books, New York, 2001.

15. Shaik MM, Gan SH, "Vitamin supplementation as possible prophylactic

treatment against migraine with aura and menstrual migraine," *BioMed Research International,* vol. 2015, article ID 469529, 2015.

16. Buse DC et al., "Chronic migraine prevalence, disability, and sociode-mographic factors: results from the American Migraine Prevalence and Prevention Study." *Headache,* 52, no. 10, pp. 1456–1470, 2012.

17. Mauskop A et al., "Intravenous magnesium sulfate relieves cluster head-aches in patients with low serum ionized magnesium levels." *Headache,* vol. 35, no. 10, pp. 597–600, 1995.

18. Mauskop A, Altura BT et al., "Intravenous magnesium sulfate rapidly alleviates headaches of various types." *Headache,* vol. 36, no. 3, pp. 154–160, 1996.

19. Crosby V, Wilcock A, Corcoran R, "The safety and efficacy of a single dose (500 mg or 1 g) of intravenous magnesium sulfate in neuropathic pain poorly responsive to strong opioid analgesics in patients with can-cer." *J Pain Symptom Management,* vol. 20, no. 1, pp. 35–39, 2000.

20. Meucci RD, Fassa AG, Faria NMX, "Prevalence of chronic low back pain: systematic review." *Revista de Saúde Pública,* vol. 49, no. 1, p. 1, 2015.

21. Yousef AA, Al-Deeb AE, "A double-blinded randomized controlled study of the value of sequential intravenous and oral magnesium therapy in patients with chronic low back pain with a neuropathic com-ponent." *Anaesthesia,* vol. 68, no. 3, pp. 260–266, 2013.

22. Sarno J. *Healing Back Pain.* Grand Central Publishing, New York, 2001.

23. www.ninds.nih.gov/disorders/tourette/detail_tourette.htm.

24. Grimaldi BL, "The central role of magnesium deficiency in Tourette's syndrome: causal relationships between magnesium deficiency, altered biochemical pathways and symptoms relating to Tourette's syndrome and several reported comorbid conditions." *Med Hypotheses,* vol. 58, no. 1, pp. 47–60, 2002.

25. Nielsen FH, Lukaski HC, "Update on the relationship between magne-sium and exercise." *Magnes Res,* vol. 19, no. 3, pp. 180–189, 2006.

26. Seelig MS, "Athletic stress, performance and magnesium in consequenc-es of magnesium deficiency on the enhancement of stress reactions; preventive and therapeutic implications: a review." *J Am Coll Nutr,* vol. 13, no. 5, pp. 429–446, 1994.

27. Blaylock RL, *Excitotoxins: The Taste That Kills.* Health Press, Santa Fe, NM, 1997.

28. Blaylock RL, *Excitotoxins: The Taste That Kills.* Health Press, Santa Fe, NM, 1997.

29. Seelig MS, "Athletic stress, performance and magnesium in consequenc-es of magnesium deficiency on the enhancement of stress reactions; preventive and therapeutic implications: a review." *J Am Coll Nutr,* vol. 13, no. 5, pp. 429–446, 1994.

30. Singh RB, "Effect of dietary magnesium supplementation in the preven-

tion of coronary heart disease and sudden cardiac death." *Magnesium Trace Elem*, vol. 9, pp. 143–151, 1990.

31. Stendig-Lindberg G, "Sudden death of athletes: is it due to long-term changes in serum magnesium, lipids and blood sugar?" *J Basic Clin Physiol Pharmacol*, vol. 3, no. 2, pp. 153–164, 1992.

Chapter 5

1. Institute of Medicine, *Dietary Reference Intake for Calcium, Phosphorus, Magnesium, Vitamin D, and Fluoride*. National Academy Press, Washington DC, 1997.
2. Durlach J et al., "Physiopathology of symptomatic and latent forms of central nervous hyperexcitability due to magnesium deficiency: a current general scheme." *Magnes Res*, vol. 13, no. 4, pp. 293–302, 2000.
3. www.adelaide.edu.au/press/titles/magnesium.
4. Cernak I et al., "Characterization of plasma magnesium concentration and oxidative stress following graded traumatic brain injury in humans." *J Neurotrauma*, vol. 17, no. 1, pp. 53–68, 2000.
5. Memon ZI et al., "Predictive value of serum ionized but not total magnesium levels in head injuries." *Scand J Clin Lab Invest*, vol. 55, no. 8, pp. 671–677, 1995.
6. Heath DL, Vink R, "Brain free magnesium concentration is predictive of motor outcome following traumatic axonal brain injury in rats." *Magnes Res*, vol. 12, no. 4, pp. 269–277, 1999.
7. Blaylock RL, *Excitotoxins: The Taste That Kills*. Health Press, Sante Fe, NM, 1997.
8. Marcus JC et al., "Serum ionized magnesium in post-traumatic headaches." *J Pediatr*, vol. 139, no. 3, pp. 459–462, 2001.
9. Personal correspondence with Dr. Russell Blaylock.
10. Altura BM, Altura BT, "Association of alcohol in brain injury, headaches, and stroke with brain-tissue and serum levels of ionized magnesium: a review of recent findings and mechanisms of action." *Alcohol*, vol. 19, no. 2, pp. 119–130, 1999.
11. Altura BM et al., "Alcohol-induced spasms of cerebral blood vessels: relation to cerebrovascular accidents and sudden death." *Science*, vol. 220, no. 4594, pp. 331–333, 1983.
12. Zhang A et al., "Chronic treatment of cultured cerebral vascular smooth cells with low concentration of ethanol elevates intracellular calcium and potentiates prostanoid-induced rises in [Ca2+]i: relation to etiology of alcohol-induced stroke." *Alcohol*, vol. 14, no. 4, pp. 367–371, 1997.
13. Altura BM, Altura BT, "Association of alcohol in brain injury, headaches, and stroke with brain-tissue and serum levels of ionized magnesium: a review of recent findings and mechanisms of action." *Alcohol*, vol. 19, no. 2, pp. 119–130, 1999.
14. Abbot L et al., "Magnesium deficiency in alcoholism: possible contribu-

tion to osteoporosis and cardiovascular disease in alcoholics." *Alcohol Clin Exp Res,* vol. 19, pp. 1076–1082, 1994.

15. Altura BM, Altura BT, "Association of alcohol in brain injury, headaches, and stroke with brain-tissue and serum levels of ionized magnesium: a review of recent findings and mechanisms of action." *Alcohol,* vol. 19, no. 2, pp. 119–130, 1999.

16. Altura BM et al., "Extracellular magnesium regulates nuclear and perinuclear free ionized calcium in cerebral vascular smooth muscle cells: possible relation to alcohol and central nervous system injury." *Alcohol,* vol. 23, no. 2, pp. 83–90, 2001.

17. Ema M et al., "Alcohol-induced vascular damage of brain is ameliorated by administration of magnesium." *Alcohol,* vol. 15, no. 2, pp. 95–103, 1998.

18. www.cdc.gov/stroke/facts.htm.

19. Yang CY, "Calcium and magnesium in drinking water and risk of death from cerebrovascular disease." *Stroke,* vol. 18, no. 8, pp. 411–414, 1998.

20. Bain LK et al., "The relationship between dietary magnesium intake, stroke and its major risk factors, blood pressure and cholesterol, in the EPIC-Norfolk cohort." *Int J Cardiol,* vol. 196, pp. 108–114, 2015.

21. Altura BT, Altura BM, "Withdrawal of magnesium causes vasospasm while elevated magnesium produces relaxation of tone in cerebral arteries." *Neurosci Lett,* vol. 20, no. 3, pp. 323–327, 1980.

22. Altura BT, Altura BM, "Interactions of Mg and K on cerebral vessels—aspects in view of stroke. Review of present status and new findings." *Magnesium,* vol. 3, nos. 4–6, pp. 195–211, 1984.

23. Li W et al., "Antioxidants prevent elevation in [Ca(2+)](i) induced by low extracellular magnesium in cultured canine cerebral vascular smooth muscle cells: possible relationship to Mg(2+) deficiency-induced vasospasm and stroke." *Brain Res Bull,* vol. 52, no. 2, pp. 151–154, 2000.

24. Blaylock RL, *Excitotoxins: The Taste That Kills.* Health Press, Sante Fe, NM, 1997, p. 181.

25. Blaylock RL, *Excitotoxins: The Taste That Kills.* Health Press, Sante Fe, NM, 1997, p. 181.

26. Altura BT et al., "Low levels of serum ionized magnesium are found in patients early after stroke which result in rapid elevation in cytosolic free calcium and spasm in cerebral vascular muscle cells." *Neurosci Lett,* vol. 230, no. 1, pp. 37–40, 1997.

27. Altura BM, Altura BT, "Association of alcohol in brain injury, headaches, and stroke with brain-tissue and serum levels of ionized magnesium: a review of recent findings and mechanisms of action." *Alcohol,* vol. 19, no. 2, pp. 119–130, 1999.

28. Li W et al., "Antioxidants prevent depletion of [Mg2+]i induced by alcohol in cultured canine cerebral vascular smooth muscle cells: possible relationship to alcohol-induced stroke." *Brain Res Bull,* vol. 55, no. 4, pp. 475–478, 2001.

29. Haley D, *Politics in Healing.* BioMed Publishing Group, 2000.
30. http://tinyurl.com/hy2qg87.
31. Horn B, "Magnesium and the cardiovascular system." *Magnesium,* vol. 6, pp. 109–111, 1987.
32. Schulz-Stubner S et al., "Magnesium as part of balanced general anaesthesia with propofol, remifentanil and mivacurium: a double-blind, randomized prospective study in 50 patients." *Eur J Anaesthesiol,* vol. 18, no. 11, pp. 723–729, 2001.
33. www.mgwater.com/rodtitle.shtml.
34. Yuen AW, Sander JW, "Can magnesium supplementation reduce seizures in people with epilepsy? A hypothesis." *Epilepsy Res,* vol. 100, nos. 1–2, pp. 152–156, 2012.
35. Pall M, "Electromagnetic fields act via activation of voltage-gated calcium channels to produce beneficial or adverse effects." *J Cell Mol Med,* vol. 17, no. 8, pp. 958–965, 2013.

Chapter 6

1. Goldberg B, *Heart Disease.* Future Medicine Publishing, Tiburon, CA, 1998.
2. Altura BT et al., "Magnesium dietary intake modulates blood lipid levels and artherogenesis." *Proc Natl Acad Sci,* vol. 87, no. 5, pp. 1840–1844, 1990.
3. Singh RB et al., "Does dietary magnesium modulate blood lipids?" *Biol Trace Elem Res,* vol. 30, pp. 50–64, 1991.
4. Corica F et al., "Effects of oral magnesium supplementation on plasma lipid concentrations in patients with non-insulin-dependent diabetes mellitus." *Magnes Res,* vol. 7, pp. 43–46, 1994.
5. Durlach J, "Commentary on recent epidemiological and clinical advances." *Magnes Res,* vol. 9, no. 2, pp. 139–141, 1996.
6. Fallon S, Enig M, *Nourishing Traditions.* Locomotion Press, Baltimore, MD, 1995.
7. Gao M et al., "Cardiovascular risk factors emerging in Chinese populations undergoing urbanization." *Hypertens Res,* vol. 22, pp. 209–215, 1999.
8. Marier JR, "Magnesium content of the food supply in the modern-day world." *Magnesium,* vol. 5, pp. 1–8, 1986.
9. Liu L et al., "Comparative studies of diet-related factors and blood pressure among Chinese and Japanese: results from the China-Japan Cooperative Research of the WHO-CARDIAC Study. Cardiovascular disease and alimentary comparison." *Hypertens Res,* vol. 23, pp. 413–420, 2000.
10. Friedland GW, Friedman M, *Medicine's 10 Greatest Discoveries.* Yale University Press, New Haven, CT, 1998.
11. Ford R, *Stale Food vs. Fresh Food: The Cause and Cure of Choked Arteries and Related Problems.* Magnolia Laboratories, Pascagoula, MS, 1969.

12. Erasmus U, *Fats That Heal, Fats That Kill.* Alive Books, Burnaby, BC, 1993, p. 64.

13. Swenson AM et al., "Magnesium modulates actin binding and ADP release in myosin motors." *J Biol Chem,* vol. 289, no. 34, pp. 23977–23991, 2014.

14. Rosanoff A, Seelig MS, "Comparison of mechanism and functional effects of magnesium and statin pharmaceuticals." *J Am Coll Nutr,* vol. 23, no. 5, pp. 501S–505S, 2004.

15. Seelig M, Rosanoff A, *The Magnesium Factor.* Avery, New York, 2003, p. 244.

16. McCully KS, "Homocysteine, folate, vitamin B$_6$, and cardiovascular disease." *JAMA,* vol. 279, no. 5, pp. 392–393, 1998.

17. McCully KS, "Vascular pathology of homocysteinemia: implications for the pathogenesis of arteriosclerosis." *Am J Pathol,* vol. 56, no. 1, pp. 111–128, 1969.

18. Eikelboom JW et al., "Homocyst(e)ine and cardiovascular disease: a critical review of the epidemiologic evidence." *Ann Intern Med,* vol. 131, no. 5, pp. 363–375, 1999.

19. Boushey CJ et al., "A quantitative assessment of plasma homocysteine as a risk factor for vascular disease. Probable benefits of increasing folic acid intakes." *JAMA,* vol. 274, no. 13, pp. 1049–1057, 1995.

20. Confalonieri M et al., "Heterozygosity for homocysteinuria: a detectable and reversible risk factor for pulmonary thromboembolism." *Monaldi Arch Chest Disease,* vol. 50, no. 2, pp. 114–115, 1995.

21. Altura B, Altura B, "Magnesium: the forgotten mineral in cardiovascular health and disease." A Gem Lecture at SUNY Downstate. *Alumni Today,* pp. 11–22, spring 2001.

22. Li W et al., "Extracellular magnesium regulates effects of vitamin B$_6$, B$_{12}$ and folate on homocysteinemia-induced depletion of intracellular free magnesium ions in canine cerebral vascular smooth muscle cells: possible relationship to [Ca2+]i, atherogenesis and stroke." *Neurosci Lett,* vol. 274, no. 2, pp. 83–86, 1999.

23. Shamsuddin AM, "Inositol phosphates have novel anti-cancer function." *J Nutr,* vol. 125 (suppl.), pp. 725S–732S, 1995.

24. Rowley KG et al., "Improvements in circulating cholesterol, antioxidants, and homocysteine after dietary intervention in an Australian Aboriginal community." *Am J Clin Nutr,* vol. 74, no. 4, pp. 442–448, 2001.

25. Tice JA et al., "Cost-effectiveness of vitamin therapy to lower plasma homocysteine levels for the prevention of coronary heart disease: effect of grain fortification and beyond." *JAMA,* vol. 286, no. 8, pp. 936–943, 2001.

26. Vollset SE et al., "Plasma total homocysteine and cardiovascular and noncardiovascular mortality: the Hordaland Homocysteine Study." *Am J Clin Nutr,* vol. 74, no. 1, pp. 130–136, 2001.

27. Batmanghelidj F, *Your Body's Many Cries for Water*. Global Health Solutions, Falls Church, VA, 1997.

28. Altura BM et al., "Hypomagnesemia and vasoconstriction: possible relationship to etiology of sudden death ischemic heart disease and hypertensive vascular diseases." *Artery*, vol. 9, no. 3, pp. 212–231, 1981.

29. Mindell E, *Prescription Alternatives*. Keats Publishing, Los Angeles, 1999.

30. Pierce JB, *Heart Healthy Magnesium: Your Nutritional Key to Cardiovascular Wellness*. Avery, New York, 1994.

31. Kisters K et al., "Hypomagnesaemia, borderline hypertension and hyperlipidaemia." *Magnesium Bull*, vol. 21, pp. 31–34, 1999.

32. Altura BM, Altura BT et al., "Magnesium deficiency and hypertension: correlation between magnesium-deficient diets and microcirculatory changes in situ." *Science*, vol. 223, no. 4642, pp. 1315–1317, 1984.

33. Resnick LM et al., "Factors affecting blood pressure responses to diet: the Vanguard study." *Am J Hypertens*, vol. 13, no. 9, pp. 956–965, 2000.

34. Altura BM, Altura BT, "Interactions of Mg and K on blood vessels—aspects in view of hypertension. Review of present status and new findings." *Magnesium*, vol. 3, nos. 4–6, pp. 175–194, 1984.

Chapter 7

1. Lukaski HC, Nielsen FH. "Dietary magnesium depletion affects metabolic responses during submaximal exercise in postmenopausal women." *J Nutr*, vol. 132, no. 5, pp. 930–935, 2002.

2. Goldberg B, *Heart Disease*. Future Medicine Publishing, Tiburon, CA, 1998.

3. Sei M et al., "Nutritional epidemiological study on mineral intake and mortality from cardiovascular disease." *Tokushima J Exp Med*, vol. 40, nos. 3–4, pp. 199–207, 1993.

4. Zwillinger L, "Effect of magnesium on the heart." *Klin Wochenschr*, vol. 14, pp. 1429–1433, 1935.

5. *MMWR*, vol. 48, no. 30, pp. 649–656, 1999.

6. Mehta LS, Beckie TM, DeVon HA, et al., "Acute myocardial infarction in women: A scientific statement from the American Heart Association." *Circulation*, vol. 134, no. 20, 2016.

7. Rademaker M, "Do women have more adverse drug reactions?" *Am J Clin Dermatol*, vol. 2, no. 6, pp. 349–351, 2001.

8. Seelig M, Rosanoff A, *The Magnesium Factor*. Avery, New York, 2003, p. 244.

9. Singh RB, "Magnesium status and risk of coronary artery disease in rural and urban populations with variable magnesium consumption." *Magnes Res*, vol. 10, no. 3, pp. 205–213, 1997.

10. Liao F, Folsom AR, "Is low magnesium concentration a risk factor for coronary heart disease? The atherosclerosis risk in communities (ARIC) study." *Am Heart J*, vol. 136, no. 3, pp. 480–490, 1998.

11. Ford ES, "Serum magnesium and ischemic heart disease: findings from a national sample of US adults." *Int J Epidemiol*, vol. 28, pp. 645–651, 1999.

12. Seelig MS, Heggtveit HA, "Magnesium interrelationships in ischemic heart disease: a review." *Am J Clin Nutr*, vol. 27, no. 1, pp. 59–79, 1974.

13. Sherer Y, Bitzur R, Cohen H, Shaish A, Varon D, Shoenfeld Y, Harats D, "Mechanisms of action of the anti-atherogenic effect of magnesium: lessons from a mouse model." *Magnes Res*, vol. 14, no. 3, pp. 173–179, 2001.

14. Morrill GA, Gupta RK, Kostellow AB, Ma GY, Zhang A, Altura BT, Altura BM, "Mg2 modulates membrane sphingolipid and lipid second messenger levels in vascular smooth muscle cells." *FEBS Lett*, vol. 440, nos. 1–2, pp. 167–171, 1998.

15. Yang ZW, Gebrewold A, et al., "Mg++-induced endothelial-dependent relaxation of blood vessels and blood pressure lowering: role of NO." *Am J Physiol Regul Integr Comp Physiol*, vol. 278, pp. R628–639, 2000.

16. Kang DH, Park SK, Lee IK, Johnson RJ, "Uric acid–induced C-reactive protein expression: implication on cell proliferation and nitric oxide production of human vascular cells." *J Am Soc Nephrol*, vol. 16, no. 12, pp. 3553–3562, 2005.

17. Shrivastava AK et al., "C-reactive protein, inflammation and coronary heart disease." *Egyptian Heart J*, vol. 67, no. 2, pp. 89–97, 2015.

18. Qu X et al., "Magnesium and the risk of cardiovascular events: a meta-analysis of prospective cohort studies." *PLoS One*, vol. 8, no. 3, p. e57720, 2013.

19. Dibaba DT et al., "Dietary magnesium intake is inversely associated with serum C-reactive protein levels: meta-analysis and systematic review." *Eur J Clin Nutr*, vol. 68, no. 4, pp. 510–516, 2014.

20. King DE, Mainous AG, Geesey ME, Egan BM, Rehman S, "Magnesium supplement intake and C-reactive protein levels in adults." *Nutr Res*, vol. 26, pp. 193–196, 2006.

21. Pierce JB, *Heart Healthy Magnesium: Your Nutritional Key to Cardiovascular Wellness*. Avery, New York, 1994.

22. Shechter M et al., "Beneficial antithrombotic effects of the association of pharmacological oral magnesium therapy with aspirin in coronary heart disease patients." *Magnes Res*, vol. 13, no. 4, pp. 275–284, 2000.

23. Zwillinger L, "Effect of magnesium on the heart." *Klin Wochenschr*, vol. 14, pp. 1429–1433, 1935.

24. Boyd LJ et al., "Magnesium sulfate in paroxysmal tachycardia." *Am J Med Sci*, vol. 206, pp. 43–48, 1943.

25. Teo KK et al., "Effects of intravenous magnesium in suspected acute myocardial infarction: overview of randomized trials." *Brit Med J*, vol. 303, pp. 1499–1503, 1991.

26. Teo KK, Yusuf S, "Role of magnesium in reducing mortality in

acute myocardial infarction. A review of the evidence." *Drugs,* vol. 46, pp. 347–359, 1993.

27. Woods KL et al., "Intravenous magnesium sulfate in suspected acute myocardial infarction: results of the second Leicester Intravenous Magnesium Intervention Trial (LIMIT-2)." *Lancet,* vol. 339, pp. 1553–1558, 1992.

28. Woods KL, Fletcher S, "Long-term outcome after intravenous magnesium sulphate in suspected acute myocardial infarction: the second Leicester Intravenous Magnesium Intervention Trial (LIMIT-2)." *Lancet,* vol. 343, pp. 816–819, 1994.

29. Ravn HB, "Pharmacological effects of magnesium on arterial thrombosis—mechanisms of action?" *Magnes Res,* vol. 12, no. 3, pp. 191–199, 1999.

30. Young IS et al., "Magnesium status and digoxin toxicity." *Br J Clin Pharmacol,* vol. 32, no. 6, pp. 717–721, 1991.

31. Lewis R et al., "Magnesium deficiency may be an important determinant of ventricular ectopy in digitalised patients with chronic atrial fibrillation." *Br J Clin Pharmacol,* vol. 31, no. 2, pp. 200–203, 1991.

32. ISIS-4 (Fourth International Study of Infarct Survival) Collaborative Group, "ISIS-4: a randomised factorial trial assessing early oral captopril, oral mononitrate, and intravenous magnesium sulphate in 58,050 patients with suspected acute myocardial infarction." *Lancet,* vol. 345, pp. 669–685, 1995.

33. Seelig MS, "Cardiovascular reactions to stress intensified by magnesium deficit in consequences of magnesium deficiency on the enhancement of stress reactions; preventive and therapeutic implications: a review." *J Am Coll Nutr,* vol. 13, no. 5, pp. 429–446, 1994.

34. Woods KL, Fletcher S, "Long-term outcome after intravenous magnesium sulphate in suspected acute myocardial infarction: the second Leicester Intravenous Magnesium Intervention Trial (LIMIT-2)." *Lancet,* vol. 343, pp. 816–819, 1994.

35. Shechter M, Shechter A, "Magnesium and myocardial infarction." *Clin Calcium,* vol. 15, no. 11, pp. 111–115, 2005.

36. Shechter M, Bairey Merz CN, Stuehlinger HG, Slany J, Pachinger O, Rabinowitz B, "Effects of oral magnesium therapy on exercise tolerance, exercise-induced chest pain, and quality of life in patients with coronary artery disease." *Am J Cardiol,* vol. 91, no. 5, pp. 517–521, 2003.

37. Shechter M, "Does magnesium have a role in the treatment of patients with coronary artery disease?" *Am J Cardiovasc Drugs,* vol. 3, no. 4, pp. 231–239, 2003.

38. Shechter M, Hod H, Rabinowitz B, Boyko V, Chouraqui P, "Long-term outcome of intravenous magnesium therapy in thrombolysis-ineligible acute myocardial infarction patients." *Cardiology,* vol. 99, no. 4, pp. 205–210, 2003.

39. Shechter M, Sharir M, Labrador MJ, Forrester J, Silver B, Bairey Merz CN, "Oral magnesium therapy improves endothelial function in patients with coronary artery disease." *Circulation*, vol. 102, no. 19, pp. 2353–2358, 2000.

40. Shechter M, Merz CN, Rude RK, Paul Labrador MJ, Meisel SR, Shah PK, Kaul S, "Low intracellular magnesium levels promote platelet-dependent thrombosis in patients with coronary artery disease." *Am Heart J*, vol. 140, no. 2, pp. 212–218, 2000.

41. Reffelmann T et al., "Low serum magnesium concentrations predict increase in left ventricular mass over 5 years independently of common cardiovascular risk factors." *Atherosclerosis*, vol. 213, no. 2, pp. 563–569, 2010.

42. Shechter M et al., "Magnesium therapy in acute myocardial infarction when patients are not candidates for thrombolytic therapy." *Am J Cardiology*, vol. 75, pp. 321–323, 1995.

43. Pierce JB, *Heart Healthy Magnesium: Your Nutritional Key to Cardiovascular Wellness.* Avery, New York, 1994.

44. Iseri LT, "Magnesium and cardiac arrhythmias." *Magnesium*, vol. 5, nos. 3–4, pp. 111–126, 1986.

45. Iseri LT, Allen BJ, "Magnesium therapy of cardiac arrhythmias in critical-care medicine." *Magnesium*, vol. 8, pp. 299–306, 1989.

46. Fox C et al., "Magnesium: its proven and potential clinical significance." *South Med J*, vol. 94, no. 12, pp. 1195–1201, 2001.

47. Perticone F et al., "Antiarrhythmic short-term protective magnesium treatment in ischemic dilated cardiomyopathy." *J Am Coll Nutr*, vol. 5, no. 3, pp. 492–499, 1990.

48. Durlach J et al., "Magnesium and ageing. II. Clinical data: aetiological mechanisms and pathophysiological consequences of magnesium deficit in the elderly." *Magnes Res*, vol. 6, no. 4, pp. 379–394, 1993.

49. Pierce JB, *Heart Healthy Magnesium: Your Nutritional Key to Cardiovascular Wellness.* Avery, New York, 1994.

50. Adameova A et al., "Role of the excessive amounts of circulating catecholamines and glucocorticoids in stress-induced heart disease." *Can J Physiol Pharmacol*, vol. 87, no. 7, pp. 493–514, 2009.

51. Boyd LJ et al., "Magnesium sulfate in paroxysmal tachycardia." *Am J Med Sci*, vol. 206, pp. 43–48, 1943.

52. Parikka HJ, Toivonen LK, "Acute effects of intravenous magnesium on ventricular refractoriness and monophasic action potential duration in humans." *Scand Cardiovasc J*, vol. 33, no. 5, pp. 300–305, 1999.

53. Thiele R, Protze F, Winnefeld K, Pfeifer R, Pleissner J, Gassel M, "Effect of intravenous magnesium on ventricular tachyarrhythmias associated with acute myocardial infarction." *Magnes Res*, vol. 13, no. 2, pp. 111–112, 2000.

54. Ceremuzynski L et al., "Hypomagnesaemia in heart failure with ven-

tricular arrhythmias. Beneficial effects of magnesium supplementation." *J Intern Med*, vol. 247, pp. 78–86, 2000.

55. Dyckner T et al., "Magnesium deficiency in congestive heart failure." *Acta Pharmacol Toxicol Copenh*, vol. 54, suppl. 1, pp. 119–123, 1984.

56. England MR et al., "Magnesium administration and dysrhythmias after cardiac surgery." *JAMA*, vol. 268, pp. 2395–2402, 1992.

57. Caspi J et al., "Effects of magnesium on myocardial function after coronary artery bypass grafting." *Ann Thorac Surg*, vol. 59, pp. 942–947, 1995.

58. Toraman F, Karabulut EH, Alhan HC, Dagdelen S, Tarcan S, "Magnesium infusion dramatically decreases the incidence of atrial fibrillation after coronary artery bypass grafting." *Ann Thorac Surg*, vol. 72, no. 4, pp. 1256–1261, 2001.

59. Onalan O et al., "Meta-analysis of magnesium therapy for the acute management of rapid atrial fibrillation." *Am J Cardiol*, vol. 99, no. 12, pp. 1726–1732, 2007.

60. Khan AM, Lubitz SA, Sullivan LM et al., "Low serum magnesium and the development of atrial fibrillation in the community: the Framingham Heart Study." *Circulation*, vol. 127, no. 1, pp. 33–38, 2013.

61. www.rnareset.com.

62. Patel NJ et al., "Contemporary trends of hospitalization for atrial fibrillation in the United States, 2000 through 2010." *Circulation*, vol. 129, pp. 2371–2379, 2014.

63. Colilla S et al., "Estimates of current and future incidence and prevalence of atrial fibrillation in the U.S. adult population." *Am J Cardiol*, vol. 112, no. 8, pp. 1142–1147, 2013.

64. www.naturalnews.com/048511_MSG_magnesium_glutamates.html.

65. http://tinyurl.com/p8lhshk.

66. www.naturalnews.com/032084_sleep_apnea_epidemic.html.

67. O'Neal WT et al., "Coronary artery calcium progression and atrial fibrillation: the Multi-Ethnic Study of Atherosclerosis." *Circ Cardiovasc Imaging*, vol. 8, no. 12, 2015.

68. www.medscape.com/viewarticle/856658.

69. Shanahan CM, "Inflammation ushers in calcification: a cycle of damage and protection?" *Circulation*, vol. 116, pp. 2782–2785, 2007.

70. McEvoy JW et al., "Coronary artery calcium progression: an important clinical measurement? A review of published reports." *J Am Coll Cardiol*, vol. 56, no. 20, 2010.

71. Puri R et al., "Impact of statins on serial coronary calcification during atheroma progression and regression." *J Am Coll Cardiol*, vol. 65, no. 13, pp. 1273–82, 2015, doi: 10.1016/j.jacc.2015.01.036.

72. Lee SY et al., "Low serum magnesium is associated with coronary artery calcification in a Korean population at low risk for cardiovascular disease." *Nutr Metab Cardiovasc Dis*, vol. 25, no. 11, pp. 1056–1061, 2015.

73. Hruby A et al., "Magnesium intake is inversely associated with coronary

artery calcification: the Framingham Heart Study." *JACC Cardiovasc Imaging*, vol. 7, no. 1, pp. 59–69, 2014.

74. Handy CE et al., "The association of coronary artery calcium with noncardiovascular disease: the Multi-Ethnic Study of Atherosclerosis." *JACC Cardiovasc Imaging*, vol. 9, no. 5, pp. 568–576, 2016.

75. Chun S, Choi Y, Chang Y, et al., "Sugar-sweetened carbonated beverage consumption and coronary artery calcification in asymptomatic men and women." *Am Heart J*, vol. 177, pp. 17–24, 2016.

76. www.msgtruth.org.

77. Seelig MS, "Review and hypothesis: might patients with the chronic fatigue syndrome have latent tetany of magnesium deficiency." *J Chron Fatigue Syndr*, vol. 4, pp. 77–108, 1998.

78. Lichodziejewsa B et al., "Clinical symptoms of mitral valve prolapse are related to hypomagnesemia and attenuated by magnesium supplementation." *Amer J Cardiol*, vol. 79, pp. 768–772, 1997.

79. Dritsa V et al., "Investigating the mechanism of aortic valve stenosis: the role of magnesium salts." *J Cardiothorac Surg*, vol. 8, suppl. 1, p. 018, 2013.

Chapter 8

1. Bastard JP et al., "Recent advances in the relationship between obesity, inflammation, and insulin resistance." *Eur Cytokine Netw*, vol. 17, no. 1, March 2006, 4–12.

2. Moslehi N et al., "Effects of oral magnesium supplementation on in-flammatory markers in middle-aged overweight women." *J Res Med Sci*, vol. 17, no. 7, pp. 607–614, 2012.

3. Cassidy A et al., "Plasma adiponectin concentrations are associated with body composition and plant-based dietary factors in female twins." *J Nutr*, vol. 139, no. 2, pp. 353–358, 2009.

4. Martinez JA et al., "Epigenetics in adipose tissue, obesity, weight loss, and diabetes." *Adv Nutr*, vol. 5, pp. 71–81, 2014.

5. Chacko SA et al., "Magnesium supplementation, metabolic and inflammatory markers, and global genomic and proteomic profiling: a randomized, double-blind, controlled, crossover trial in overweight individuals." *Am J Clin Nutr*, vol. 93, no. 2, pp. 463–473, 2011.

6. Seelig M, Rosanoff A, *The Magnesium Factor*. Avery, New York, 2003.

7. Nielsen FH, "Magnesium, inflammation and obesity in chronic disease." *Nutr Rev*, vol. 68, no. 6, pp. 333–340, 2010.

8. Singh RB, "Association of low plasma concentrations of antioxidant vitamins, magnesium and zinc with high body fat per cent in Indian men." *Magnes Res*, vol. 11, no. 1, pp. 3–10, 1998.

9. Ma J et al., "Associations of serum and dietary magnesium with cardio-vascular disease, hypertension, diabetes, insulin, and carotid arterial wall thickness; the ARIC study, Artherosclerosis Risk in Communities Study." *J Clin Epidemiol*, vol. 48, pp. 927–940, 1995.

10. Humphries S et al., "Low dietary magnesium is associated with insulin resistance in a sample of young, non-diabetic black Americans." *Am J Hypertens,* vol. 12, no. 8, pt. 1, pp. 747–756, 1999.

11. Alzaid AA et al., "Effects of insulin on plasma magnesium in non-insulin-dependent diabetes mellitus: evidence for insulin resistance." *J Clin Endocrinol Metab,* vol. 80, no. 4, pp. 1376–1381, 1995.

12. Barbagallo M et al., "Altered cellular magnesium responsiveness to hyperglycemia in hypertensive subjects." *Hypertension,* vol. 38, no. 3, pt. 2, pp. 612–615, 2001.

13. Dominguez LJ et al., "Magnesium responsiveness to insulin and insulin-like growth factor I in erythrocytes from normotensive and hypertensive subjects." *J Clin Endocrinol Metab,* vol. 83, no. 12, pp. 4402–4407, 1998.

14. Resnick LM, "Cellular ions in hypertension, insulin resistance, obesity, and diabetes: a unifying theme." *J Am Soc Nephrol,* vol. 3, suppl. 4, pp. 578–585, 1992.

15. Karppanen H, Neuvonen PJ, "Ischaemic heart-disease and soil magnesium in Finland: water hardness and magnesium in heart muscle." *Lancet,* Dec. 15, 1973.

16. Resnick LM, "Ionic basis of hypertension, insulin resistance, vascular disease, and related disorders. The mechanism of Syndrome X." *Am J Hypertens,* vol. 6, no. 5, pt. 1, pp. 413–417, 1993.

17. Resnick LM, "The cellular ionic basis of hypertension and allied clinical conditions." *Prog Cardiovasc Dis,* vol. 42, pp. 1–22, 1999.

18. Resnick LM et al., "Hypertension and peripheral insulin resistance. Possible mediating role of intracellular free magnesium." *Am J Hypertens,* vol. 3, no. 5, pt. 1, pp. 373–379, 1990.

19. He K, Liu K, Daviglus ML, Morris SJ, Loria CM, Van Horn L, Jacobs DR, Savage PJ, "Magnesium intake and incidence of metabolic syndrome among young adults." *Circulation,* vol. 113, no. 13, pp. 1675–1682, 2006.

20. Paolisso G et al., "Low fasting and insulin-mediated intracellular magnesium accumulation in hypertensive patients with left ventricular hypertrophy; role of insulin resistance." *Hypertension,* vol. 9, pp. 199–203, 1995.

21. Nadler JL et al., "Magnesium deficiency produces insulin resistance and increased thromboxane synthesis." *Hypertension,* vol. 21, no. 6, pt. 2, pp. 1024–1029, 1993.

22. Chacko SA et al., "Magnesium supplementation, metabolic and inflammatory markers, and global genomic and proteomic profiling: a randomized, double-blind, controlled, crossover trial in overweight individuals.," *Am J Clin Nutr,* vol. 93, no. 2, pp. 463–473, 2011.

23. Bardicef M et al., "Extracellular and intracellular magnesium depletion in pregnancy and gestational diabetes." *Am J Obstet Gynecol,* vol. 172, no. 3, pp. 1009–1013, 1995.

24. Resnick LM et al., "Intracellular and extracellular magnesium depletion in type 2 (non-insulin-dependent) diabetes mellitus." *Diabetologia*, vol. 36, no. 8, pp. 767–770, 1993.

25. Chrysant SG, Chrysant GS. "Usefulness of the polypill for the prevention of cardiovascular disease and hypertension." *Curr Hypertens Rep*, vol. 18, no. 2, p. 14, 2016.

26. Gommers LM et al., "Hypomagnesemia in type 2 diabetes: a vicious circle?" *Diabetes*, vol. 65, no. 1, pp. 3–13, 2016.

27. Kao WH et al., "Serum and dietary magnesium and the risk for type 2 diabetes mellitus: the Atherosclerosis Risk in Communities Study." *Arch Intern Med*, vol. 159, no. 18, pp. 2151–2159, 1999.

28. Lima M de L, "The effect of magnesium supplementation in increasing doses on the control of type 2 diabetes." *Diabetes Care*, vol. 83, no. 5, pp. 682–686, 1998.

29. Paolisso G, Barbagallo M, "Hypertension, diabetes mellitus, and insulin resistance: the role of intracellular magnesium." *Am J Hypertens*, vol. 10, no. 3, pp. 346–355, 1997.

30. Kim DJ et al., "Magnesium intake in relation to systemic inflammation, insulin resistance, and the incidence of diabetes." *Diabetes Care*, vol. 33, pp. 2604–2610, 2010.

31. Yokota K et al., "Clinical efficacy of magnesium supplementation in patients with type 2." *J Am Coll Nutr*, vol. 23, no. 5, pp. 506S–509S, 2004.

32. Yokota K et al., "Clinical efficacy of magnesium supplementation in patients with type 2." *J Am Coll Nutr*, vol. 23, no. 5, pp. 506S–509S, 2004.

33. Kishimoto Y et al., "Effects of magnesium on postprandial serum lipid responses in healthy human subjects." *Br J Nutr*, vol. 103, pp. 469–472, 2010.

34. Mooren FC et al., "Oral magnesium supplementation reduces insulin resistance in non-diabetic subjects—a double-blind, placebo-controlled, randomized trial." *Diabetes Obes Metab*, vol. 13, no. 3, pp. 281–284, 2011.

35. Guerrero-Romero F, Rodriguez-Moral M, "Magnesium improves the beta-cell function to compensate variation of insulin sensitivity: double-blind, randomized clinical trial." *Eur J Clin Invest*, vol. 41, no. 4, pp. 405–410, 2011.

36. Lu J et al., "Serum magnesium concentration is inversely associated with albuminuria and retinopathy among patients with diabetes." *J Diabetes Res*, 1260141, 2016.

37. Veronese N et al., "Effect of magnesium supplementation on glucose metabolism in people with or at risk of diabetes: a systematic review and meta-analysis of double-blind randomized controlled trials." *Eur J Clin Nutr*, doi: 10.1038/ejcn.2016.154. [Epub ahead of print]

38. Bherwani S et al., "Hypomagnesaemia: a modifiable risk factor of diabetic nephropathy." *Horm Mol Biol Clin Investig*, 2016, doi: 10.1515/hmbci-2016-0024. [Epub ahead of print]

39. Barbagallo M, Dominguez LJ, "Magnesium and type 2 diabetes." *World J Diabetes*, vol. 6, no. 10, pp. 1152–1157, 2015.

40. Guerrero-Romero F et al., "Oral magnesium supplementation improves glycemic status in subjects with prediabetes and hypomagnesaemia: a double-blind placebo-controlled randomized trial." *Diabetes Metab*, vol. 41, no. 3, pp. 202–207, 2015.

41. Dabelea D et al., "Prevalence of type 1 and type 2 diabetes among children and adolescents from 2001 to 2009." *JAMA*, vol. 311, no. 17, pp. 1778–1786, 2014.

42. Huerta MG et al., "Magnesium deficiency is associated with insulin resistance in obese children." *Diabetes Care*, vol. 28, no. 5, pp. 1175–1181, 2005.

43. Merz CN et al., "Oral magnesium supplementation inhibits platelet-dependent thrombosis in patients with coronary artery disease." *Am J Cardiol*, vol. 84, pp. 152–156, 1999.

44. Lima M de L, "The effect of magnesium supplementation in increasing doses on the control of type 2 diabetes." *Diabetes Care*, vol. 83, no. 5, pp. 682–686, 1998.

45. Engelen W, Bouten A, De Leeuw I, De Block C, "Are low magnesium levels in type 1 diabetes associated with electromyographical signs of polyneuropathy?" *Magnes Res*, vol. 13, no. 3, pp. 197–203, 2000.

46. Djurhuus MS et al., "Effect of moderate improvement in metabolic control on magnesium and lipid concentrations in patients with type 1 diabetes." *Diabetes Care*, vol. 22, no. 4, pp. 546–554, 1999.

47. Squires S, "The amazing statistics and dangers of soda pop." *Washington Post*, February 27, 2001.

48. Ludwig DS et al., "Relation between consumption of sugar-sweetened drinks and childhood obesity: a prospective, observational analysis." *Lancet*, vol. 357, no. 9255, pp. 505–508, 2001.

49. Bellisle F, Rolland-Cachera MF, "How sugar-containing drinks might increase adiposity in children." *Lancet*, vol. 357, no. 9255, pp. 490–491, 2001.

50. Malik VS et al., "Sugar-sweetened beverages and weight gain in children and adults: a systematic review and meta-analysis." *Am J Clin Nutr*, vol. 98, no. 4, pp. 1084–1102, 2013.

51. Bernstein J et al., "Depression of lymphocyte transformation following oral glucose ingestion." *Am J Clin Nutr*, vol. 30, p. 613, 1977.

52. Sanchez A et al., "Role of sugars in human neutrophilic phagocytosis." *Am J Clin Nutr*, vol. 26, no. 11, pp. 1180–1184, 1973.

53. Kijak E et al., "Relationship of blood sugar level and leukocytic phago-cytosis." *S Calif State Dent Assoc J*, vol. 32, no. 9, 1964.

54. Campbell-McBride N, *Gut and Psychology Syndrome*. Medinform, Cambridge, UK, 2010.

55. Lima M de L, "The effect of magnesium supplementation in increas-

ing doses on the control of type 2 diabetes." *Diabetes Care,* vol. 83, no. 5, pp. 682–686, 1998.

56. Yang CY et al., "Magnesium in drinking water and the risk of death from diabetes mellitus." *Magnes Res,* vol. 12, no. 2, pp. 131–137, 1999.

57. Zhao HX et al., "Drinking water composition and childhood-onset type 1 diabetes mellitus in Devon and Cornwall, England." *Diabet Med,* vol. 18, no. 9, pp. 709–717, 2001.

58. Howard JMH, "Magnesium deficiency in peripheral vascular disease." *J Nutritional Med,* vol. 1, p. 39, 1990.

Chapter 9

1. Werbach M, "Premenstrual syndrome: magnesium." *Townsend Letter for Doctors,* June 1995, p. 26.

2. Sherwood RA et al., "Magnesium and the premenstrual syndrome." *Ann Clin Biochem,* vol. 23, no. 6, pp. 667–670, 1986.

3. Posaci C et al., "Plasma copper, zinc and magnesium levels in patients with premenstrual tension syndrome." *Acta Obstet Gynecol Scand,* vol. 73, no. 6, pp. 452–455, 1994.

4. Facchinetti F et al., "Oral magnesium successfully relieves premenstrual mood changes." *Obstet Gynecol,* vol. 78, no. 2, pp. 177–181, 1991.

5. Somer E, *The Essential Guide to Vitamins and Minerals.* HarperCollins, New York, 1995.

6. Murray M, *Encyclopedia of Natural Medicine,* 2nd ed. Prima, Rocklin, CA, 1998.

7. Muneyvirci-Delale O et al., "Sex steroid hormones modulate serum ionized magnesium and calcium levels throughout the menstrual cycle in women." *Fertil Steril,* vol. 69, no. 5, pp. 58–62, 1998.

8. Li W et al., "Sex steroid hormones exert biphasic effects on cytosolic magnesium ions in cerebral vascular smooth muscle cells: possible relationships to migraine frequency in premenstrual syndromes and stroke incidence." *Brain Res Bull,* vol. 54, no. 1, pp. 83–89, 2001.

9. Marz R, *Medical Nutrition from Marz,* 2nd ed. Omni Press, Portland, OR, 1997.

10. Benassi L et al., "Effectiveness of magnesium pidolate in the prophylactic treatment of primary dysmenorrhea." *Clin Exp Obstet Gynecol,* vol. 19, no. 3, pp. 176–179, 1992.

11. Fontana-Klaiber H, Hogg B, "Therapeutic effects of magnesium in dysmenorrhea." *Schweiz Rundsch Med Prax,* vol. 79, no. 16, pp. 491–494, 1990.

12. Seifert B et al., "Magnesium—a new therapeutic alternative in primary dysmenorrhea." *Zentralbl Gynakol,* vol. 111, no. 11, pp. 755–760, 1989.

13. Muneyvirci-Delale O et al., "Divalent cations in women with PCOS: implications for cardiovascular disease." *Gynecol Endocrinol,* vol. 15, no. 3, pp. 198–201, 2001.

Chapter 10

1. Goldberg B, *Alternative Medicine Guide: Women's Health Series 1*. Future Medicine, Tiburon, CA, 1998.

2. Franz KB, "Magnesium intake during pregnancy." *Magnesium*, vol. 6, pp. 18–27, 1987.

3. Dalton LM et al., "Magnesium in pregnancy." *Nutr Rev*, vol. 74, no. 9, pp. 549–557, 2016.

4. Edorh AP, Tachev K, Hadou T, Gbeassor M, Sanni A, Creppy EE, Le Faou A, Rihn BH, "Magnesium content in seminal fluid as an indicator of chronic prostatitis." *Cell Mol Biol*, vol. 49, pp. 419–423, 2003.

5. Jafrin W et al., "An evaluation of serum magnesium status in preeclampsia compared to the normal pregnancy." *Mymensingh Medicine J*, vol. 23, no. 4, pp. 649–653, 2014.

6. Conradt A, Weidinger AH, "The central position of magnesium in the management of fetal hypotrophy—a contribution to the pathomechanism of utero-placental insufficiency, prematurity and poor intrauterine fetal growth as well as pre-eclampsia." *Magnesium Bull*, vol. 4, pp. 103–124, 1982.

7. Handwerker SM et al., "Ionized serum magnesium levels in umbilical cord blood of normal pregnant women at delivery: relationship to calcium, demographics, and birthweight." *Am J Perinatol*, vol. 10, no. 5, pp. 392–397, 1993.

8. Handwerker SM, Altura BT, Altura BM, "Serum ionized magnesium and other electrolytes in the antenatal period of human pregnancy." *J Am Coll Nutr*, vol. 15, no. 1, pp. 36–43, 1996.

9. Almonte RA et al., "Gestational magnesium deficiency is deleterious to fetal outcome." *Biol Neonate*, vol. 76, no. 1, pp. 26–32, 1999.

10. Seelig MS, "Toxemias of pregnancy, postpartum cardiomyopathy and SIDS in consequences of magnesium deficiency on the enhancement of stress reactions; preventive and therapeutic implications: a review." *J Am Coll Nutr*, vol. 13, no. 5, pp. 429–446, 1994.

11. Lazard EM, "A preliminary report on the intravenous use of magnesium sulphate in puerperal eclampsia." *Am J Obst Gynec*, vol. 9, pp. 178–188, 1925.

12. Seelig MS, *Magnesium Deficiency in the Pathogenesis of Disease: Early Roots of Cardiovascular, Skeletal, and Renal Abnormalities*. Plenum, New York, 1980.

13. Seelig MS, "Prenatal and neonatal mineral deficiencies: magnesium, zinc and chromium." In *Clinical Disorders in Pediatric Nutrition*, Marcel Dekker, New York, pp. 167–196, 1982.

14. Seelig MS, "Magnesium in pregnancy: special needs for the adolescent mother." *J Am Coll Nutr*, vol. 10, p. 566, 1991.

15. Caddell JL, "Magnesium deficiency promotes muscle weakness, con-

tributing to the risk of sudden infant death (SIDS) in infants sleeping prone." *Magnes Res*, vol. 14, nos. 1–2, pp. 39–50, 2001.

16. Caddell JL, "A triple-risk model for the sudden infant death syndrome (SIDS) and the apparent life-threatening episode (ALTE): the stressed magnesium deficient weanling rat." *Magnes Res*, vol. 14, no. 3, pp. 227–238, 2001.

17. Durlach J et al., "Magnesium and thermoregulation. I. Newborn and infant. Is sudden infant death syndrome a magnesium-dependent disease of the transition from chemical to physical thermoregulation?" *Magnes Res*, vol. 4, pp. 137–152, 1991.

18. Nelson KB et al., "Can magnesium sulfate reduce the risk of cerebral palsy in very low birth weight infants?" *Pediatrics*, vol. 95, no. 2, 1995.

19. Schendel D et al., "Prenatal magnesium sulfate exposure and the risk for cerebral palsy or mental retardation among very low birth-weight children aged 3–5 years." *JAMA*, vol. 276, pp. 1805–1810, 1996.

20. Dedhia HV, Banks DE, "Pulmonary response to hyperoxia: effects of magnesium." *Environ Health Perspect*, vol. 102, suppl. 10, pp. 101–105, 1994.

21. Oorschot DE, "Cerebral palsy and experimental hypoxia-induced perinatal brain injury: is magnesium protective?" *Magnes Res*, vol. 13, no. 4, pp. 265–273, 2000.

22. Bara M, Guiet-Bara A, "Magnesium regulation of Ca2+ channels in smooth muscle and endothelial cells of human allantochorial placental vessels." *Magnes Res*, vol. 14, nos. 1–2, pp. 11–18, 2001.

Chapter 11

1. Brown S, *Better Bones, Better Body.* Keats, New Canaan, CT, 1996.

2. Thomas AJ et al., "Ca, Mg and P status of elderly inpatients: dietary intake, metabolic balance studies and biochemical status." *Br J Nutr*, vol. 62, pp. 211–219, 1989.

3. Bunker VW, "Osteoporosis in the elderly." *Br J Biomed Sci*, vol. 51, no. 3, pp. 228–240, 1994.

4. Morehouse-Grand K, Grand S. "Can vegans have healthy bones? A literature review." *Topics in Integrative Health Care*, vol. 5, no. 4, ID 5.4003, 2014.

5. The National Institutes of Health Osteoporosis Prevention, Diagnosis, and Therapy Consensus Statement, Mar. 2000.

6. Zheng J et al., "Association between serum level of magnesium and postmenopausal osteoporosis: a meta-analysis." *Biol Trace Elem Res*, vol. 159, nos. 1–3, pp. 8–14, 2014.

7. Belluci MM et al., "Magnesium deficiency results in an increased formation of osteoclasts." *J Nutr Biochem*, vol. 24, no. 8, pp. 1488–1498, 2013.

8. Rude RK, "Magnesium deficiency-induced osteoporosis in the rat:

uncoupling of bone formation and bone resorption." *Magnes Res,* vol. 12, no. 4, pp. 257–267, 1999.

9. Rude RK et al., "Magnesium deficiency induces bone loss in the rat." *Miner Electrolyte Metab,* vol. 24, no. 5, pp. 314–320, 1998.

10. Brodowski J, "Levels of ionized magnesium in women with various stages of postmenopausal osteoporosis progression evaluated on the basis of densitometric examinations." *Przegl Lek,* vol. 57, no. 12, pp. 714–716, 2000.

11. Sojka JE, Weaver CM, "Magnesium supplementation and osteoporosis." *Nutr Rev,* vol. 53, p. 71, 1995.

12. Goldberg B, *Alternative Medicine Guide: Women's Health Series 2.* Future Medicine, Tiburon, CA, 1998.

13. Goldberg B, *Alternative Medicine Guide: Women's Health Series 2.* Future Medicine, Tiburon, CA, 1998.

14. Abraham GE, Grewal HA, "Total dietary program emphasizing magnesium instead of calcium: effect on the mineral density of calcaneous bone in postmenopausal women on hormonal therapy." *J Reprod Med,* vol. 35, no. 5, pp. 503–507, 1990.

15. Seelig MS, "Increased magnesium need with use of combined estrogen and calcium for osteoporosis." *Magnes Res,* vol. 3, pp. 197–215, 1990.

16. Goldberg B, *Alternative Medicine Guide: Women's Health Series 2.* Future Medicine, Tiburon, CA, 1998.

17. Brown S, *Better Bones, Better Body.* Keats, New Canaan, CT, 1996.

18. Compston J et al., "Diagnosis and management of osteoporosis in postmenopausal women and older men in the UK: National Osteoporosis Guideline Group (NOGG) update 2013." *Maturitas,* vol. 75, no. 4, 392–396, 2013.

19. Maggio M et al., "Magnesium and anabolic hormones in older men." *Int J Androl,* vol. 34, no. 6, part 2, pp. e594–e600, 2011.

20. Cinar V et al., "Effects of magnesium supplementation on testosterone levels of athletes and sedentary subjects at rest and after exhaustion." *Biol Trace Elem Res,* vol. 140, no. 1, pp. 18–23, 2011.

21. Rotter I et al., "Relationship between serum magnesium concentration and metabolic and hormonal disorders in middle-aged and older men." *Magnes Res,* vol. 28, no. 3, pp. 99–107, 2015.

22. Stafford RS et al., "National trends in osteoporosis visits and osteoporosis treatment, 1988–2003." *Arch Intern Med,* vol. 164, pp. 1525–1530, 2004.

23. Abrams SA et al., "Magnesium metabolism in 4-year-old to 8-year-old children." *J Bone Miner Res,* vol. 29, no, 1, pp. 118–122, 2014.

24. Tucker KL et al., "Potassium, magnesium, and fruit and vegetable intakes are associated with greater bone mineral density in elderly men and women." *Am J Clin Nutr,* vol. 69, no. 4, pp. 727–736, 1999.

25. Curfman G, "FDA strengthens warning that NSAIDs increase heart

attack and stroke risk." *Harvard Health Blog*, July 13, 2015, www
.patienteducationcenter.org/fda-strengthens-warning-that-nsaids
-increase-heart-attack-and-stroke-risk-3.

26. Schmidt M et al., "Non-steroidal anti-inflammatory drug use and risk of
atrial fibrillation or flutter: population based case-control study," *BMJ*,
vol. 343, d3450, 2011.

27. Li Y, Yue J, Yang C. "Unraveling the role of Mg++ in osteoarthritis."
Life Sci, vol. 147, pp. 24–29, 2016.

28. Zeng C et al., "Relationship between serum magnesium concentration and radiographic knee osteoarthritis." *J Rheumatol*, vol. 42, no. 7,
pp. 1231–1236, 2015.

29. Hall WD et al., "Risk factors for kidney stones in older women in the
southern United States." *Am J Med Sci*, vol. 322, no. 1, pp. 12–18, 2001.

30. http://lowoxalateinfo.com/guide-to-low-oxalate-greens.

31. Milne DB, Nielsen FH, "The interaction between dietary fructose and
magnesium adversely affects macromineral homeostasis in men." *J Am
Coll Nutr*, vol. 19, no. 1, pp. 31–37, 2000.

32. Institute of Medicine, *Dietary Reference Intake for Calcium, Phosphorus, Magnesium, Vitamin D, and Fluoride*. National Academy Press, Washington DC,
1997.

33. Milne D, Nielsen F, "Too much soda may take some fizz out of the
bones." *Proc ND Acad Sci*, vol. 51, p. 212, 1998.

34. Bunce GE et al., "Distribution of calcium and magnesium in rat kidney
homogenate fractions accompanying magnesium deficiency induced
nephrocalcinosis." *Exp Mol Pathol*, vol. 21, no. 1, pp. 16–28, 1974.

35. Johansson G et al., "Effects of magnesium hydroxide in renal stone
disease." *J Am Coll Nutr*, vol. 1, no. 2, 1982.

36. Prien EL, "Magnesium oxide–pyridoxine therapy for recurring calcium
oxalate urinary calculi." *J Urology*, vol. 112, pp. 509–551, 1974.

37. Johannson G et al., "Biochemical and clinical effects of prophylactic
treatment of renal calcium stones with magnesium hydroxide." *J Urol*,
vol. 124, pp. 770–774, 1980.

38. Driessens FC, Verbeeck RM, "On the prevention and treatment of calcification disorders of old age." *Med Hypotheses*, vol. 3, pp. 131–137, 1988.

39. Labeeuw M et al., "Role of magnesium in the physiopathology and
treatment of calcium renal lithiasis." *Presse Med*, vol. 16, no. 1, pp. 25–
27, 1987.

40. Massey L, "Magnesium therapy for nephrolithiasis." *Magnes Res*, vol. 18,
no. 12, pp. 123–126, 2005.

41. Jeppesen BB, "Greenland, a soft-water area with a low incidence of
ischemic heart death." *Magnesium*, vol. 6, no. 6, pp. 307–313, 1987.

42. Loh AH, Cohen AH. "Drug-induced kidney disease—pathology and
current concepts." *Ann Acad Med Singapore*, vol. 38, no. 3, pp. 240–250,
2009.

43. www.empowher.com/kidney-failure/content/top-ten-drugs-cause-kidney-damage.

44. Xie Y et al., "Proton pump inhibitors and risk of incident CKD and progression to ESRD." *J Am Soc Nephrol*, vol. 27, no. 10, pp. 3153–3163, 2016.

45. Thongprayoon C et al., "High mortality risk in chronic kidney disease and end stage kidney disease patients with clostridium difficile infection: a systematic review and meta-analysis." *J Nature Sci*, vol. 1, no. 4, p. e85, 2015.

46. Geiger H, Wanner C. "Magnesium in disease." *Clin Kidney J*, vol. 5, suppl. 1, pp. i25–i38, 2012.

47. Jahnen-Dechent W, Ketteler M. "Magnesium basics." *Clin Kidney J*, vol. 5, suppl. 1, pp. i3–i14, 2012.

48. "Magnesium—a versatile and often overlooked element: New perspectives with a focus on chronic kidney disease." *Clin Kidney J*, vol. 5, suppl. 1, 2012.

49. Alhosaini M et al., "Magnesium and dialysis: the neglected cation." *Am J Kidney Dis*, vol. 66, no. 3, pp. 523–531, 2015.

50. Markell MS, Altura BT, et al. "Deficiency of serum ionized magnesium in patients receiving hemodialysis or peritoneal dialysis." *ASAIO J*, vol. 39, no. 3, pp. M801–M804, 1993.

51. Alhosaini M et al., "Magnesium and dialysis: the neglected cation." *Am J Kidney Dis*, vol. 66, no. 3, pp. 523–531, 2015.

52. Demer LL, Tintut Y. "Vascular calcification: pathobiology of a multifaceted disease." *Circulation*, vol. 117, no. 22, pp. 2938–2948, 2008.

53. McCarty MF, Dinicolantonio JJ, "The molecular biology and pathophysiology of vascular calcification." *Postgrad Med*, vol. 126, no. 2, pp. 54–64, 2014.

Part Three

1. www.mgwater.com/cancer.shtml.

2. www.mgwater.com/rodtitle.shtml.

3. Daniel D et al., "Magnesium intake and incidence of pancreatic cancer: the Vitamins and Lifestyle Study." *Br J Cancer*, vol. 113, no. 11, pp. 1615–1621, 2015.

4. Ma E et al., "High dietary intake of magnesium may decrease risk of colorectal cancer in Japanese men." *J Nutr*, vol. 140, pp. 779–785, 2010.

5. Kuno T et al., "Organomagnesium suppresses inflammation-associated colon carcinogenesis in male Crj: CD-1 mice." *Carcinogenesis*, vol. 34, no. 2, pp. 361–369, 2013.

6. Tao MH et al., "Associations of intakes of magnesium and calcium and survival among women with breast cancer: results from Western New York Exposures and Breast Cancer (WEB) Study." *Am J Cancer Res*, vol. 6, no. 1, pp. 105–113, 2015.

7. Piovesan D et al., "The human 'magnesome': detecting magnesium binding sites on human proteins." *BMC Bioinformatics,* vol. 13, suppl. 14, p. S10, 2012.

8. www.mgwater.com/rodtitle.shtml.

Chapter 12

1. Goldstein JA, ed., *Chronic Fatigue Syndromes: The Limbic Hypothesis.* Haworth Press, New York, 1993.

2. Seelig MS, "Review and hypothesis: might patients with the chronic fatigue syndrome have latent tetany of magnesium deficiency." *J Chron Fatigue Syndr,* vol. 4, pp. 77–108, 1998.

3. Papadopol V, Tuchendria E, Palamaru I, "Magnesium and some psychological features in two groups of pupils (magnesium and psychic features)." *Magnes Res,* vol. 14, nos. 1–2, pp. 27–32, 2001.

4. Durlach V et al., "Neurotic, neuromuscular and autonomic nervous form of magnesium imbalance." *Magnes Res,* vol. 10, pp. 169–195, 1997.

5. Cox IM, "Red blood cell magnesium and chronic fatigue syndrome." *Lancet,* vol. 337, pp. 757–760, 1991.

6. Goldberg B, *Chronic Fatigue, Fibromyalgia and Environmental Illness: 26 Doctors Show You How They Reverse These Conditions with Clinically Proven Alternative Therapies.* Future Medicine, Tiburon, CA, 1998.

7. Goldberg B, *Chronic Fatigue, Fibromyalgia and Environmental Illness: 26 Doctors Show You How They Reverse These Conditions with Clinically Proven Alternative Therapies.* Future Medicine, Tiburon, CA, 1998.

8. Seelig MS, "Athletic stress, performance and magnesium in consequences of magnesium deficiency on the enhancement of stress reactions; preventive and therapeutic implications: a review." *J Am Coll Nutr,* vol. 13, no. 5, pp. 429–446, 1994.

9. Abraham GE, Flechas JD, "Management of fibromyalgia: rationale for the use of magnesium and malic acid." *P J Nutr Med,* vol. 3, pp. 49–59, 1992.

Chapter 13

1. Rogers S. *Detoxify or Die.* Sand Key, Sarasota, FL, 2002.

2. "CDC releases most extensive assessment to date of Americans' exposure to environmental chemicals," Centers for Disease Control and Prevention telebriefing, January 31, 2003, www.cdc.gov/media/transcripts /t030131.htm.

3. "GAO finds that USDA, EPA have neglected pledge to cut pesticide use," U.S. General Accounting Office, U.S. Newswire, Sept. 27, 2001, http://leahy.senate.gov/press/200109/010927.html.

4. www.cdc.gov/exposurereport.

5. www.texascenter.org/almanac/Waste/MUNICIPALCH8P2.HTML.

6. Kreutzer R et al., "Prevalence of people reporting sensitivities to

chemicals in a population-based survey." *Am J Epidemiol*, vol. 150, no. 1, pp. 1–12, 1999.

7. "Everyday carcinogens: stopping cancer before it starts." Workshop on Primary Cancer Prevention, McMaster University, Hamilton, Ontario, Canada, March 26–27, 1999.

8. Goering PL et al., "Toxicity assessment of mercury vapor from dental amalgams." *Fundam Appl Toxicol*, vol. 19, no. 3, pp. 319–329, 1992.

9. Halbach S, "Amalgam tooth fillings and man's mercury burden. Review." *Hum Exp Toxicol*, vol. 13, no. 7, pp. 496–501, 1994.

10. Lorscheider FL et al., "Mercury exposure from 'silver' tooth fillings: emerging evidence questions a traditional dental paradigm." *FASEB J*, vol. 9, no. 7, pp. 504–508, 1995.

11. Arenholt-Bindslev D, Larsen AH, "Mercury levels and discharge in waste water from dental clinics." *Water Air Soil Pollut*, vol. 86, nos. 1–4, pp. 93–99, 1996.

12. Drasch G et al., "Comparison of the body burden of the population of Leipzig and Munich with the heavy metals cadmium, lead and mercury—a study of human organ samples." *Gesundheitswesen*, vol. 56, no. 5, pp. 263–267, 1994.

13. Liu XY, Jin TY, Nordberg GF, "Increased urinary calcium and magnesium excretion in rats injected with mercuric chloride." *Pharmacol Toxicol*, vol. 68, no. 4, pp. 254–259, 1991.

14. Durlach J, "Diverse applications of magnesium therapy." In *Handbook of Metal-Ligand Interactions in Biological Fluids—Bioinorganic Medicine*, vol. 2, Marcel Dekker, New York, 1995.

15. Kedryna T et al., "Effect of environmental fluorides on key biochemical processes in humans." *Folia Med Cracov*, vol. 34, no. 1–4, pp. 49–57, 1993.

16. Semczuk M, Semczuk-Sikora A, "New data on toxic metal intoxication (Cd, Pb, and Hg in particular) and Mg status during pregnancy. Review." *Med Sci Monit*, vol. 7, no. 2, pp. 332–340, 2001.

17. Semczuk M, Semczuk-Sikora A, "New data on toxic metal intoxication (Cd, Pb, and Hg in particular) and Mg status during pregnancy. Review." *Med Sci Monit*, vol. 7, no. 2, pp. 332–340, 2001.

18. Durlach J et al., "Magnesium: a competitive inhibitor of lead and cadmium. Ultrastructure studies of the human amniotic epithelial cell." *Magnes Res*, vol. 3, pp. 31–36, 1990.

19. Soldatovic D et al., "Contribution to interaction between magnesium and toxic metals: the effect of prolonged cadmium intoxication on magnesium metabolism in rabbits." *Magnes Res*, vol. 11, no. 4, pp. 283–288, 1998.

20. Allen VG, "Influence of aluminum on magnesium metabolism." In Altura BM, Durlach J, Seelig MS, eds., *Magnesium in Cellular Processes and Medicine*, Krager, Basel, 1987, pp. 50–66.

21. Rogers S, *The EI Syndrome: An Rx for Environmental Illness,* rev. ed. Sand Key, Sarasota, FL, 1995.

Chapter 14

1. Seelig M, "Consequences of magnesium deficiency on the enhancement of stress reactions; preventive and therapeutic implications (a review)." *J Am Coll Nutr,* vol. 13, no. 5, pp. 429–446, 1994.
2. *Physicians' Desk Reference,* 56th ed., Medical Economics, Oradell, NJ, 2002.
3. Gurkan F et al., "Intravenous magnesium sulphate in the management of moderate to severe acute asthmatic children nonresponding to conventional therapy." *Eur J Emerg Medicine,* vol. 6, no. 3, pp. 201–205, 1999.
4. Ciarallo L et al., "Intravenous magnesium therapy for moderate to severe pediatric asthma: results of a randomized, placebo-controlled trial." *J Pediatr,* vol. 129, pp. 809–814, 1996.
5. Dominguez LJ et al., "Bronchial reactivity and intracellular magnesium: a possible mechanism for the bronchodilating effects of magnesium in asthma." *Clin Sci (Colch),* vol. 95, no. 2, pp. 137–142, 1998.
6. Britton J, "Dietary magnesium, lung function, wheezing and airway hyperreactivity in a random population sample." *Lancet,* vol. 344, pp. 357–362, 1994.
7. Kew KM et al., "Intravenous magnesium sulfate for treating adults with acute asthma in the emergency department." *Cochrane Database Syst Rev,* vol. 5, CD010909, 2014.
8. Santi M et al., "Magnesium in cystic fibrosis: Systematic review of the literature." *Pediatr Pulmonol,* vol. 51, no. 2, pp. 196–202, 2016.

Chapter 15

1. Barbagallo M et al., "Cellular ionic alterations with age: relation to hypertension and diabetes." *J Am Geriatr Soc,* vol. 48, no. 9, pp. 1111–1116, 2000.
2. Barbagallo M, "Diabetes mellitus, hypertension and ageing: the ionic hypothesis of ageing and cardiovascular-metabolic diseases." *Diabetes Metab,* vol. 23, no. 4, pp. 281–294, 1997.
3. Hartwig A, "Role of magnesium in genomic stability." *Mutat Res,* vol. 18, no. 475 (1–2), pp. 113–121, 2001.
4. Worwag M et al., "Prevalence of magnesium and zinc deficiencies in nursing home residents in Germany." *Magnes Res,* vol. 12, no. 3, pp. 181–189, 1999.
5. Paolisso G et al., "Mean arterial blood pressure and serum levels of the molar ratio of insulin-like growth factor-1 to its binding protein-3 in centenarians." *J Hypertens,* vol. 17, pp. 67–73, 1999.
6. Durlach J et al., "Magnesium and ageing. II. Clinical data: aetiological mechanisms and pathophysiological consequences of magnesium deficit in the elderly." *Magnes Res,* vol. 6, no. 4, pp. 379–394, 1993.

7. Leone N et al., "Zinc, copper and magnesium and risks for all-cause, cancer, and cardiovascular mortality." *Epidemiology,* vol. 17, no. 3, pp. 308–314, 2006.

8. Guasch-Ferre M et al., "Dietary magnesium intake is inversely associated with mortality in adults at high cardiovascular disease risk." *J Nutr,* vol. 144, no. 1, pp. 55–60, 2014.

9. Wolf F, Hilewitz A. Hypomagnesaemia in patients hospitalised in internal medicine is associated with increased mortality. *Int J Clin Pract,* vol. 68, no. 1, pp. 111–116, 2014.

10. Li W et al., "Antioxidants prevent elevation in [Ca(2+)](i) induced by low extracellular magnesium in cultured canine cerebral vascular smooth muscle cells: possible relationship to Mg(2+) deficiency-induced vasospasm and stroke." *Brain Res Bull,* vol. 52, no. 2, pp. 151–154, 2000.

11. Hartwig A, "Role of magnesium in genomic stability." *Mutat Res,* vol. 18, no. 475 (1–2), pp. 113–121, 2001.

12. Blaylock RL, *Excitotoxins: The Taste That Kills.* Health Press, Sante Fe, NM, 1997.

13. Wolf FI, Trapani V, et al., "Magnesium deficiency affects mammary epithelial cell proliferation: involvement of oxidative stress." *Nutr Cancer,* vol. 61, no. 1, pp. 131–136, 2009.

14. Wolf FI et al., "TRPM7 and magnesium, metabolism, mitosis: An old path with new pebbles." *Cell Cycle,* vol. 9, no. 17, p. 3399, 2010.

15. Laires MJ et al., "Role of cellular magnesium in health and human disease." *Front Biosci,* vol. 1, no. 9, pp. 262–276, 2004.

16. Giovanni G et al., "Molecular mechanism of endothelial and vascular aging: implications for cardiovascular disease." *Eur Heart J,* vol. 36, no. 48, pp. 3392–3403, 2015.

17. Liu G, Slutsky I, "Magnesium may reverse middle-age memory loss." *MIT Tech Talk,* vol. 49, no. 12, December 8, 2004.

18. Abumaria N et al., "Effects of elevation of brain magnesium on fear conditioning, fear extinction, and synaptic plasticity in the infralimbic prefrontal cortex and lateral amygdala." *J Neurosci,* vol. 31, no. 42, pp. 14871–14881, 2011.

19. Shah NC et al., "Short-term magnesium deficiency downregulates telomerase, upregulates neutral sphingomyelinase and induces oxidative DNA damage in cardiovascular tissues: relevance to atherogenesis, cardiovascular diseases and aging." *Int J Clin Exp Med,* vol. 7, no. 3, pp. 497–514, 2014.

20. Rowe WJ, "Correcting magnesium deficiency may prolong life." *Clin Interv Aging,* vol. 7, pp. 51–54, 2012.

21. Blaylock RL, *Excitotoxins: The Taste That Kills.* Health Press, Sante Fe, NM, 1997.

22. Rondeau V et al., "Aluminum in drinking water and cognitive decline

in elderly subjects: the Paquid cohort." *Am J Epidemiol*, vol. 154, no. 3, pp. 288–290, 2001.

23. Rondeau V et al., "Relation between aluminum concentrations in drinking water and Alzheimer's disease: an 8-year follow-up study." *Am J Epidemiol*, vol. 152, pp. 59–66, 2000.

24. Durlach J. "Magnesium depletion and pathogenesis of Alzheimer's disease." *Magnes Res*, vol. 3, no. 3, pp. 217–218, 1990.

25. Foster HD, "How aluminum causes Alzheimer's disease: the implications for prevention and treatment of Foster's multiple antagonist hypothesis." *J Ortho Mol Med*, vol. 15, 2000. www.orthomolecular.org/library/jom/2000/articles/2000-v15n01-p021.shtml.

26. Andrasi E et al., "Disturbances of magnesium concentrations in various brain areas in Alzheimer's disease." *Magnes Res*, vol. 13, no. 3, pp. 189–196, 2000.

27. Durlach J, "Diverse applications of magnesium therapy." In *Handbook of Metal-Ligand Interactions in Biological Fluids—Bioinorganic Medicine*, vol. 2, Marcel Dekker, New York, 1995.

28. Barbagallo M et al., "Altered ionized magnesium levels in mild-to-moderate Alzheimer's disease." *Magnes Res*, vol. 24, no. 3, pp. S115–S121, 2011.

29. Cherbuin N et al., "Dietary mineral intake and risk of mild cognitive impairment: the PATH Through Life Project." *Front Aging Neurosci*, vol. 6, no. 4, p. 4, 2014.

30. Andrási E, Igaz S, Molnár Z, Makó S, "Disturbances of magnesium concentrations in various brain areas in Alzheimer's disease." *Magnes Res*, vol. 13, pp. 189–196, 2000.

31. Xu ZP et al., "Magnesium protects cognitive functions and synaptic plasticity in streptozotocin-induced sporadic Alzheimer's model." *PLoS One*, vol. 9, no. 9, p. e108645, 2014.

32. Li W et al., "Elevation of brain magnesium prevents synaptic loss and reverses cognitive deficits in Alzheimer's disease mouse model." *Mol Brain*, vol. 7, 65, 2014.

33. de Baaij JHF et al., "Magnesium in man: implications for health and disease." *Physiol Rev*, vol. 95, no. 1, pp. 1–46, 2015.

34. Yasui M et al., "Calcium, magnesium and aluminum concentrations in Parkinson's disease." *Neurotoxicology*, vol. 13, no. 3, pp. 593–600, 1992.

35. Yasui M, "Calcium, magnesium and aluminum concentrations in Parkinson's disease." *Neurotoxicology*, vol. 13, no. 3, pp. 593–600, 1992.

36. Blaylock RL, *Excitotoxins: The Taste That Kills*. Health Press, Sante Fe, NM, 1997.

37. Nelson L, "Pesticides and Parkinson's disease." American Academy of Neurology 52nd Annual Meeting, San Diego, CA, April 29–May 6, 2000.

38. Blaylock RL, *Excitotoxins: The Taste That Kills*. Health Press, Sante Fe, NM, 1997.
39. www.psychologytoday.com/basics/dopamine.
40. Blaylock RL, *Excitotoxins: The Taste That Kills*. Health Press, Sante Fe, NM, 1997.

Chapter 16

1. Altura BM, Altura BT, "Role of magnesium in patho-physiological processes and the clinical utility of magnesium ion selective electrodes." *Scand J Clin Lab Invest Suppl*, vol. 224, pp. 211–234, 1996.
2. Altura BT, Altura BM, "A method for distinguishing ionized, complexed and protein-bound Mg in normal and diseased subjects." *Scand J Clin Lab Invest Suppl*, vol. 217, pp. 83–87, 1994.
3. Altura BT et al., "Comparative findings on serum IMg2+ of normal and diseased human subjects with the NOVA and KONE ISE's for Mg2+." *Scand J Clin Lab Invest Suppl*, vol. 217, pp. 77–81, 1994.
4. Altura BT et al., "Characterization of a new ion selective electrode for ionized magnesium in whole blood, plasma, serum, and aqueous samples." *Scand J Clin Lab Invest Suppl*, vol. 217, pp. 21–36, 1994.
5. Altura BT et al., "A new method for the rapid determination of ionized Mg2 in whole blood, serum and plasma." *Methods and Findings in Exp Clin Pharmacol*, vol. 4, pp. 297–304, 1992.
6. Altura BT, Altura BM, "Measurement of ionized magnesium in whole blood, plasma and serum with a new ion-selective electrode in healthy and diseased human subjects." *Magnes Trace Elem*, vol. 10, nos. 2–4, pp. 90–98, 1991–1992.
7. Altura BT, Altura BM, "A method for distinguishing ionized, complexed and protein-bound Mg in normal and diseased subjects." *Scand J Clin Lab Invest Suppl*, vol. 217, pp. 83–87, 1994.
8. Altura BM, Altura BT, "Role of magnesium in patho-physiological processes and the clinical utility of magnesium ion selective electrodes." *Scand J Clin Lab Invest Suppl*, vol. 224, pp. 211–234, 1996.
9. Altura BM, Altura BT, "Role of magnesium in patho-physiological processes and the clinical utility of magnesium ion selective electrodes." *Scand J Clin Lab Invest Suppl*, vol. 224, pp. 211–234, 1996.
10. Personal communication with Burton Altura, November 2001.
11. Altura BT et al., "Clinical studies with the NOVA ISE for IMg2+." *Scand J Clin Lab Invest Suppl*, vol. 217, pp. 53–67, 1994.
12. Marcus JC, Altura BT, Altura BM, "Serum ionized magnesium in post-traumatic headaches." *J Pediatr*, vol. 139, no. 3, pp. 459–462, 2001.
13. Muneyvirci-Delale O et al., "Divalent cations in women with PCOS: implications for cardiovascular disease." *Gynecol Endocrinol*, vol. 3, pp. 198–201, 2001.

14. Marcus JC et al., "Serum ionized magnesium in premature and term infants." *Pediatr Neurol*, vol. 4, pp. 311–314, 1998.

15. Scott VL et al., "Ionized hypomagnesemia in patients undergoing orthotopic liver transplantation: a complication of citrate intoxication." *Liver Transpl Surg*, vol. 2, no. 5, pp. 343–347, 1996.

16. Altura BT et al., "Low levels of serum ionized magnesium are found in patients early after stroke which result in rapid elevation in cytosolic free calcium and spasm in cerebral vascular muscle cells." *Neurosci Lett*, vol. 230, no. 1, pp. 37–40, 1997.

17. Handwerker SM, Altura BT, Altura BM, "Serum ionized magnesium and other electrolytes in the antenatal period of human pregnancy." *J Am Coll Nutr*, vol. 15, no. 1, pp. 36–43, 1996.

18. Memon ZI et al., "Predictive value of serum ionized but not total magnesium levels in head injuries." *Scand J Clin Lab Invest*, vol. 55, no. 8, pp. 671–677, 1995.

19. Handwerker SM, Altura BT, Altura BM, "Ionized serum magnesium and potassium levels in pregnant women with preeclampsia and eclampsia." *J Reprod Medicine*, vol. 40, no. 3, pp. 201–208, 1995.

20. Ismail Y et al., "The underestimated problem of using serum magnesium measurements to exclude magnesium deficiency in adults: a health warning is needed for 'normal' results." *Clin Chem Laboratory*, vol. 48, no. 3, pp. 323–327, 2010.

21. Mircetic RN, Dodig S, Raos M, Petres B, Cepelak I, "Magnesium concentration in plasma, leukocytes and urine of children with intermittent asthma." *Clin Chim Acta*, vol. 312, nos. 1–2, pp. 197–203, 2001.

22. www.spectracell.com/clinicians/products/mnt.

23. www.exatest.com.

24. Ryzen E et al., "Parenteral magnesium tolerance testing in the evaluation of magnesium deficiency." *Magnesium*, vol. 4, pp. 137–147, 1985.

25. Burton Altura, personal communication, November 2001.

26. Seelig MS, "The requirement of magnesium by the normal adult." *Am J Clin Nutr*, vol. 14, pp. 342–390, 1964.

27. Seelig MS, "Magnesium requirements in human nutrition." *Magnes Bull*, vol. 3, no. 1A, pp. 26–47, 1981.

28. Franz KB, "Magnesium intake during pregnancy." *Magnesium*, vol. 6, pp. 18–27, 1987.

29. Seelig MS, "The requirement of magnesium by the normal adult." *Am J Clin Nutr*, vol. 14, pp. 342–390, 1964.

30. Seelig MS, "Magnesium requirements in human nutrition." *Magnes Bull*, vol. 3, no. 1A, pp. 26–47, 1981.

31. Glei M et al., "Magnesium content of foodstuffs and beverages and magnesium intake of adults in Germany." *Magnes Bull*, vol. 17, pp. 22–28, 1995.

32. Cashman KD et al., "Optimal nutrition: calcium, magnesium and phosphorus." *Proc Nutr Soc,* vol. 58, pp. 477–487, 1999.

Chapter 17

1. Durlach J, Bac P, Bara M, Guiet-Bara A, "Cardiovasoprotective foods and nutrients: possible importance of magnesium intake." *Magnes Res,* vol. 12, no. 1, pp. 57–61, 1999.
2. Murray M, *Encyclopedia of Nutritional Supplements.* Prima, Rocklin, CA, 1996.
3. Wood M, *Seven Herbs: Plants as Teachers.* North Atlantic Books, Berkeley, CA, 1987.
4. Weed S, *Healing Wise: The Wise Woman Herbal.* Ash Tree Publishing, Woodstock, NY, 1989.
5. Duke JA, *The Green Pharmacy.* St. Martin's Press, New York, 1998.
6. Chevallier A, *The Encyclopedia of Medicinal Plants.* DK Publishing, New York, 1996.
7. Jiang L et al., "Magnesium levels in drinking water and coronary heart disease mortality risk: a meta-analysis." *Nutrients,* vol. 8, no. 1, 2016.
8. Marx A et al., "Magnesium in drinking water and ischemic heart disease." *Epidemiol Rev,* vol. 19, pp. 258–272, 1997.
9. Von Wiesenberger A, *The Pocket Guide to Bottled Water.* Contemporary Books, Chicago, 1991.

Chapter 18

1. Laires MJ et al., "Role of cellular magnesium in health and human disease." *Front Biosci,* vol. 9, pp. 262–276, 2004.
2. Durlach J, *Magnesium in Clinical Practice.* Libbey, London, 1988.
3. Fehlinger R, "Therapy with magnesium salts in neurological diseases." *Magnes Bull,* vol. 12, pp. 35–42, 1990.
4. Ducroix T, "L'enfant spasmophile—Aspects diagnostiques et thérapeutiques." *Magnes Bull,* vol. 1, pp. 9–15, 1984.
5. Seelig MS, "Athletic stress, performance and magnesium in consequences of magnesium deficiency on the enhancement of stress reactions; preventive and therapeutic implications: a review." *J Am Coll Nutr,* vol. 13, no. 5, pp. 429–446, 1994.
6. Slutsky I et al., "Enhancement of learning and memory by elevating brain magnesium." *Neuron,* vol. 65, no. 2, pp. 165–177, 2010.
7. www.adelaide.edu.au/press/titles/magnesium.
8. Chazov EI, Malchikova LS, Lipina NV, Asafov GB, Smirnov VN, "Taurine and electrical activity of the heart." *Circ Res,* vol. 35, suppl. 3, pp. 11–21, 1974.
9. Chahine R, Feng J, "Protective effects of taurine against reperfusion-induced arrhythmias in isolated ischemic rat heart." *Arzneimittelforschung,* vol. 48, no. 4, pp. 360–364, 1998.

10. Johnson S, "The multifaceted and widespread pathology of magnesium deficiency." *Med Hypotheses,* vol. 56, no. 2, pp. 163–170, 2001.

11. Rude RK et al., "Low serum concentrations of 1,25-dihydroxyvitamin D in human magnesium deficiency." *J Clin Endocrinol Metab,* vol. 61, pp. 833–940, 1985.

12. Fuss M et al., "Correction of low circulating levels of 1,25-dihydroxy-vitamin D by 25-hydroxyvitamin D during reversal of hypomagnesaemia." *Clinical Endocrinol Oxf,* vol. 31, pp. 31–38, 1989.

13. Manuel y Keenoy B, Moorkens G, Vertommen J, Noe M, Neve J, De Leeuw I, "Magnesium status and parameters of the oxidant-antioxidant balance in patients with chronic fatigue: effects of supplementation with magnesium." *J Am Coll Nutr,* vol. 19, no. 3, pp. 374–382, 2000.

14. Boericke OE, *Pocket Manual of Homeopathic Materia Medica,* 9th ed. Boericke & Runyon, Philadelphia, 1927.

Index

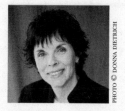

PHOTO © DONNA DIETRICH

DR. CAROLYN DEAN is a medical doctor and naturopathic doctor on the cutting edge of the natural medicine revolution since 1979. She holds a medical license in California and is a graduate of the Ontario Naturopathic College and a former board member of the Canadian College of Naturopathic Medicine.

Dr. Dean is the author of 33 health books and 113 Kindle books including *Atrial Fibrillation: ReMineralize Your Heart, Invisible Minerals Parts I and II, Death by Modern Medicine, IBS for Dummies, Future Health Now Encyclopedia,* and *Hormone Balance.* Dr. Dean has accumulated close to 1,000 articles and interviews in various print and online health magazines, radio, and television. She has a weekly radio show, an online blog, and a two-year online wellness program called Completement Now!

Dr. Dean is on the Medical Advisory Board of the nonprofit educational site Nutritional Magnesium Association (www .nutritionalmagnesium.org). Her magnesium outreach has won her an award from the Heart Rhythm Society in the United Kingdom for Outstanding Medical Contribution to Cardiac Rhythm Management, 2012. Find out more about Dr. Dean at www.DrCarolynDean.com. As a reader of this book, you can use the following URL to claim free gifts from Dr. Dean: http:// bit.ly/mg-miracle-gift. On www.RnAReSet.com you can reset your ailing body with Dr. Dean's Total Body ReSet using her unique Completement Formulas: ReMag (magnesium), ReMag Lotion, ReMyte (multiple minerals), ReCalcia (calcium), Re-Aline (detox), RnA Drops (cell enhancer), ReNew (skin serum), and ReStructure (protein powder).

drcarolyndean.com
Facebook.com/carolyn.dean.56
Twitter: @DrCarolynDean